Clinical Issues, Diagnosis and Management of Bladder Diseases

Clinical Issues, Diagnosis and Management of Bladder Diseases

Editor: William Miller

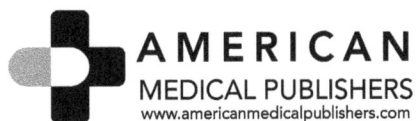

AMERICAN
MEDICAL PUBLISHERS
www.americanmedicalpublishers.com

AMERICAN
MEDICAL PUBLISHERS
www.americanmedicalpublishers.com

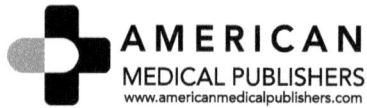

Cataloging-in-Publication Data

Clinical issues, diagnosis and management of bladder diseases / edited by William Miller.
    p. cm.
Includes bibliographical references and index.
ISBN 978-1-63927-996-8
1. Bladder--Diseases. 2. Bladder--Diseases--Diagnosis. 3. Bladder--Diseases--Treatment.
4. Bladder--Examination. I. Miller, William.
RC919 .C55 2023
616.62--dc23

American Medical Publishers,
41 Flatbush Avenue,
1st Floor, New York,
NY 11217, USA

ISBN 978-1-63927-996-8 (Hardback)

Contents

Preface

Bladder is a hollow organ in the lower abdomen. Its main function is to store urine and it can be affected by a variety of conditions. The most common types of bladder diseases include overactive bladder, cystitis, bladder cancer, urinary incontinence and interstitial cystitis. There are several signs and symptoms of bladder diseases, such as cloudy urine, blood in the urine, bladder leakage, urinating frequently in small amounts, pain during sexual intercourse, etc. The risk factors associated with bladder diseases include birth control, hormonal changes, hysterectomy, obesity, autoimmune disorders and medical conditions like diabetes. The diagnosis of bladder diseases is accomplished through various tests. These consist of using cystoscope for inspection of the bladder wall, urine tests and X-rays. The treatment is determined by the cause of the issue and can include medications, and in extreme circumstances surgery can also be done. This book covers new techniques for the clinical diagnosis and management of bladder diseases. A number of latest researches have been included to keep the readers up-to-date with the global concepts on this medical condition.

This book unites the global concepts and researches in an organized manner for a comprehensive understanding of the subject. It is a ripe text for all researchers, students, scientists or anyone else who is interested in acquiring a better knowledge of this dynamic field.

I extend my sincere thanks to the contributors for such eloquent research chapters. Finally, I thank my family for being a source of support and help.

Editor

Progressive bladder remodeling due to bladder outlet obstruction: A systematic review of morphological and molecular evidences in humans

Ferdinando Fusco[1][*] [iD], Massimiliano Creta[1], Cosimo De Nunzio[2], Valerio Iacovelli[3], Francesco Mangiapia[1], Vincenzo Li Marzi[4] and Enrico Finazzi Agrò[3]

Abstract

Background: Bladder outlet obstruction is a common urological condition. We aimed to summarize available evidences about bladder outlet obstruction-induced molecular and morphological alterations occurring in human bladder.

Methods: We performed a literature search up to December 2017 including clinical and preclinical basic research studies on humans. The following search terms were combined: angiogenesis, apoptosis, bladder outlet obstruction, collagen, electron microscopy, extracellular matrix, fibrosis, hypoxia, histology, inflammation, innervation, ischemia, pressure, proliferation, remodeling, suburothelium, smooth muscle cells, stretch, urothelium.

Results: We identified 36 relevant studies. A three-stages model of bladder wall remodeling can be hypothesized involving an initial hypertrophy phase, a subsequent compensation phase and a later decompensation. Histological and molecular alterations occur in the following compartments: urothelium, suburothelium, detrusor smooth muscle cells, detrusor extracellular matrix, nerves. Cyclic stretch, increased hydrostatic and cyclic hydrodynamic pressure and hypoxia are stimuli capable of modulating multiple signaling pathways involved in this remodeling process.

Conclusions: Bladder outlet obstruction leads to progressive bladder tissue remodeling in humans. Multiple signaling pathways are involved.

Keywords: Bladder outlet obstruction, Bladder remodeling, Systematic review

Background

Bladder outlet obstruction (BOO), clinically defined as high-pressure/low-flow micturition pattern at urodynamic investigations, is a common urological condition in humans with benign prostatic obstruction (BPO) being the most frequent causative factor. It represents a key pathophysiological link between benign prostate enlargement (BPE) and lower urinary tract symptoms (LUTS) [1–3]. Besides symptoms, BOO can also lead to progressive tissue remodeling of the bladder and of the upper urinary tract with subsequent serious

functional impairments [1–4]. Based on the results from studies on animal models exposed to experimental partial outlet obstruction, the remodeling of the bladder involves the modulation of several signaling pathways as well as histological alterations occurring in almost all cellular compartments [5]. These changes are described to progress through three sequential stages: hypertrophy, compensation and decompensation [6]. In the hypertrophy stage, mechanical stress activates early signals that mediate bladder wall hypertrophy. At the same time, due to the occurrence of focal area of hypoxia, angiogenesis is stimulated thus enabling blood flow to increase relative to bladder mass [6]. In the compensated stage bladder growth and angiogenesis stop. At some point, if obstruction persists, the bladder shifts to a decompensated state as a result of cyclical

* Correspondence: ferdinando-fusco@libero.it
[1]Dipartimento di Neuroscienze e Scienze Riproduttive ed Odontostomatologiche, Università Degli Studi Di Napoli Federico II, Via Pansini, 5, 80131 Naples, Italy
Full list of author information is available at the end of the article

ischemia-reperfusion injury occurring during the micturition phase that leads to the activation of pathways involved in the progressive loss of smooth muscle, deposition of extracellular matrix and neuronal loss [6]. The duration of these stages varies considerably according to the experimental models and is unpredictably. Data about the reversibility of these alterations are also lacking. Human detrusor differs significantly from animal models and most of the species used for research don't suffer from naturally occurring outflow obstruction [7]. *The aim of the present study was to summarize available evidences about BOO-induced morphological and molecular alterations occurring in the various compartments of human bladder.*

Methods

We performed a systematic review using the Preferred Reporting Items for Systematic Reviews and Meta-Analyses Statement as a guideline in the development of the study protocol and the report of the current study [8]. In December 2017 we used the National Library of Medicine PubMed search engine, the Scopus database, and the ISI Web of Knowledge official website to search for all published studies evaluating morphological and molecular alterations involved in BOO-induced bladder wall remodeling. The following search terms were combined: angiogenesis, apoptosis, bladder outlet obstruction, collagen, electron microscopy, extracellular matrix, fibrosis, hypoxia, histology, inflammation, innervation, ischemia, pressure, proliferation, remodeling, suburothelium, smooth muscle cells, stretch, urothelium. We included publications that met the following criteria: reporting original in vitro and in vivo research; English language; human studies. Reference lists in relevant articles and reviews were also screened for additional studies.

Results

The search strategy revealed a total of 159 results. Screening of the titles and abstracts revealed 44 papers eligible for inclusion. Further assessment of eligibility, based on full-text papers, led to the exclusion of 8 papers. This left 36 papers meeting our criteria for inclusion [9–44] (Fig. 1).

Alterations occurring in the urothelium and suburothelium

We identified one study describing BOO-induced alterations occurring in the context of urothelium and suburothelium [9]. Bladder biopsies were obtained from 33 men with urodynamic proven BOO and 10 control subjects. Authors demonstrated the occurrence of significant urothelial dysfunction and alterations of urothelial signaling and sensory transduction pathways in patients with BOO. In detail, the following alterations were found: significantly lower expression of the adhesion protein E-cadherin and of the muscarinic receptor M3, and significantly higher expression of the purinergic receptor P2X3 and of the muscarinic receptor M2. Interestingly, patients with detrusor underactivity had a significantly lower expression of E-cadherin and of inducible nitric oxide synthase as well as a significantly higher expression of β3 adrenoreceptors than patients with detrusor overactivity/ hypersensitive bladder. Clinically, lower expression of E-cadherin was associated with lower voided volumes thus suggesting a more severe or decompensated status with more severe urothelial dysfunction. Alterations found in the suburothelium of BOO patients included: inflammation, with a significantly increased level of activated mast cells, and increased apoptosis.

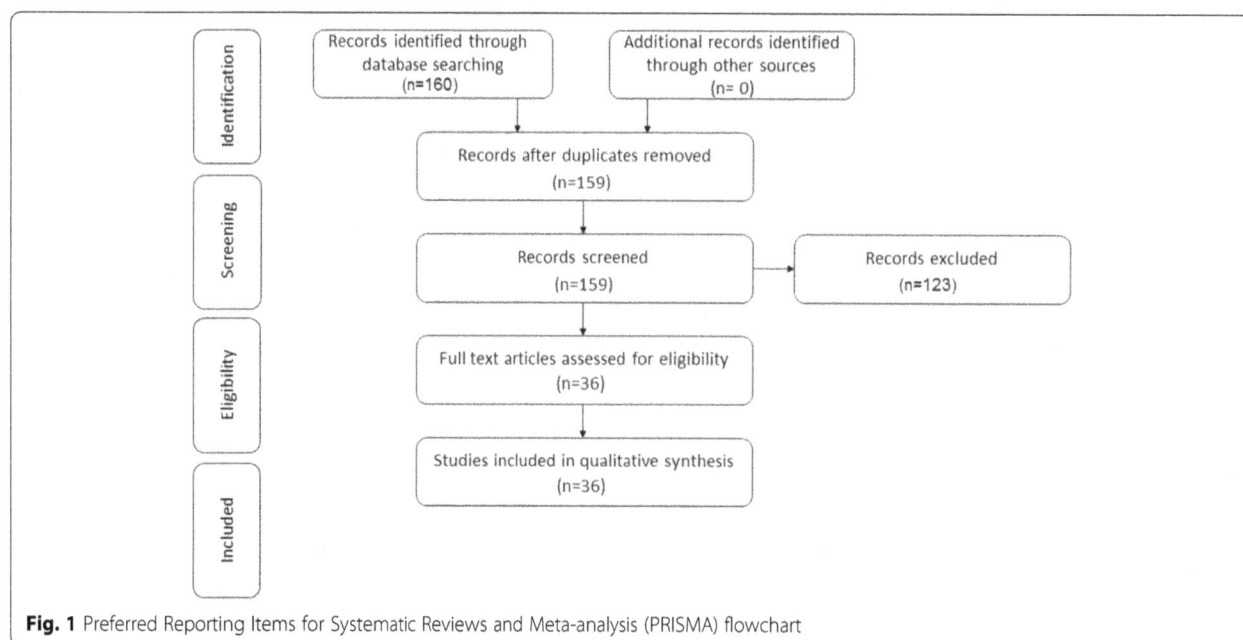

Fig. 1 Preferred Reporting Items for Systematic Reviews and Meta-analysis (PRISMA) flowchart

Alterations occurring in the detrusor muscle: morphological aspects

The detrusor muscle represents the bladder compartment more extensively investigated. Studies describing BOO-induced morphological alterations occurring in the detrusor are summarized in Table 1. Significant alterations involving both smooth muscle cells (SMCs) and extracellular matrix (ECM) have been demonstrated using light and electron microscopy studies.

SMCs alterations

Detrusor SMCs hypertrophy represents the most relevant morphological alteration occurring in BOO patients. Gilpin et al. compared the morphological and morphometric characteristics of detrusor specimens from patients with unequivocal urodynamic BOO accompanied by evidence of severe bladder trabeculation at cystoscopy and subjects with normal urodynamic assessment and absent trabeculation [10]. Although authors did not find morphological evidences of SMCs hyperplasia, the mean profile

Table 1 Summary of studies describing BOO-induced detrusor morphological alterations

Author, year	Study design	Subjects in the case group (n)	Main findings
Gosling, 1980 [15]	Case control	9	• ↑ intrafascicular and interfascicular collagen • ↓ SMCs diameter
Gilpin, 1985 [10]	Case control	14	• ↑connective tissue infiltration of some smooth muscle bundles in 12/14 patients • ↑ SMCs mean profile area
Elbadawi, 1993 [12]	Case control	7	• ↓ intermediate cell junctions • ↑intrafascicular collagen and elastic fibers • ↑ SMCs hypertrophy • ↑ SMCs and axons degeneration in patients with impaired detrusor contractility
Inui, 1999 [19]	Case control	26	• Significant positive linear relationship between C/M and estimated bladder weight in patients with bladder weight ≥ 60 g • ↑ C/M in patients with bladder weight ≥ 60 g
Tse, 2000 [13]	Case control	9	• Myohypertrophy pattern in all cases
Brierly, 2003 [14]	Case control	12	• Myohypertrophy pattern in 8/10 BOO patients. • Degenerative pattern in 4/10 BOO patients.
Holm, 2003 [22]	Case control	25	• Significant correlation between intra- and interfascicular elastin and BOO degree
Mirone, 2004 [15]	Case control	36	• ↑collagen content in BPO patients with respect to controls • ↑collagen content in patients with severe symptoms
Horn, 2004 [44]	Observational	54	• Correlation between abnormal morphology and impaired bladder compliance and decreased capacity
Collado, 2006 [11]	Case control	33	• ↑ intrafascicular and interfascicular collagen • ↑ intrafascicular fibrosis in BOO patients with history of AUR • ↑ SMCs diameter in BOO patients with respect to controls • Not significant differences in terms of SMCs diameter between BOO patients with and without AUR history • Positive correlation between SMCs diameter and symptoms duration
Rubinstein, 2007 [18]	Case control	10	• ↑ collagen and elastic fibers
Blatt, 2012 [16]	Case control	17	• Poor post-TURP voiding outcome in patients with detrusor ultrastructural pattern characterized by variable muscle cell size, muscle cell shape, abnormal fascicle arrangement and collagenosis.
Bellucci, 2017 [21]	Case control	19	• ↑ C/M • Significant negative correlation between C/M and bladder compliance • Significant correlation between the probability of urinary retention and C/M
Averbeck, 2017 [20]	Observational	38	• ↑ C/M in patients with PVR ≥ 200 mL and in those with reduced bladder compliance

AUR acute urinary retention, *BOO* bladder outlet obstruction, *C/M* connective tissue-to-smooth muscle ratio, *PVR* post void residual volume, *SMCs* smooth muscle cells, *TURP* trans urethral resection of the prostate

area of SMCs was higher in BOO patients due to hypertrophy. Similarly, Collado et al. demonstrated that detrusor SMCs diameter was significantly higher in BOO patients with respect to controls [11]. Authors found a positive correlation between SMCs diameter and symptoms duration but no statistically significant differences between BOO patients with and without history of Acute Urinary Retention (AUR). Electron microscopy studies also confirmed the evidence of SMCs hypertrophy in many cases. Elbadawi et al. investigated the ultrastructural basis of obstructive detrusor dysfunction in a prospective case-control study enrolling 35 elderly subjects [12]. Authors described the "myohypertrophy" structural pattern in patients with urodynamic proven BOO. This pattern was characterized by 4 distinctive features, including SMCs hypertrophy, marked widening of intercellular spaces with reduced normal intermediate cell junctions, increased deposition of collagen and elastin between SMCs, and patchy distribution of the preceding features in various muscle fascicles. This ultrastructural pattern was confirmed by other authors in patients with urodynamic evidence of BOO [13, 14]. Of note, the evidence of SMCs hypertrophy has not been confirmed in all patients. In their light microscopy study, Gosling et al. failed to found evidences of SMCs hypertrophy or hyperplasia in a subset of patients with unequivocal BPO accompanied by trabeculated urinary bladder [15]. On the contrary, authors identified some muscle bundles containing SMCs characterized by a small diameter [15]. Elbadawi et al. showed degeneration of SMCs in the specimens of patients who had impaired detrusor contractility [12]. The degenerative pattern was confirmed by Brierly et al. in BOO patients with high post void residual volume [14].

ECM alterations

Detrusor ECM remodeling is characterized by increased accumulation of collagen and elastic fibers in both the interfascicular and intrafascicular compartments. This finding has been confirmed in several studies using both light and electron microscopy techniques [10, 11, 15–21]. Interestingly, Gilpin et al. found that patients with evidence of interfascicular connective tissue infiltration had the highest levels of SMCs mean profile area thus leading the authors to hypothesize that the deposition of connective tissue occurs at a later stage with respect to onset of SMCs hypertrophy [10]. This hypothesis has been confirmed by other studies. Inui et al. investigated the relationship between the amount of detrusor connective tissue in patients with BPH and the degree of bladder hypertrophy evaluated by ultrasound estimated bladder weight. In detail, authors compared the ratio of connective tissue-to-smooth muscle (C/M) between controls and BPE cases [19]. The study failed to found statistically significant differences between the two groups

(27.3% in BPE patients and 24.7% in controls). However, a significant positive linear relationship between C/M and estimated bladder weight was evident in all BPE patients with estimated bladder weight ≥ 60 g [19]. Interestingly, 30% of BPE patients had C/M < 20% compared to only 7.7% of controls. Author hypothesized that the increase in ultrasound estimated bladder weight is caused at early stages by hyperplasia and/or hypertrophy of detrusor SMCs leading to a lower C/M and later to the additional increase of connective tissue with higher C/M. Other studies confirmed the occurrence of increased detrusor ECM accumulation with more advanced stages within the natural history of BOO. Collado et al. compared detrusor C/M of patients with urodynamic BOO and no history of AUR, patients with urodynamic BOO and history of AUR and non-obstructed controls [11]. Patients with BOO (obstruction and AUR groups) had a significantly higher intrafascicular and interfascicular collagen content than the control group. Patients with history of AUR had statistically significant higher levels of intrafascicular collagen than BOO patients without history of AUR. Moreover, authors found a statistically significant correlation between the amount of intrafascicular fibrosis and detrusor pressure at maximum urinary flow as well as with the Abrams-Griffiths number in BOO patients without history of AUR at pre-operative urodynamics. Additionally, a statistically significant negative correlation was found between intrafascicular fibrosis and postoperative bladder compliance in the same group of patients. Finally, a positive and significant correlation was found between intrafascicular fibrosis and both detrusor pressure at maximum urinary flow and the Abrams-Griffiths number in BOO patients with history of AUR at postoperative urodynamic evaluation [11]. Averbeck et al. evaluated the collagen content in the bladder wall of men undergoing open prostate surgery. Although BOO was not a predictor of increased collagen deposition, patients with reduced bladder compliance and those with a PVR ≥ 200 mL showed a significantly higher C/M [20]. Similarly, Bellucci et al. found a significant negative correlation between C/M and bladder compliance [21]. Moreover, the probability of urinary retention increased significantly with the C/M. Mirone et al. found higher detrusor collagen content in patients with BPO and severe symptoms with respect to patients with moderate symptoms [22]. Blatt et al. investigated the correlation between detrusor ultrastructural features of patients with urodynamic BOO or a hypocontractile detrusor and clinical outcomes after transurethral resection of the prostate [16]. Authors found that the morphological pattern characterized by variable SMCs size, SMCs shape, abnormal fascicle arrangement and collagenosis correlated with poor postoperative voiding outcome. Holm et al. investigated the correlation between ultrastructural findings and urodynamic parameters in patients with BOO [17]. SMCs hypertrophy, occurrence of abnormal cell junctions and configurations, variation in intercellular distances, and intracellular changes were investigated. The increase in intra- and interfascicular elastin was only parameter which was found to relate to the degree of obstruction in BOO patients.

Alterations occurring in the detrusor muscle: molecular aspects and signaling pathways

Data about molecular aspects and signaling pathways involved in BOO-induced detrusor remodeling mainly derive from in vitro cell culture models of human bladder SMCs (HBSMCs) exposed to stressful stimuli such as cyclic mechanical stretch, increased hydrostatic (HP) or cyclic hydrodynamic pressure (CHP), and hypoxia. Further evidences derive from genetic and molecular studies on tissue specimens from BOO patients. Table 2 summarizes evidences from these studies.

Effects of cyclic stretch

Yang et al. investigated the effects of cyclic stretch on HBSMCs gene expression [23]. Authors identified multiple mechano-responsive genes encoding *cytokine, growth-related factors, adhesive molecules, signal transduction molecules, cytoskeleton and extracellular matrix proteins, developmental, differentiation, and inflammatory factors*. Twelve of proteins encoded by these genes had interacting partners in the vascular system and were functionally involved in multiple aspects of angiogenesis and vascular development such as endothelial cell proliferation and migration, SMCs differentiation, and arterial-venous differentiation.

Effects of increased pressure

The effects of increased pressure on HBSMCs has been investigated by many authors. These studies demonstrated the existence of multiple pressure-dependent pathways involved into cellular processes such as adhesion, proliferation, inflammation, and ECM remodeling.

Effects of increased pressure on cell adhesion

Wang et al. demonstrated a significant decreased expression of the gap junction connexin 43 under hydrostatic pressures > 60 cm H_2O for 24 h or pressures > 40 cm H_2O for 72 h [24].

Effects of increased pressure on cell hypertrophy and hyperplasia

Lee et al. investigated the effects of HP on HBSMCs in terms of cell hypertrophy and hyperplasia and the potential role of muscarinic receptors [26]. HBSMCs proliferation and hypertrophy were measured by 3H-thymidine

and leucine incorporation assays, respectively [25]. 3H-thymidine incorporation increased by 16.7, 25.9 and 39.4% after exposure to acetylcholine, 40 cmH₂O HP, and both, respectively. Similarly, leucine incorporation increased by 66.5, 66.5 and 81.8%, after exposure to acetylcholine, 40 cmH₂O HP, and both, respectively. These findings were consistent with increased proliferation and hypertrophy, respectively. Antimuscarinic agents determined a dramatic decrease in thymidine and leucine incorporation for cells exposed to increased HP, most pronounced when both M2 and M3 receptor antagonist were applied. In a subsequent study, authors found that M2 and M3 receptor expression increases in a time- and pressure-dependent manner in isolated HBSMCs [26]. Preis et al. investigated the role of platelet derived growth factor (PDGF) pathway in pressure-induced proliferation [27]. Exposure of HBSMCs to HP induced proliferation in a time dependent manner. Moreover, HBSMCs showed increased PDGF receptor (PDGFR) α and β expression. Interestingly, DNA synthesis in cells with intact PDGFR α was increased after short-term HP but cells lacking PDGFR α did not proliferate. All studies evaluating the effects of CHP on HBSMCs demonstrated increased proliferation under CHP > 100 cmH₂O. Involved signaling pathways include: phosphoinositide 3-kinase/serum-glucocorticoid regulated kinase 1, S-phase kinase-associated protein 2, p27, Ras-related C3 botulinum toxin substrate 1, miR-3180-5p and miR 4323 [28–32]. MiR-3180-5p promotes HBSMCs proliferation by the activation of the pro-proliferative cyclin-dependent kinase 2 pathway [29]. On the other hand, miR 4323 can promote HBSMCs proliferation by inhibiting LYN expression and activating the Erk1/2 pathway, also known as the mitogen activated protein kinase signaling pathway [30].

Effects of increased pressure on inflammatory pathways

Liang et al. investigated the effects of HP and acetylcholine on the release of inflammatory cytokines in HBSMCs to test the hypothesis that mechanical force and muscarinic receptors have pro-inflammatory effect in obstructed bladder [33]. HP produced a significant time-dependent and pressure-dependent increase in expressions of inflammatory genes. HP of 200 cm H_2O for 24 h was associated with a statistically significant increase of monocyte chemoattractant protein, IL-6, and RANTES. Both NFκB and ERK1/2 pathways were proved to be involved in pressure-induced inflammation.

Effects of increased pressure on ECM remodeling

Backhaus et al. applied HP to HBSMCs to determine the effect on matrix metalloproteinases (MMPs) and tissue inhibitors of metalloproteinases (TIMP) [34]. Exposure of HBSMCs to a sustained HP of 20 cm H_2O for 7 h

Table 2 Summary of studies evaluating BOO-induced molecular alterations and related cellular events in human detrusor

Author, year	Experimental conditions	Molecular alteration	Cellular events
Backhaus, 2002 [34]	HBSMCs exposed to HP (0.3, 20 and 40 cm H_2O) for 1, 3, 7 and 24 h	$\downarrow$ MMP-1, 2, 9 after exposure to 20 cm H_2O for 7 h $\uparrow$TIMP-1 after exposure to 40 cm H_2O 3, 7 and 24 h	
Wang, 2013 [24]	HBSMCs exposed to HP (0, 20, 40, 60, 80 and 100 cm H_2O) for 6, 12, 24 and 72 h	$\downarrow$expression of the gap junction connexin 43 under HP > 60 cm H_2O for 24 h or HP > 40 cm H_2O for 72 h.	
Chen, 2012 [28]	HBSMCs exposed to CHP (0, 100, 200, and 300 cm H_2O)	$\uparrow$ SGK1 expression and activity	$\uparrow$ proliferation in the 200 and 300 cm H_2O groups
Chen, 2014 [32]	HBSMCs exposed to CHP (0, 100, 200, and 300 cm H_2O)	$\uparrow$ Skp2 expression and $\downarrow$ p27 expression under 200 and 300 cmH_2O CHP	
Wu, 2012 [31]	HBSMCs exposed to CHP (static, 100, 200, and 300 cm H_2O)	Ras-related C3 botulinum toxin substrate 1, mitogen-activated protein kinase kinase 1/2 and extracellular regulated protein kinases 1/2 activated by 200 and 300 cmH_2O CHP	$\uparrow$proliferation under 200 and 300 cmH_2O CHP
Preis, 2015 [27]	HBSMCs exposed to HP of 136 cm H_2O for 1 h	$\uparrow$ expression of PDGFR α and β	$\uparrow$ proliferation
Sun, 2016 [29]	HBSMCs exposed to CHP up to 200 cm H_2O	$\uparrow$ miR-3180-5p	$\uparrow$ proliferation
Sun, 2017 [30]	HBSMCs exposed to CHP up to 200 cm H_2O	$\uparrow$ miR 4323	$\uparrow$ proliferation
Lee, 2006 [25]	HBSMCs exposed to HP (40 cm H_2O) and/or acetylcholine for 24 h	Activation of muscarinic receptors	$\uparrow$ proliferation $\uparrow$ hypertrophy
Lee, 2008 [26]	HBSMCs exposed to acetylcholine in the presence or absence of HP (10, 20, and 40 cm H_2O)	$\uparrow$ M2 and M3 receptors expression	$\uparrow$ proliferation $\uparrow$ hypertrophy
Yang, 2008 [23]	HBSMCs exposed to cyclic stretch with maximum of 15% strain magnitude at a frequency of 0.3 Hz for either 1 h or 24 h.	30 genes upregulated and 59 downregulated after 1 h exposure 59 genes upregulated and 27 downregulated after 24 h exposure	
Backhaus, 2002 [34]	HBSMCs exposed to HP (0.3, 20 and 40 cm H_2O)	$\downarrow$ MMP-1, 2, 9 $\uparrow$TIMP-1	
Liang, 2017 [33]	HBSMCs exposed to HP (100, 200, or 300 cm H_2O) and/or acetylcholine	$\uparrow$ IL-6, monocyte chemoattractant protein, and RANTES	
Galvin, 2004 [7]	HBSMCs exposed to 1% O_2 tension for 24, 48, 72, and 96 h	$\uparrow$ HIF-1α $\uparrow$ VEGF $\uparrow$ p27^{kip1}	$\downarrow$ proliferation
Wiafe, 2017 [35]	HBSMCs exposed to 3% O_2 tension for 2, 24, 48, and 72 h	$\uparrow$ HIF1α, HIF2α, and HIF3α $\uparrow$VEGF $\uparrow$TGFβ1 $\uparrow$CTGF $\uparrow$ collagens 1, 2, 3, 4 $\uparrow$ fibronectin $\uparrow$aggrecan $\uparrow$TIMP $\uparrow$ α-smooth muscle actin $\uparrow$vimentin, $\uparrow$desmin $\uparrow$TNFα, IL 1β, and IL 6 $\downarrow$ IL-10	
Boopathi , 2011 [38]		$\uparrow$ expression of GATA-6 in cases	

Table 2 Summary of studies evaluating BOO-induced molecular alterations and related cellular events in human detrusor *(Continued)*

Author, year	Experimental conditions	Molecular alteration	Cellular events
	Bladder samples from subjects with BOO and controls	↓ Caveolin-1 expression	
Koritsiadis, 2008 [36]	Bladder samples from subjects scheduled for BPE-surgery and controls	↑ HIF-1α expression in stromal cells between muscle bundles and in connective tissue beneath the mucosal layer	
Barbosa, 2017 [37]	Bladder samples from subjects with obstructive BPE and controls	↑ collagens I and III ↓ MMP-9 and TIMP-1 ↑VEGF ↓ CD105	
Gheinani, 2017 [43]	Bladder samples from subjects with different states of urodynamic defined BOO-induced bladder dysfunction	Progressive increase in the number of altered mRNA and miRNAs from the detrusor overactive to the obstruction group to the underactive detrusor groups	

BOO bladder outlet obstruction, *BPE* benign prostatic enlargement, *CHP* cyclic hydrodynamic pressure, *CTGF* connective tissue transforming growth factor, *HBSMCs* human bladder smooth muscle cells, *HIF* hypoxia inducible factor, *HP* hydrostatic pressures, *IL* interleukin, *MMP* matrix metalloproteinases, *PDGFR* platelet derived growth factor receptor, *SGK1* serum-glucocorticoid regulated kinase 1, *Skp2* S-phase kinase-associated protein 2, *TGF* transforming growth factor, *TIMP* tissue inhibitor *of* metalloproteinases, *TNF* tumor necrosis factor, *VEGF* vascular endothelial growth factor

resulted in a significant time dependent decrease in MMP-1, 2 and 9 activities compared to controls maintained at atmospheric pressure. TIMP-1 levels increased an average of 10% after exposure to 20 cm H_2O. These changes became statistically significant when the cells were exposed to 40 cm H_2O.

Effects of hypoxia
Available evidences demonstrate that hypoxia can modulate signaling pathways involved in angiogenesis, proliferation and ECM remodeling.

Effects of hypoxia on hypoxia inducible factor and vascular endothelial growth factor
Galvin et al. demonstrated significant time-dependent upregulation of hypoxia inducible factor (HIF)-1α and vascular endothelial growth factor (VEGF) in HBSMCs exposed to hypoxia [7]. HIF-1α expression was maximal at 72 h while a twofold increase in VEGF production was evident after 24 h of hypoxia and this increase continued in a time-dependent manner. Wiafe et al. investigated the effects of hypoxia on HIF1α, HIF2α, HIF3α and VEGF expression [35]. Transcription of HIF1α and HIF2α demonstrated a time-dependent increased expression and were transiently upregulated in response to short-term hypoxia (2–24 h). HIF3α genes and protein were significantly expressed after 72 h of hypoxia when HIF1 and HIF2α proteins had resumed normoxic control levels. VEGF mRNA increased significantly after 24 and 72 h. The up-regulation of HIF and VEGF has been confirmed in bladder specimens from LUTS/BPE subjects. Koritsiadis et al. compared the expression of HIF-1alpha and carbonic anhydrase IX, a further cellular marker of hypoxia, in detrusor tissue retrieved from

patients scheduled for surgery to treat BPE and controls [36]. The mean number of total cells immunoreactive to HIF-1α in the study group was significantly higher with respect to the control group. HIF-1α was expressed mainly in stromal cells between muscle bundles and in connective tissue beneath the mucosal layer, while urothelium and detrusor had no immunoreactivity [36]. Interestingly, the HIF-1α response was limited in a time-dependent manner. Indeed, the probability of HIF-1α immunoreactivity was four times greater in men with BOO for < 10 years, than in those with BOO for > 10 years with an odds ratio of 4.25 thus suggesting that the bladder can compensate for the first few years after that the adaptive response declines [36]. Moreover, the risk of identifying a high expression of HIF-1α was four times higher in patients with urinary retention [36]. Barbosa et al. compared the gene expression of the angiogenic growth factor VEGF in bladder specimens from patients with obstructive BPH with grade IV or higher BOO as per Schäfer criteria and age-matched controls [37]. Patients with BOO presented a statistically significant overexpression of VEGF. Interestingly, upregulation of VEGF was particularly evident in subjects with risk factors for atherosclerosis.

Effects of hypoxia on HBSMCs proliferation
Galvin et al. demonstrated that HBSMCs exposed to hypoxia maintain their cell viability in culture and do not undergo cell death when placed under hypoxic conditions [7]. However, hypoxia significantly reduces the rate of proliferation in a time-dependent manner, associated with an increase in the cell cycle inhibitor p27^{kip1} [7].

Effects of hypoxia on HBSMCs differentiation

Wiafe et al. found evidences in favor of HBSMCs dedifferentiation, as demonstrated by the increased expression of α-smooth muscle actin, vimentin, and desmin, and acquisition of a profibrotic phenotype [35]. Pro-fibrotic changes included the upregulation of SMAD 2, SMAD 3, and connective tissue growth factor (CTGF) genes as well as collagens 1, 2, 3, and 4, fibronectin, aggrecan, and TIMP-1 transcripts [35]. Collagen 1 transcripts exhibited a consistent increase over the entire time course, with a 3.4-fold increase after 2 h eventually reaching a maximum fold increase of 12 by 72 h. Collagen 2 transcript levels showed a 4-fold increase by 72 h; collagen 3 exhibited a similar increase, although a 5-fold increase was evident at 48 and 72 h. Collagen 4 transcripts rose by almost 8-fold following 72 h hypoxia. Total secreted collagen remained at control values until 24 h at which point levels rose by 100% and values remained consistently elevated during prolonged hypoxia. Fibronectin transcripts showed a consistent increase from 1.9 to 3.9-fold for values between 24 and 72 h.

Effects of hypoxia on inflammatory pathways

Wiafe et al. demonstrated that hypoxia can produce a robust inflammatory response in isolated HBSMCs [35]. Indeed, hypoxia induced increased expression of TNFα, IL 1β, and IL 6 which are all part of the acute phase proteins secreted in response to inflammation. Transcript levels of the anti-inflammatory cytokine, IL-10 exhibited a consistent decline [35].

Other SMCs molecular alterations

Boopathi et al. demonstrated the loss of caveolin-1, a protein that has a pivotal role in regulating SMCs contractile activity, in bladder wall smooth muscle from BPO subjects [38].

Alterations occurring in the neuronal compartment

We identified four studies describing BOO-induced morphological alterations involving bladder innervation and two studies investigating the potential role of tissue nerve growth factor (Table 3). Golsin et al. found a 56% reduction in the number of acetylcholine-positive nerves in the specimens from obstructed bladder with respect to controls [39]. Cumming et al. confirmed the significant reduction of detrusor innervation in bladder biopsies from patients with urodynamic confirmed BOO [40]. Interestingly, innervation level was normalized in 80% of patients after BOO relief. Chapple et al. demonstrated a reduction in the density of innervation by vasoactive intestinal polypeptide, calcitonin gene-related peptide, substance P and somatostatin-immunoreactive but not neuropeptide Y-immunoreactive nerve fibers in bladder specimens from BOO patients [41]. Elbadawi et al. showed axon degeneration at electron microscopy in

Table 3 Summary of studies evaluating BOO-induced neuronal alterations

Author, year	Study design	Subjects in the cases group (n)	Findings
Gosling, 1986 [39]	Case-control	19	↓ autonomic nerve supply
Chapple, 1992 [41]	Case-control	19	↓ density of innervation by vasoactive intestinal polypeptide, calcitonin gene-related peptide, substance P and somatostatin immunoreactive nerve fibers in the obstructed bladder.
Cumming, 1992 [40]	Case-control	10	↓innervation
Elbadawi, 1993 [12]	Case control	7	↑axon degeneration in patients with impaired detrusor contractility
Steers, 1991 [42]	Case-control	–	↑ NGF in grossly hypertrophied human bladders
Barbosa, 2017 [37]	Case-control	43	↑ NGF receptor expression in smokers and dyslipidemic patients

NGF nerve growth factor

specimens of patients who had impaired detrusor contractility [12]. The role of tissue nerve growth factor, a key signal in the regulation of nerve physiology, is controversial. Steers et al. found that the amount of nerve growth factor in grossly hypertrophied human bladders exceeded that in non-hypertrophied samples [42]. In the study by Barbosa et al. the levels of nerve growth factor and of nerve growth factor receptor in bladder tissue from the overall BPO population were not different with respect to controls [37]. However, the levels of nerve growth factor receptors were higher in the subgroup of smokers and dyslipidemic BPO patients [37].

Discussion

To our knowledge, we performed the first systematic review of studies investigating BOO-induced morphological and molecular alterations in human bladder. Data summarized demonstrate the occurrence of a remodeling process involving multiple cellular compartments, namely urothelium, suburothelium, detrusor SMCs, detrusor ECM, and neurons. Based on evidences from in-vitro HBSMCs cultures, cyclical stretch, increased pressure and hypoxia can modulate several signaling pathways potentially involved in this process. Taken together, these data support the hypothesis that the natural history of BOO may be characterized, also in humans, by three morpho-functional stages: an initial hypertrophy phase, a subsequent compensation, and a late decompensation (Fig. 2). Increased intravescical pressure during bladder voiding, the pathognomonic urodynamic feature of BOO, can be considered the "primum movens". Indeed, it can stimulate compensatory SMCs hypertrophy and proliferation as demonstrated by in vitro studies. Tissue hypoxia subsequently intervenes as further critical stress factor. It is due to the imbalance between increased oxygen demand and lower oxygen delivery and may arise early in the natural history of BOO-induced bladder remodeling. Clinically, detrusor hypoxia has been confirmed in studies on human subjects with evidence of BOO [45–47]. Compensatory responses to hypoxia have been demonstrated in several human tissues, including the bladder. These include hypoxia-induced pathways such as HIF and VEGF. Available data suggest that, similar to animal models, these adaptive responses may counteract hypoxia only for a limited period of time. Persistent hypoxia also inhibits HBSMCs proliferation thus favoring the transition from the hypertrophy to the compensation phase, and activates signaling involved in ECM remodeling and collagen accumulation that characterize the transition from compensation to decompensation. Indeed, increased deposition of collagen and elastin in the interfascicular and intrafascicular detrusor compartments can alter the bio-mechanical properties of the bladder causing decreased compliance and impaired voiding function, which are feature considered by some authors as clinical marker of decompensation. Results from the present review have relevant clinical implications. In recent years evidences have emerged demonstrating that LUTS/BPO represent a progressive disorder in many patients [48–50]. Progression, however, has been defined based on clinical parameters such as deterioration of symptoms and health-related quality of life, decreased urinary peak flow rate, increased prostate size, and unfavorable outcomes such as AUR and BPE-related surgery [48–50]. Based on the results from the present study, clinicians should be aware of the fact that, beyond subjective symptoms, BPO also causes progressive morphological remodeling of the bladder with potential serious functional impairments. Consequently, this aspect should be carefully taken in account in the management of these patients and therapeutic outcomes should include not only the improvement of subjective symptoms but also the prevention of pathologic bladder remodeling. Evidences summarized in the present review suggest the existence of multiple signaling pathways that can represent potential targets for future therapies. Meantime, increased bladder pressure is the only pathophysiological mechanism that can be realistically improved in everyday clinical practice. Although multiple treatment options are available to treat LUTS/BPO, only surgery, alpha-1 adrenergic antagonists and 5-alpha reductase inhibitors have been reported to improve BOO by reducing bladder pressures. The progressive model of bladder remodeling

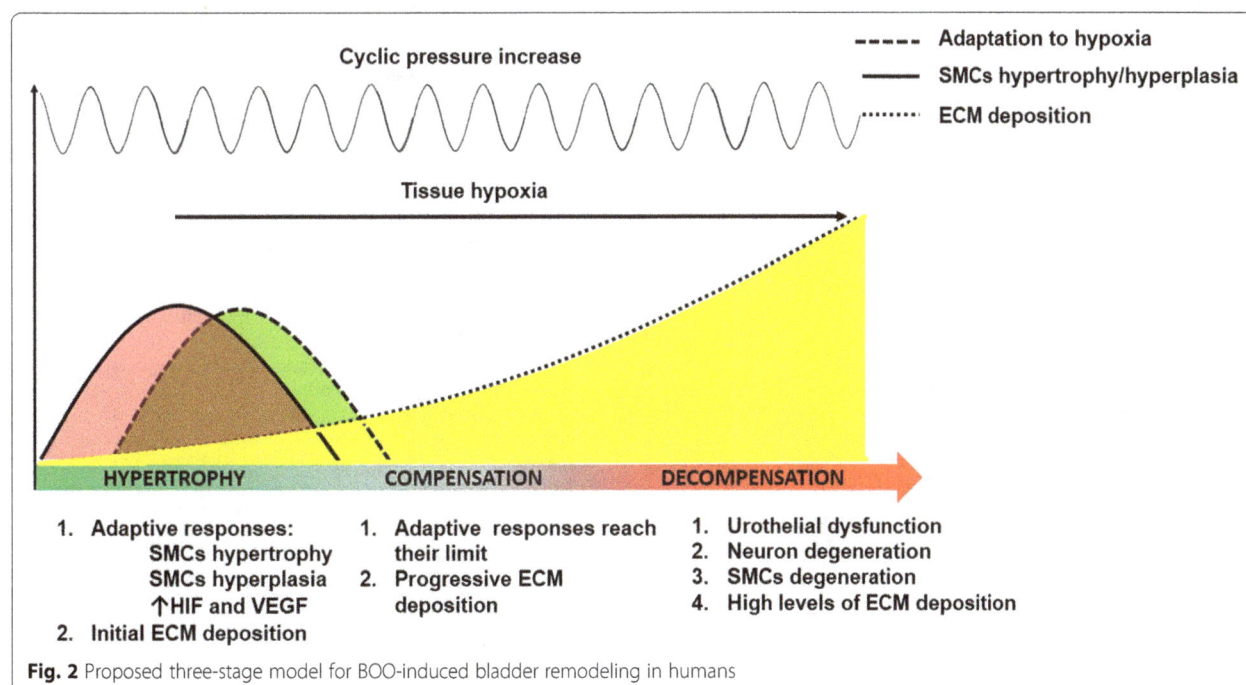

Fig. 2 Proposed three-stage model for BOO-induced bladder remodeling in humans

emerged from evidences summarized in the present study also contributes to explain the failures of surgical and medical therapies when prescribed later in the natural history of BOO and suggests to intervene early [48–50]. Although adherence to medical therapy for LUTS/BPO has been reported to prevent clinical disease progression the advantages in terms of morphological remodeling deserve further investigations [51]. At time, only few clinical markers of morphological bladder remodeling are available including increased estimated bladder weight and endoscopic evidence of bladder trabeculation. The role of bladder biopsies is controversial [44]. Results from the present study provide the basis for future investigations about urinary and/or serum markers of bladder remodeling. Some limits of the present study should be acknowledged: studies included are often outdated and enrolled a limited number of patients. Cultured cells may differ from fresh detrusor tissues as potential interactions among various compartments are not considered and cells are simply exposed to a single stress factor. Consequently, the molecular mechanism of bladder remodeling in BOO remains unclear and it remains difficult to establish an integrated signaling pathway. Further issues deserving investigations are the timing and the reversibility of BOO-induced bladder remodeling.

Conclusions

Evidences from available studies on human tissues demonstrate that BOO induces molecular and morphological alterations in multiple bladder compartments, namely urothelium, suburothelium, detrusor SMCs, detrusor ECM, and neurons. Cyclic stretch, increased pressure and hypoxia have been demonstrated to modulate multiple signaling pathways involved in these processes. A three-stages model can be hypothesized to characterize BOO-induced bladder remodeling also in humans: hypertrophy, compensation, decompensation.

Abbreviations
AUR: Acute urinary retention; BOO: Bladder outlet obstruction; BPE: Benign prostatic enlargement; BPO: Benign prostatic obstruction; C/M: Connective Tissue-to-Smooth Muscle Ratio; CHP: Chronic hydrostatic pressure; CTGF: Connective tissue growth factor; ECM: Extracellular matrix; HBSMCs: Human bladder smooth muscle cells; HIF: Hypoxia inducible factor; HP: Hydrostatic pressure; IL: Interleukin; LUTS: Lower urinary tract symptoms; MMPs: Matrix metalloproteinases; PDGF: Platelet derived growth factor; SMCs: Smooth Muscle Cells; TIMP: Tissue inhibitors of metalloproteases; TNF: Tumor necrosis factor; VEGF: Vascular endothelial growth factor

Acknowledgements
All authors belong to the Italian Society of Urodynamics (SIUD) Publication Group.

Authors' contributions
Conception and design: FF, MC, EFA. Drafting of the manuscript: MC, FF, VLM, VI. Analysis and interpretation of data: FM, CDN, VI. Supervision: EFA, FM, CDN. We confirm that all authors read and approved the final manuscript.

Author details
[1]Dipartimento di Neuroscienze e Scienze Riproduttive ed Odontostomatologiche, Università Degli Studi Di Napoli Federico II, Via Pansini, 5, 80131 Naples, Italy. [2]Dipartimento di Urologia, Ospedale Sant'Andrea, Università Degli Studi di Roma "La Sapienza", Rota, Italy. [3]Dipartimento di Medicina Sperimentale e Chirurgia, Università Degli Studi di Roma "Tor Vergata", Roma, Italy. [4]Dipartimento di Urologia, Ospedale Careggi, Università Degli Studi di Firenze, Firenze, Italy.

References
1. Fusco F, Creta M, Imperatore V, Longo N, Imbimbo C, Lepor H, et al. Benign prostatic obstruction relief in patients with lower urinary tract symptoms suggestive of benign prostatic enlargement undergoing endoscopic surgical procedures or therapy with alpha-blockers: a review of urodynamic studies. Adv Ther. 2017;34(4):773–83.
2. Fusco F, Palmieri A, Ficarra V, Giannarini G, Novara G, Longo N, et al. α1-blockers improve benign prostatic obstruction in men with lower urinary tract symptoms: a systematic review and meta-analysis of urodynamic studies. Eur Urol. 2016;69(6):1091–101.
3. Creta M, Bottone F, Sannino S, Maisto E, Franco M, Mangiapia F, et al. Effects of alpha1-blockers on urodynamic parameters of bladder outlet obstruction in patients with lower urinary tract symptoms suggestive of benign prostatic enlargement: a review. Minerva Urol Nefrol. 2016;68(2):209–21.
4. Mirone V, Imbimbo C, Longo N, Fusco F. The detrusor muscle: an innocent victim of bladder outlet obstruction. Eur Urol. 2007;51(1):57–66.
5. Komninos C, Mitsogiannis I. Obstruction-induced alterations within the urinary bladder and their role in the pathophysiology of lower urinary tract symptomatology. Can Urol Assoc J. 2014;8(7–8):E524–30.
6. Levin R, Chichester P, Levin S, Buttyan R. Role of angiogenesis in bladder response to partial outlet obstruction. Scand J Urol Nephrol Suppl. 2004;215:37–47.
7. Galvin DJ, Watson RW, O'Neill A, Coffey RN, Taylor C, Gillespie JI, et al. Hypoxia inhibits human bladder smooth muscle cell proliferation: a potential mechanism of bladder dysfunction. Neurourol Urodyn. 2004;23(4):342–8.
8. Moher D, Liberati A, Tetzlaff J, Altman DG. PRISMA Group Preferred reporting items for systematic reviews and meta-analyses: the PRISMA statement. BMJ. 2009;339:2535.
9. Jiang YH, Lee CL, Kuo HC. Urothelial dysfunction, suburothelial inflammation and altered sensory protein expression in men with bladder outlet obstruction and various bladder dysfunctions: correlation with Urodynamics. J Urol. 2016;196(3):831–7.
10. Gilpin SA, Gosling JA, Barnard RJ. Morphological and morphometric studies of the human obstructed, trabeculated urinary bladder. Br J Urol. 1985;57(5):525–9.
11. Collado A, Batista E, Gelabert-Más A, Corominas JM, Arañó P, Villavicencio H. Detrusor quantitative morphometry in obstructed males and controls. J Urol. 2006;176(6 Pt 1):2722–8.
12. Elbadawi A, Yalla SV, Resnick NM. Structural basis of geriatric voiding dysfunction. IV. Bladder outlet obstruction. J Urol. 1993;150(5 Pt 2):1681–95.
13. Tse V, Wills E, Szonyi G, Khadra MH. The application of ultrastructural studies in the diagnosis of bladder dysfunction in a clinical setting. J Urol. 2000;163(2):535–9.
14. Brierly RD, Hindley RG, McLarty E, Harding DM, Thomas PJ. A prospective evaluation of detrusor ultrastructural changes in bladder outlet obstruction. BJU Int. 2003;91(4):360–4.
15. Gosling JA, Dixon JS. Structure of trabeculated detrusor smooth muscle in cases of prostatic hypertrophy. Urol Int. 1980;35(5):351–5.
16. Blatt AH, Brammah S, Tse V, Chan L. Transurethral prostate resection in patients with hypocontractile detrusor–what is the predictive value of ultrastructural detrusor changes? J Urol. 2012;188(6):2294–9.
17. Holm NR, Horn T, Smedts F, Nordling J, de la Rossette J. The detrusor muscle cell in bladder outlet obstruction–ultrastructural and morphometric findings. Scand J Urol Nephrol. 2003;37(4):309–15.
18. Rubinstein M, Sampaio FJ, Costa WS. Stereological study of collagen and elastic system in the detrusor muscle of bladders from controls and patients with infravesical obstruction. Int Braz J Urol. 2007;33(1):33–9.
19. Inui E, Ochiai A, Naya Y, Ukimura O, Kojima M. Comparative morphometric study of bladder detrusor between patients with benign prostatic hyperplasia and controls. J Urol. 1999;161(3):827–30.

20. Averbeck MA, De Lima NG, Motta GA, Beltrao LF, Abboud Filho NJ, Rigotti CP, et al. Collagen content in the bladder of men with LUTS undergoing open prostatectomy: a pilot study. Neurourol Urodyn. 2017;25 https://doi.org/10.1002/nau.23418.

21. Bellucci CHS, Ribeiro WO, Hemerly TS, de Bessa J Jr, Antunes AA, Leite KRM, et al. Increased detrusor collagen is associated with detrusor overactivity and decreased bladder compliance in men with benign prostatic obstruction. Prostate Int. 2017;5(2):70–4.

22. Mirone V, Imbimbo C, Sessa G, Palmieri A, Longo N, Granata AM, et al. Correlation between detrusor collagen content and urinary symptoms in patients with prostatic obstruction. J Urol. 2004;172(4 Pt 1):1386–9.

23. Yang R, Amir J, Liu H, Chaqour B. Mechanical strain activates a program of genes functionally inolved in paracrine signaling of angiogenesis. Physiol Genomics. 2008;36(1):1–14.

24. Wang Y, Wang K, Li H, Chen L, Xu F, Wu T. Effects of different sustained hydrostatic pressures on connexin 43 in human bladder smooth muscle cells. Urol Int. 2013;90(1):75–82.

25. Lee SD, Akbal C, Jung C, Kaefer M. Intravesical pressure induces hyperplasia and hypertrophy of human bladder smooth musclecells mediated by muscarinic receptors. J Pediatr Urol. 2006;2(4):271–6.

26. Lee SD, Misseri R, Akbal C, Jung C, Rink RC, Kaefer M. Muscarinic receptor expression increases following exposure to intravesical pressures of < or =40 cm-H2O: a possible mechanism for pressure-induced cell proliferation. World J Urol. 2008;26(4):387–93.

27. Preis L, Herlemann A, Adam RM, Dietz HG, Kappler R, Stehr M. Platelet Derived Growth Factor Has a Role in Pressure Induced Bladder Smooth Muscle CellHyperplasia and Acts in a Paracrine Way. J Urol. 2015;194(6):1797–805.

28. Chen L, Wei TQ, Wang Y, Zhang J, Li H, Wang KJ. Simulated bladder pressure stimulates human bladder smooth muscle cell proliferation via the PI3K/SGK1 signaling pathway. J Urol. 2012;188(2):661–7.

29. Sun Y, Luo DY, Zhu YC, Zhou L, Yang TX, Tang C, et al. MiR 3180 5p promotes proliferation in human bladder smooth muscle cell by targeting PODN under hydrodynamic pressure. Sci Rep 2016; 9. 6:33042.

30. Sun Y, Luo D, Zhu Y, Wang K. MicroRNA 4323 induces human bladder smooth muscle cell proliferation under cyclic hydrodynamic pressure by activation of erk1/2 signaling pathway. Exp Biol Med (Maywood) 2017; 242(2):169–176.

31. Wu T, Chen L, Wei T, Wang Y, Xu F, Wang K. Effect of cyclic hydrodynamic pressure-induced proliferation of human bladder smooth muscle through Ras-related C3 botulinum toxin substrate 1, mitogen-activated protein kinase kinase 1/2 and extracellular regulated protein kinases 1/2. Int J Urol. 2012;19(9):867–74.

32. Chen L, Wu T, Wei TQ, Wei X, Li SF, Wang KJ, et al. Skp2-mediated degradation of p27 regulates cell cycle progression in compressed human bladder smooth muscle cells. Kaohsiung J Med Sci. 2014;30(4):181–6.

33. Liang Z, Xin W, Qiang L, Xiang C, Bang-Hua L, Jin Y, et al. Hydrostatic pressure and muscarinic receptors are involved in the release of inflammatory cytokines in human bladder smooth muscle cells. Neurourol Urodyn. 2017;36(5):1261–9.

34. Backhaus BO, Kaefer M, Haberstroh KM, Hile K, Nagatomi J, Rink RC, et al. Alterations in the molecular determinants of bladder compliance at hydrostatic pressures lessthan 40 cm. H2O. J Urol. 2002;168(6):2600–4.

35. Wiafe B, Adesida A, Churchill T, Adewuyi EE, Li Z, Metcalfe P. Hypoxia-increased expression of genes involved in inflammation, dedifferentiation, pro-fibrosis, and extracellular matrix remodeling of human bladder smooth muscle cells. In Vitro Cell Dev Biol Anim. 2017;53(1):58–66.

36. Koritsiadis G, Stravodimos K, Koutalellis G, Agrogiannis G, Koritsiadis S, Lazaris A, et al. Immunohistochemical estimation of hypoxia in human obstructed bladder and correlation with clinical variables. BJU Int. 2008; 102(3):328–32.

37. Barbosa JABA, Reis ST, Nunes M, Ferreira YA, Leite KR, Nahas WC, et al. The obstructed bladder: expression of collagen, matrix metalloproteinases, muscarinic receptors, and Angiogenic and neurotrophic factors in patients with benign prostatic hyperplasia. Urology. 2017;106:167–72.

38. Boopathi E, Gomes CM, Goldfarb R, John M, Srinivasan VG, Alanzi J, et al. Transcriptional repression of Caveolin-1 (CAV1) gene expression by GATA-6 in bladder smoothmuscle hypertrophy in mice and human beings. Am J Pathol. 2011;178(5):2236–51.

39. Gosling JA, Gilpin SA, Dixon JS, Gilpin CJ. Decrease in the autonomic innervation of human detrusor muscle in outflow obstruction. J Urol. 1986;136(2):501–4.

40. Cumming JA, Chisholm GD. Changes in detrusor innervation with relief of outflow tract obstruction. Br J Urol. 1992;69(1):7–11.

41. Chapple CR, Milner P, Moss HE, Burnstock G. Loss of sensory neuropeptides in the obstructed human bladder. Br J Urol. 1992;70(4):373–81.

42. Steers WD, Kolbeck S, Creedon D, Tuttle JB. Nerve growth factor in the urinary bladder of the adult regulates neuronal form and function. J Clin Invest. 1991;88(5):1709–15.

43 Gheinani AH, Kiss B, Moltzahn F, Keller I, Bruggmann R, Rehrauer H, et al. Characterization of miRNA-regulated networks, hubs of signaling, and biomarkers in obstruction-induced bladder dysfunction. JCI Insight. 2017;2(2):e89560.

44 Horn T, Kortmann BB, Holm NR, Smedts F, Nordling J, Kiemeney LA, et al. Routine bladder biopsies in men with bladder outlet obstruction? Urology. 2004;63(3):451–6.

45 Belenky A, Abarbanel Y, Cohen M, Yossepowitch O, Livne PM, Bachar GN. Detrusor resistive index evaluated by Doppler ultrasonography as a potential indicator of bladder outlet obstruction. Urology. 2003;62(4): 647–50.

46 Farag FF, Meletiadis J, Saleem MD, Feitz WF, Heesakkers JP. Near-infrared spectroscopy of the urinary bladder during voiding in men with lower urinary tractsymptoms: a preliminary study. Biomed Res Int. 2013;2013:452857.

47 Macnab AJ, Shadgan B, Stothers L, Afshar K. Ambulant monitoring of bladder oxygenation and hemodynamics using wireless near-infraredspectroscopy. Can Urol Assoc J. 2013;7(1–2):E98–E104.

48 Roehrborn CG. 5-alpha-reductase inhibitors prevent the progression of benign prostatic hyperplasia. Rev Urol. 2003;5(Suppl 5):S12–21.

49 Roehrborn CG. Alfuzosin 10 mg once daily prevents overall clinical progression of benign prostatic hyperplasia but not acute urinary retention: results of a 2-year placebo-controlled study. BJU Int. 2006;97(4):734–41.

50 Fusco F, Arcaniolo D, Creta M, Piccinocchi G, Arpino G, Laringe M, et al. Demographic and comorbidity profile of patients with lower urinary tract symptoms suggestive of benign prostatic hyperplasia in a real-life clinical setting: are 5-alpha-reductase inhibitor consumers different? World J Urol. 2015;33(5):685–9.

51 Cindolo L, Pirozzi L, Fanizza C, Romero M, Tubaro A, Autorino R, et al. Drug adherence and clinical outcomes for patients under pharmacological therapy for lower urinary tract symptoms related to benign prostatic hyperplasia: population-based cohort study. Eur Urol. 2015 Sep;68(3):418–25.

2

The unveiling of a new risk factor associated with bladder cancer

Sally Temraz, Yolla Haibe, Maya Charafeddine, Omran Saifi, Deborah Mukherji and Ali Shamseddine[*] iD

Abstract

Background: No accurate evaluation of smoking and water pollution on bladder cancer has been conducted in the Lebanese population. Our aim is to examine the significance of smoking and one of the main water pollutants Trihalomethanes (THM) on bladder cancer risk.

Methods: Population Attributable Fraction (PAF) was used to quantify the contribution of the risk factors smoking and THMs on bladder cancer in Lebanon. To calculate PAF for each risk factor, we used the proportion of the population exposed and the relative risk for each risk factor. Relative risks for each risk factor were obtained from published meta-analyses. The population at risk values were obtained from a report on chronic disease risk factor surveillance in Lebanon which was conducted by the World Health Organization between 2008 and 2009 and a national study by Semerjian et al. that conducted a multipathway exposure assessment of selected public drinking waters of Lebanon for the risk factors smoking and THMs, respectively.

Results: Bladder cancer cases that were the result of smoking in Lebanon among males and females are 33.4 and 18.6%, respectively. Cases attributed to mid-term exposure to THM contamination of drinking water is estimated at 8.6%.

Conclusion: This paper further highlights the negative impact of smoking on bladder cancer risk and adds an overlooked and often underestimated risk that THMs have on this type of cancer. Thus, it is imperative that a national based study which assesses THM exposure by gender and smoking status be implemented to determine the real risk behind this byproduct.

Keywords: Bladder cancer, Smoking, Trihalomethanes, Lebanon, Water pollution

Background

Bladder cancer is the ninth most common cancer among both sexes combined, accounting for 3.1% of all cancer cases in the world [1]. Incidence rates vary from 10 to 30 cases/100,000 for men and 1–6 cases/100,000 in women [2]. In addition to the well-known risk factors including advanced age, male gender and white race, environmental risk factors have significantly influenced incidence rates among exposed individuals [2, 3]. The International Agency for Research on Cancer (IARC) identified smoking as one of the causes of bladder cancer in both men and women [4]. Moreover, two large cohort studies conducted in Europe and the USA found that cigarette smoking is an important risk factor for

bladder cancer [5, 6]. Another potential risk factor for cancer is the production of chlorination by-products which are introduced during water treatment [7]. Naturally occurring humic and fluvic acids in water from decomposed plant and organic chemical interact with chlorine to form hundreds of halogenated chemical species, including trihalomethanes (THM), other haloalkanes, haloalkenes, haloacetic acids, other haloacids, haloacetonitriles, haloketones, haloaldehydes, and others [8]. The most commonly found and studied are trihalomethanes, with the highest concentration of chloroform, this chemical interaction occurs at the first stage of chlorination until distribution. THMs and other haloacetate byproducts were found carcinogenic in animal models and mutagenic in bacterial systems [8]. Two meta-analyses reported an association between THMs ingestion and bladder cancer risk [9, 10] and several case-control studies

* Correspondence: as04@aub.edu.lb
Department of Internal Medicine, American University of Beirut Medical Center, P.O.Box: 11-0236, Riad El Solh, Riad El Solh, Beirut 110 72020, Lebanon

supported this association [11–14]. Although some reported a modest association via the ingestion route [14], the main discrepancies in results were related to those reporting an association between THMs exposure through shower, swimming pools and inhalation and bladder cancer risk [15, 16]. The IARC classified THMs as Group 3 carcinogens concluding that there was inadequate evidence for their carcinogenicity to humans from the ecological and death certificate studies.

Recent data from the Lebanese National Cancer Registry (NCR) revealed that bladder cancer was the second most common cancer in males in 2008 after prostate. In fact it has the highest incidence rate in the Arab World, reaching 34 cases per 100,000 [1, 17]. This rate is expected to increase to 41/100,000 by 2018 considering the increasing number elderly and the high smoking levels [17].

Smoking remains the most well established risk factor in respiratory cancers and bladder cancer. Additional risk factors including water pollution have been studied to explain the rise in bladder cancer in specific areas among non-smokers. However, no accurate evaluation of smoking and water pollution on bladder cancer has been conducted in the Lebanese population. Our aim is to examine the significance of smoking and water pollution on the incidence of bladder cancer in Lebanon.

Methods

In this retrospective data analysis, the exposure to the risk is examined in relation to bladder cancer occurrence. The population attributable fraction (PAF) was used to estimate the role of THM on bladder cancer incidence in Lebanon. To quantify the contribution of a risk factor to cancer, two main components are needed; the proportion of the population subjected to the risk and the relative risk of cancer associated with that risk factor. Cancers that are the consequence of exposure to a risk factor are usually the result of an accumulation to that exposure over many years; a latent period of 10 years is viewed as satisfactory for most risk factors [18].

Prevalence of risk factors

In order to study the impact of smoking and water pollution on bladder cancer in the Lebanese population, we relied on population based reports or studies involving a representative sample of the Lebanese population that identifies the proportion of the population at risk. We used a report on chronic disease risk factor surveillance in Lebanon which was conducted by the World Health Organization between 2008 and 2009. The report involved subjects aged 25–64 years that were randomly selected using Lebanese Governorates strata [19]. From this report, data on behavioral factors such as tobacco smoking, physical activity and alcohol consumption were obtained as well as body mass index (BMI), age and gender [19]. We also studied the effect of the carcinogen THM found in water samples in Lebanon. For data on THM contamination of drinking water, we relied on a report published by Semergian et al. [20], where they found that an average of 94.7% of investigated networks in Lebanon exceeded the set United States Environmental Protection Agency (USEPA) range of concern for increased carcinogenic risk from THM. [21]. According to the Central Administration for Statistics (CAS), the only sources of drinking water are underground water or surface water. Thus bottled water, which is derived from either ground or surface water, is a representation of both.

To complete the analysis, relative risks were retrieved for each risk factor from meta-analyses from epidemiological studies, as shown in Table 1.

Risk factor: Smoking

We estimated the proportion of bladder cancer cases that were the result of smoking (including smokers and previous smokers). Data were stratified as: smokers, ex-smokers and non-smokers for all age and gender categories. The role of smoking on bladder cancer was calculated for each age and gender separately, aggregating the smokers and ex-smokers in one category in the final analysis. Noting that the relative risk (RR) for smokers and ex-smokers differ, calculations for each category were carried out separately first.

The RRs for smokers and ex-smokers were retrieved from a large meta-analysis in Korea [22], in which the population smoking habits and behavior is similar to our population.

Risk factor: THM

To obtain the RR of THM on bladder cancer risk, we relied on a study by Semerjian et al. that conducted a

Table 1 Showing population at risk and relative risk for each risk factor associated with bladder cancer in Lebanon

Risk factor	Population at risk		Reference	Relative risk		Reference
	Males	Females	[19]	Males	Females	[22]
Smoking						
Ex-smokers	6.9%	3.3%		1.5	0.92	
Current smokers	46.8%	31.6%		2	1.73	
Trihalomethanes	94.7%		[20]	1.1–1.4		[9, 20]

multipathway exposure assessment of selected public drinking waters of Lebanon based on the concentrations of THM within water distribution systems [20]. We also relied on a meta-analysis which involved six case-control studies (6084 incident bladder cancer cases, 10,816 controls) and two cohort studies (124 incident bladder cancer cases) [9]. The combined OR for mid-term exposure in both genders was 1.10 (95% CI 1.0 to 1.2) and for long term exposure was 1.4 (95% CI 1.2 to 1.7). Consistent results were shown in the Semergian study that noted an increased cancer risk for the spring season ranging between 1.19–1.39 folds [20]. The meta-analysis used a combination of RR and ORs. Noting that when the incidence of the outcome is low, such as in this case, it is safe to assume that the OR reported by Villanueva et al's metanalysis is equal to the RR.

Statistical method

To estimate the contribution of a risk factor to disease burden, this is expressed in the percentage of disease that is caused by a specific risk factor. The attributable risk in a population depends on the prevalence of the risk factor and the strength of its association (relative risk) with the disease. The formula is

$$PAF = Pe \, (RRe\text{-}1)/[1 + Pe \, (RRe\text{-}1)]$$

where Pe is the prevalence of the exposure and RRe is the relative risk of bladder cancer due to that exposure.In the case where the risk factor presents more than one exposure level, such as in tobacco smoking (ex-smokers, current smokers), a modified formula of the Levin formula was adopted as follows [23]:

$$PAF = P_1(RR_1\text{-}1) + P_2(RR_2\text{-}1)/1 + (P_1(RR_1\text{-}1) + P_2(RR_2\text{-}1))$$

We thus applied this formula to obtain the PAR for each of the above mentioned risk factors.

Results

We applied the formula for each of the risk factors and results are reported in Table 2.

Smoking:
By applying the modified Levin formula, we used as P_1 the percent of males that were current smokers (46.8%)

Table 2 Percentage attributable risk of smoking, THM on bladder cancer cases in Lebanon

Formula application	Gender	25–34	35–44	45–54	55–64	ALL
Smoking	M	29.5%	34.3%	37.5%	34.7%	33.4%
	F	11.2%	19.2%	24.7%	24.2%	18.6%
Trihalomethanes	Both	NA	NA	NA	NA	8.65%

NA not available

and RR_1 the relative risk due to smoking which is 2 and used as P_2 the percent of males that were ex-smokers (6.9%) and RR_2 the relative risk due to ex-smoking which is 1.5. Bladder cancer cases that were the result of smoking in Lebanon among males were 33.4% of cases for all age groups. Similarly, we applied the formula for females and found that bladder cancer cases that were the result of smoking among females were 18.6% of cases for all age groups if we consider the smokers percentage in 2009 and its implication by 2018. The risk impact is not immediate; we need a 10-year lag to draw any conclusions. For specific age groups of males and females, the percent of smokers and ex-smokers for each age category were obtained from the WHO's Chronic Disease Risk Factor Surveillance data for Lebanon [19] and formula applied. Results are shown in Table 2.

THM contamination:
Chlorination is the most adopted method of water sanitization in Lebanon, it is economical, quick and accessible. To calculate the percentage of bladder cancer cases attributed to mid-term exposure to THM contamination of drinking water we used the value of 94.7% for the Pe and value of 1.1 for RR since exposure to THM in Lebanon is midterm exposure. By applying the formula, we found that around 8.6% of bladder cancer cases in Lebanon could be attributed to THMs.

Discussion

Our results reveal that the proportion of bladder cancer cases in the Lebanese population which could be attributed to smoking are 33.4% in males and 18.6% in females. The prevalence of smoking in Lebanon is on the rise where adult smoking is estimated at 38.5% (males at 46% and females at 31%) and youth smoking is highest worldwide (65.8% for boys and 54.1% for girls) [24], with waterpipe smoking the major form of smoking (33.9%) followed by cigarette smoking (8.6%) [24]. Cancer incidence studies and the NCR consistently showed that bladder cancer has been distinctively high compared to regional and international rates [17, 25, 26]. We estimate that over a hundred case control and cohort studies have evaluated the risk attributed to smoking on bladder cancer. An analysis performed by Freedman et al. in 2011 which included 467,528 men and women found that compared to non-smokers, former and current smokers had a two- and a four-fold increased risk of bladder cancer, respectively [6]. The population risk of bladder cancer attributable to smoking was approximately 50% for both men and women [6].

Chlorination of water before it reaches the consumer is highly prevalent in Lebanon and our results show that THM contamination of drinking water could be responsible for 8.6% of bladder cancer cases. Initially, water chlorination played an essential role in reducing mortality rates due to water contamination with pathogens. Chlorination was seen as a miraculous public health solution in the early twentieth century when concerns were restricted to the presence of pathogens in water. The first potential hazards of chlorination were introduced in 1974 linking a toxic byproduct of this chlorination with organic matter to cancer risk [27]. The summary of the results of a meta analysis that evaluated the association between chlorinated drinking water and different cancer sites showed that it only affects the bladder ($P < 0.001$) and rectum ($P = 0.04$), whereas it showed no significant results in all of other sites including gastrointestinal sites, breast, and respiratory sites [7].

Our analysis was calculated for mid-term exposure since chlorination has not been used for a long time in Lebanon. However, within 20 years, the exposure would be long term and the risks are anticipated to be higher. A meta-analysis investigating the role of long term exposure of over 40 years to chlorinated drinking water in six case-control studies, revealed that it was associated with an increased risk of bladder cancer in men (combined OR = 1.4, 95% CI 1.1 to 1.9) and women (combined OR = 1.2, 95%CI 0.7 to 1.8, 9]. Another meta-analysis by Costet et al. reported a significant odds-ratio for men exposed to an average residential THM level > 50 µg/L (OR = 1.47) when compared to men exposed to levels ≤5 µg/L. The risk was not significant in females or through cumulative exposure through ingestion [10].

In addition to water ingestion, the high volatility and permeability of some disinfection by-products suggests that they can get into human bodies through bathing, washing vegetables, and swimming [27]. Following the solid waste management and landfill scandal in Lebanon, marine pollution gained major media attention and warned swimmers of accessing coastal areas in the summer. This news led a large proportion of swimmers to escape sea water pollution and opt for resort swimming pools instead. However, it was revealed that the chlorine concentration levels in these pools are high and uncontrollable as it is added arbitrarily in any of the private beach resorts thus increasing the exposure of the people to THM.

A case-control study conducted in Spain by Villanueva et al. tackling all entry routes of THMs, showed that individuals with long term exposure to THMs were twice as likely to have bladder cancer, OR = 2.10 (95% confidence interval: 1.09, 4.02) for average household THM levels of > 49 versus < 8 µg/L. When compared to controls, subjects who were drinking chlorinated water with a total THM exposure > 35 µg/day had an odds ratio of 1.35 (95% CI: 0.92, 1.99). On the other hand, the odds ratio attributed to exposure to highest compared to lowest quartile THM exposure through duration of shower or bath was calculated at 1.83 (95% CI: 1.17, 2.87). The odds ratio attributed to swimming in pools was 1.57 (95% CI: 1.18, 2.09) [28]. On the other hand, a recent case control study by Freeman et al. reported significant adjusted ORs for bladder cancer comparing participants with exposure above the 95th percentile with those in the lowest quartile of daily exposure to brominated THMs [OR = 1.98 (95% CI: 1.19, 3.29), p - trend = 0.03] and cumulative exposure to brominated THMS 1.78 (95% CI: 1.05, 3.00), p - trend = 0.02 but was not significant for chlorinated THMs. Moreover, Freeman et al. did not find any association between swimming pool use and bladder cancer contrary to what Villanueva et al. reported. Thus, the association between THMs and bladder cancer risk is still inconclusive but seems to be more in favor of the ingestion route of THMs than exposure through skin.

Several limitations in our study should be noted. First, we have no national based data on THM concentrations in drinking water as we have for smoking. This deficiency of exposure to THM by age, and gender limited our calculation to a general estimate of the exposure for all population. Socio economic and geographical differences were not accounted for while they can affect drinking water availability and exposure to contaminated water. Our results are therefore general estimates and not an actual representation of the water quality in Lebanon. Moreover, the risk calculated for THM included both smokers and non-smokers since our data source had limited information on the subject and did not stratify according to smoker and non-smokers. Although estimates, the figures reported reveal a possible problem in the drinking waters of Lebanon and risk of bladder cancer which was not previously accounted for. Our underground waters have been compromised with sewage and solid waste. It is thus imperative that a national based study be conducted to assess all sources of drinking water in Lebanon and a framework be placed to prevent further contamination and corrective measures be taken where possible.

Conclusions

Our results have highlighted the impact of smoking on bladder cancer risk as have many previous reports all over the world. In our report, there were 33.4% of male cases of bladder cancers and 18.6% of female cases attributed to smoking. This paper adds an overlooked risk affecting bladder cancer that is the impact that THMs and have on bladder cancer risk. We estimated the risk from THM exposure to be 8.65%. A national based study to assess THM exposure by gender and smoking status is highly needed to determine the risk of this contaminant on bladder cancer.

Abbreviations

BMI: Body mass index; CAS: Central Administration for Statistics; CC: Chronic cystitis; IARC: The International Agency for Research on Cancer; LARI: Lebanese Agricultural Research Institute; NCR: National Cancer Registry; PAF: Population attributable fraction; TCC: Transition cell cancer; THM: Trihalomethanes; USEPA: United States Environmental Protection Agency

Acknowledgements

Not applicable.

Authors' contributions

ST conceived of the study and wrote the paper. DM revised and edited the paper. MC analyzed and interpreted the results. YH and OS helped in acquisition of data. AS conceived, designed and revised the paper. All authors have read and approved the final manuscript.

References

1. Ferlay J, Soerjomataram I, Dikshit R, Eser S, Mathers C, Rebelo M, et al. Cancer incidence and mortality worldwide: sources, methods and major patterns in GLOBOCAN 2012. Int J Cancer. 2015;136:E359–86.
2. Jankovic S, Radosavljevic V. Risk factors for bladder cancer. Tumori. 2007;93: 4–12.
3. Malats N, Real FX. Epidemiology of bladder cancer. Hematol Oncol Clin North Am. 2015;29:177–89 vii.
4. IARC Monographs on the Evaluation of Carcinogenic Risks to Humans. Personal Habits and Indoor Combustions, vol. 100. E. Lyon, France: International Agency for Research on Cancer; 2012.
5. Bjerregaard BK, Raaschou-Nielsen O, Sorensen M, Frederiksen K, Christensen J, Tjonneland A, et al. Tobacco smoke and bladder cancer-- in the European prospective investigation into Cancer and nutrition. Int J Cancer. 2006;119:2412–6.
6. Freedman ND, Silverman DT, Hollenbeck AR, Schatzkin A, Abnet CC. Association between smoking and risk of bladder cancer among men and women. JAMA. 2011;306:737–45.
7. Morris RD. Drinking water and cancer. Environ Health Perspect. 1995; 103(Suppl 8):225–31.
8. Cantor KP. Drinking water and cancer. Cancer Causes Control. 1997;8: 292–308.
9. Villanueva C, Fernandez F, Malats N, Grimalt J, Kogevinas M. Meta-analysis of studies on individual consumption of chlorinated drinking water and bladder cancer. J Epidemiol Community Health. 2003;57:166–73.
10. Costet N, Villanueva CM, Jaakkola JJ, Kogevinas M, Cantor KP, King WD, et al. Water disinfection by-products and bladder cancer: is there a European specificity? A pooled and meta-analysis of European case-control studies. Occup Environ Med. 2011;68:379–85.
11. Cantor KP, Lynch CF, Hildesheim ME, Dosemeci M, Lubin J, Alavanja M, et al. Drinking water source and chlorination byproducts. I. Risk of bladder cancer. Epidemiology. 1998;9:21–8.
12. King WD, Marrett LD. Case-control study of bladder cancer and chlorination by-products in treated water (Ontario, Canada). Cancer Causes Control. 1996;7:596–604.
13. Bove GE Jr, Rogerson PA, Vena JE. Case-control study of the effects of trihalomethanes on urinary bladder cancer risk. Arch Environ Occup Health. 2007;62:39–47.
14. Beane Freeman LE, Cantor KP, Baris D, Nuckols JR, Johnson A, Colt JS, et al. Bladder Cancer and water disinfection by-product exposures through multiple routes: a population-based case-control study (New England, USA). Environ Health Perspect. 2017;125:067010.
15. Amado RG, Wolf M, Peeters M, Van Cutsem E, Siena S, Freeman DJ, et al. Wild-type KRAS is required for panitumumab efficacy in patients with metastatic colorectal cancer. J Clin Oncol. 2008;26:1626–34.
16. Villanueva CM, Cantor KP, Grimalt JO, Malats N, Silverman D, Tardon A, et al. Bladder cancer and exposure to water disinfection by-products through ingestion, bathing, showering, and swimming in pools. Am J Epidemiol. 2007;165:148–56.
17. Shamseddine A, Saleh A, Charafeddine M, Seoud M, Mukherji D, Temraz S, et al. Cancer trends in Lebanon: a review of incidence rates for the period of 2003-2008 and projections until 2018. Popul Health Metrics. 2014;12:4.
18. Parkin DM, Boyd L, Walker LC. 16. The fraction of cancer attributable to lifestyle and environmental factors in the UK in 2010. Br J Cancer. 2011; 105(Suppl 2):S77–81.
19. Sibai A, Hwala N: WHO steps chronic disease risk factor surveillance: data book for Lebanon, 2009. American University of Beirut; 2010.
20. Semerjian L, Dennis J. Multipathway risk assessment of trihalomethane exposure in drinking water of Lebanon. J Water Health. 2007;5:511–22.
21. Semerjian LA. Quality assessment of various bottled waters marketed in Lebanon. Environ Monit Assess. 2011;172:275–85.
22. Park S, Jee SH, Shin HR, Park EH, Shin A, Jung KW, et al. Attributable fraction of tobacco smoking on cancer using population-based nationwide cancer incidence and mortality data in Korea. BMC Cancer. 2014;14:406.
23. Hanley JA. A heuristic approach to the formulas for population attributable fraction. J Epidemiol Community Health. 2001;55:508–14.
24. Saade G, Warren CW, Jones NR, Asma S, Mokdad A. Linking global youth tobacco survey (GYTS) data to the WHO framework convention on tobacco control (FCTC): the case for Lebanon. Prev Med. 2008;47(Suppl 1):S15–9.
25. Shamseddine A, Sibai AM, Gehchan N, Rahal B, El-Saghir N, Ghosn M, et al. Cancer incidence in postwar Lebanon: findings from the first national population-based registry, 1998. Ann Epidemiol. 2004;14:663–8.
26. Kulhanova I, Bray F, Fadhil I, Al-Zahrani AS, El-Basmy A, Anwar WA, et al. Profile of cancer in the eastern Mediterranean region: the need for action. Cancer Epidemiol. 2017;47:125–32.
27. Villanueva CM, Cantor KP, Cordier S, Jaakkola JJ, King WD, Lynch CF, et al. Disinfection byproducts and bladder cancer: a pooled analysis. Epidemiology. 2004;15:357–67.
28. Villanueva CM, Cantor KP, Grimalt JO, Castano-Vinyals G, Malats N, Silverman D, et al. Assessment of lifetime exposure to trihalomethanes through different routes. Occup Environ Med. 2006;63:273–7.

3

Prognosis and risk factors of patients with upper urinary tract urothelial carcinoma and postoperative recurrence of bladder cancer in central China

Qingwei Wang[1]*(iD), Tao Zhang[1], Junwei Wu[1], Jianguo Wen[1,2], Deshang Tao[1], Tingxiang Wan[1] and Wen Zhu[1]

Abstract

Background: To investigate the prognostic risk factors and postoperative recurrence of bladder cancer in patients with upper urinary tract urothelial carcinomas (UTUCs).

Methods: Data of 439 UTUC patients were retrospectively analyzed. Follow-up and analysis of smoking effects, consumption of traditional Chinese medicine containing aristolochic acid, history of bladder cancer, age, sex, presence or absence of diabetes mellitus (DM), metformin use, tumor characteristics (number, location, stage, grade), and open or laparoscopic surgery on the prognosis of UTUCs were performed. Cox proportional hazard regression analysis was performed to analyze the relationship between various factors and the postoperative survival rate. The survival rate was analyzed using the Kaplan-Meier method. Moreover, logistic regression analysis was performed to analyze the relationship between the above mentioned factors and postoperative recurrence of bladder cancer.

Results: Overall, 439 patients met, including 236 males (53.7%) and 203 females (46.3%), the criteria for the final statistical analysis, and the average age was 66.7 years. The 1-, 3-, and 5-year overall survival rates of 439 UTUC patients were 90.0, 76.4, and 67.7%, respectively. The 5-year survival rates of T1, T2, T3, and T4 patients were 90.2%, 78%, 43.8%, and 18.5%, respectively. Factors influencing the long-term survival rate of UTUC patients were smoking, taking traditional Chinese medicine containing aristolochic acid, history of bladder cancer, age, tumor size, tumor stage, tumor grade, and lymph node metastasis. The risk factors related to postoperative bladder cancer recurrence were advanced tumor stage, high grade tumor, preoperative ureteroscopy, ureteral urothelial carcinoma, no postoperative bladder perfusion chemotherapy and DM without metformin use.

Conclusions: Advanced tumor stage and presence of a high-grade tumor were risk factors for not only poor UTUC prognosis but also BC recurrence. In addition, preoperative ureteroscopy, ureteral urothelial carcinoma and DM without metformin use were high risk factors for BC recurrence, whereas regular postoperative bladder perfusion chemotherapy was a protective factor.

Keywords: Upper urinary tract urothelial carcinoma, Survival analysis, Bladder cancer recurrence, Prognostic factor, Risk factor

---

* Correspondence: qwwang@zzu.edu.cn
[1]Department of Urology, The First Affiliated Hospital of Zhengzhou University, Zhengzhou 450052, Henan, China
Full list of author information is available at the end of the article

Background

Upper urinary tract urothelial carcinoma (UTUC) is a relatively rare tumor, accounting for approximately 10% of all renal tumors and only 5% of all urothelial carcinomas [1, 2], with an estimated annual incidence of almost two cases per 100,000 inhabitants in Western countries. The epidemiology and disease presentation of UTUCs in the Chinese population, however, are quite different from those in Western populations. First, UTUCs account for 20–30% of all transitional cell carcinomas (TCCs) in China, which is more common than that in Western countries [3, 4]. Second, UTUCs are more common in women than in men, with a ratio of 1.3:1 [4]. Third, the incidence of renal pelvis urothelial carcinoma is twice more among Chinese populations than among Western populations. TCC of the ureter accounts for more than half of UTUCs [5, 6] and about 25% of all renal carcinomas in China [3]. Finally, contrary to findings in Western countries, UTUC with an advanced stage, large tumor size, and lymph node metastasis (LNM) are less likely to progress in female Chinese patients than in male Chinese patients [7]. This may be associated with diverse environmental factors, such as pure-arsenic exposure in drinking water and consumption of aristolochic acid in Chinese herbs [3, 8].

However, the epidemiology and biological characteristics of UTUCs in the Chinese population have not gained research focus, and data are limited. Moreover, it remains unclear whether the following factors are related to prognosis and postoperative recurrence of bladder cancer (BC) in UTUC patients: diabetes mellitus (DM), metformin use in DM patients, preoperative ureteroscopy, and location of UTUC. Currently, radical nephroureterectomy (RNU) is the gold standard for treating UTUCs [9]. The incidence of intravesical tumor recurrence after operation is 20–50% [10]. Notably, 44% of patients with BC recurrence have invasive disease (≥pT1 stage), and 82–89% of BC recurrences occur within 2 years after RNU [11]. Hence, identifying high risk factors of BC recurrence after RNU is a major concern for UTUC patients.

Although a few studies have assessed predictive or risk factors of UTUCs and/or BC recurrence in Chinese people [3, 12], data were mainly obtained from the population of the North and Southeast of China, not from the central areas of China. Since the epidemiology and disease characteristics may be related to different areas, along with factors influencing survival and tumor recurrence remain controversial, we developed a database of UTUC in our region to investigate the prognostic risk factors of UTUC and BC recurrence in central China. We hope that our research will contribute to UTUC treatment options and reduce the risk of recurrence of BC after RNU.

Methods

Subjects

Data of patients with upper urinary tract tumors (UUTTs) from the Department of Urology of our hospital (the largest hospital in China, located in central China) were collected from March 2011 to February 2017. The inclusion criteria were as follows: 1. patients with unilateral UTUCs; 2. those who underwent RNU; 3. those with postoperative pathological confirmation of UTUC; and 4. those with complete clinical data and follow-up. The exclusion criteria were as follows: 1. patients with bilateral UTUC; 2. those with a history of UTUC awaiting renal transplantation; 3. those who received conservative treatment or simple nephrectomy; and 4. those with incomplete or missing clinical data.

Finally, 481 patients with UUTTs were selected. Among them, 12 patients did not undergo RNU, 8 had incomplete clinical data, 11 were lost to follow-up, 5 had squamous cell carcinoma, 4 had adenocarcinoma, and 2 were diagnosed with sarcoma. Finally, 439 patients with UTUC were included in this study. All patients underwent RNU with bladder cuff resection, and each patient was confirmed as having UTUC based on pathological reports.

Data records

The collected clinical data of UTUC patients included smoking status, history of taking Chinese herbs containing aristolochic acid, history of BC, DM, and DM with/without metformin use, age, sex, tumor characteristics (number, location, stage, grade, type), operation method, preoperative ureteroscopy, postoperative bladder perfusion chemotherapy, and BC recurrence (Table 1).

The criteria for identifying the influencing factors were as follows: a smoking index (number of cigarettes per day×years of smoking) above 200 was considered smoking. A history of taking Chinese medicine containing aristolochic acid was considered if at least 1 of the following criteria were met: 1) taking Chinese herbal medicine or Chinese patent medicine containing caulis aristolochiae manshuriensis; the duration of ingestion included the continuous use of caulis aristolochiae manshuriensis for > 15 days or the discontinuous use for > 2 months and 2) the continuous or intermittent use of other types of Chinese herbal or proprietary medicines containing aristolochic acid ingredients for > 6 months. Those aged > 50 years were considered as advanced in age. A low tumor location indicated ureteral urothelial carcinoma (UUC). The tumor clinical staging was performed according to the American Joint Committee on Cancer (AJCC) 2002; the tumor grading was assessed based on the WHO pathological grading system of malignant urothelial cancer 2004.

Table 1 The related prognostic influencing factors of UTUCs and the risk factors of bladder cancer recurrence in this study

Influential factors	Classification	No. of patients (%)
Sex	Male	236(53.7%)
	Female	203(46.3%)
Age	<50 yr	132(30.1%)
	≥50 yr	307(69.9%)
Smoking	Yes	204(46.5%)
	No	235(53.5%)
TCHAA	Yes	173(39.4%)
	No	166(60.6%)
History of BC	Yes	95(9.2%)
	No	344(90.8%)
DM	Yes	133(30.3%)
	No	306(69.7%)
DM + metformin use	Yes	53(39.8%)
	No	80(60.2%)
Number of tumors	Single	278(63.3%)
	Multiple	161(36.7%)
Tumor location	Renal pelvis	253(57.6%)
	Ureter	140(42.4%)
Tumor stage	T1-T2	246(56.0%)
	T3-T4	193(44.0%)
Tumor size	<3 cm	255(58.1%)
	≥3 cm	184(41.9%)
Tumor grade	G1-G2	352(80.2%)
	G3	87(19.8%)
LNM	Yes	86(19.6%)
	No	353(80.4%)
Preoperative Ureteroscopy	Yes	139(31.7%)
	No	300(68.3%)
Operation mode	Laparoscopic surgery	312(71.1%)
	Open surgery	127 (28.9%)
BC recurrence		89(20.3%)
	Renal pelvis carcinoma	30(33.7%)
	Ureteral carcinoma	59(66.3%)
	242 cases of PBPC	28(11.6%)
	197 cases of no PBPC	61(31.0%)
	DM	63(70.9%)
	DM with Metformin use	15(16.9%)
	DM without metformin use	48(53.9%)

THCAA taking Chinese herbs containing aristolochic acid, *LNM* lymph node metastasis, *PBPC* postoperative bladder perfusion chemotherapy, *DM* diabetes mellitus, *BC* bladder cancer

Follow-up

All patients were followed up regularly by telephone or internet contact, which was recorded in the electronic medical records (EMR) system of our hospital. Full-time urologists were responsible for following up patients according to the UTUC guidelines, and the patients were urged to undergo their medical examinations on time. All examination results during the follow-up period were recorded in detail. Postoperatively, cystoscopy was performed every 3 months within 2 years to assess for recurrence, then once every 6 months in the 3rd–4th year, and then once a year thereafter. During the follow-up time, other routine examinations, including blood routine tests, liver and kidney function tests, abdominal B-scan ultrasonography, chest X-ray every 6 months, and abdominal computed tomography (CT) once a year, were performed. Based on the treatment guidelines for UTUCs and patients' wishes, bladder perfusion chemotherapy following RNU for patients with UTUC was not a compulsory treatment. Depending on whether bladder instillation was performed after the operation, patients were divided into two groups: the perfusion group and the non-perfusion group. Perfusion was performed once a week for a maximum of 8 weeks and then once a month for 1 year following the operation. All data were recorded and monitored using the Jiahe EMR System. The survival rate, BC recurrence rate, and risk factors of BC recurrence were analyzed. The mortality and cause of death in the follow-up period were assessed based on data obtained from the family members, and the remaining data were obtained from the EMR system or the attending doctor.

Statistical analysis

Each influencing clinical factor was quantified (Table 1). A Cox proportional hazard regression model was used to evaluate the relationship between the risk factors and postoperative survival rate. Survival time was defined as the difference between follow-up time and operative time in months. The Kaplan-Meier method was used to analyze the survival rate. Furthermore, factors affecting postoperative BC recurrence were analyzed using a logistic regression model. SPSS 20.0 software was used to analyze the data, and a P value < 0.05 was considered statistically significant.

Results

Overall, 439 patients were included in the final statistical analysis. Among the 439 patients, 236 were males (53.7%) and 203 were females (46.3%), and the average age was 66.7 years. The follow-up period ranged from 18 to 84 months, with an average of 62.5 months. Factors included in the analysis are shown in Table 1. Tumor-associated death, BC recurrence rate, survival rate, risk factors for UTUCs, and BC recurrence were analyzed to predict the prognosis of patients with UTUC.

Survival rate

The 1-, 3-, and 5-year overall survival rates of the 439 patients were 90.0, 76.4, and 67.7%, respectively. The 5-year survival rates of patients with T1, T2, T3, and T4 were 90.2, 78, 43.8, and 18.5%, respectively (Fig. 1).

Effects of cox regression analysis on the prognosis of UTUCs

Cox regression analysis was performed to eliminate confounding factors. Eight factors, namely smoking, consumption of Chinese medicine containing aristolochic acid, history of BC, age, tumor stage, tumor grade, tumor size, and LNM, had a significant effect on survival and were identified as prognostic factors ($P < 0.05$). This suggested that smoking, taking Chinese medicine containing aristolochic acid, history of BC, older age, advanced tumor stage, high-grade tumors, larger tumors, and presence of LNM were risk factors of UTUC patients with poor prognosis. Sex, number of tumors, tumor location, DM, and mode of operation had no effect on the prognosis ($P > 0.05$). The results of the analysis of factors influencing survival time and prognosis are shown in Table 2.

Analysis of risk factors of postoperative BC recurrence

Among the 439 patients, 89 (20.3%) had BC recurrence, and their data were analyzed using the binary logistic regression model. We found that advanced tumor stage, presence of a high-grade tumor, preoperative ureteroscopy, DM without metformin use, and UUC were risk factors of postoperative BC recurrence. Patients with 1 or more than 1 of the risk factors were more likely to experience BC recurrence. Furthermore, regular postoperative bladder perfusion chemotherapy was a protective factor for recurrent BC. The results of the analysis of high risk factors for postoperative BC recurrence are shown in Table 3.

Discussion

In this study, we found that smoking, consuming Chinese medicine containing aristolochic acid, history of BC, old age, advanced tumor stage, presence of high-grade tumor, larger tumor size, and LNM were predictive factors for worse survival of UTUC. In addition, tumor stage, tumor grade, preoperative ureteroscopy, UUC, and DM without metformin use were risk factors of BC recurrence, whereas regular postoperative bladder perfusion chemotherapy and DM with metformin use were protective factors for BC relapse. Because the accurate prediction of the prognosis of UTUC patients could contribute to risk stratification and devising therapeutic options for urologists or oncologists, we analyzed each predictor in detail.

The incidence of UTUCs has been increasing each year, and 60% of UTUCs are found to have already

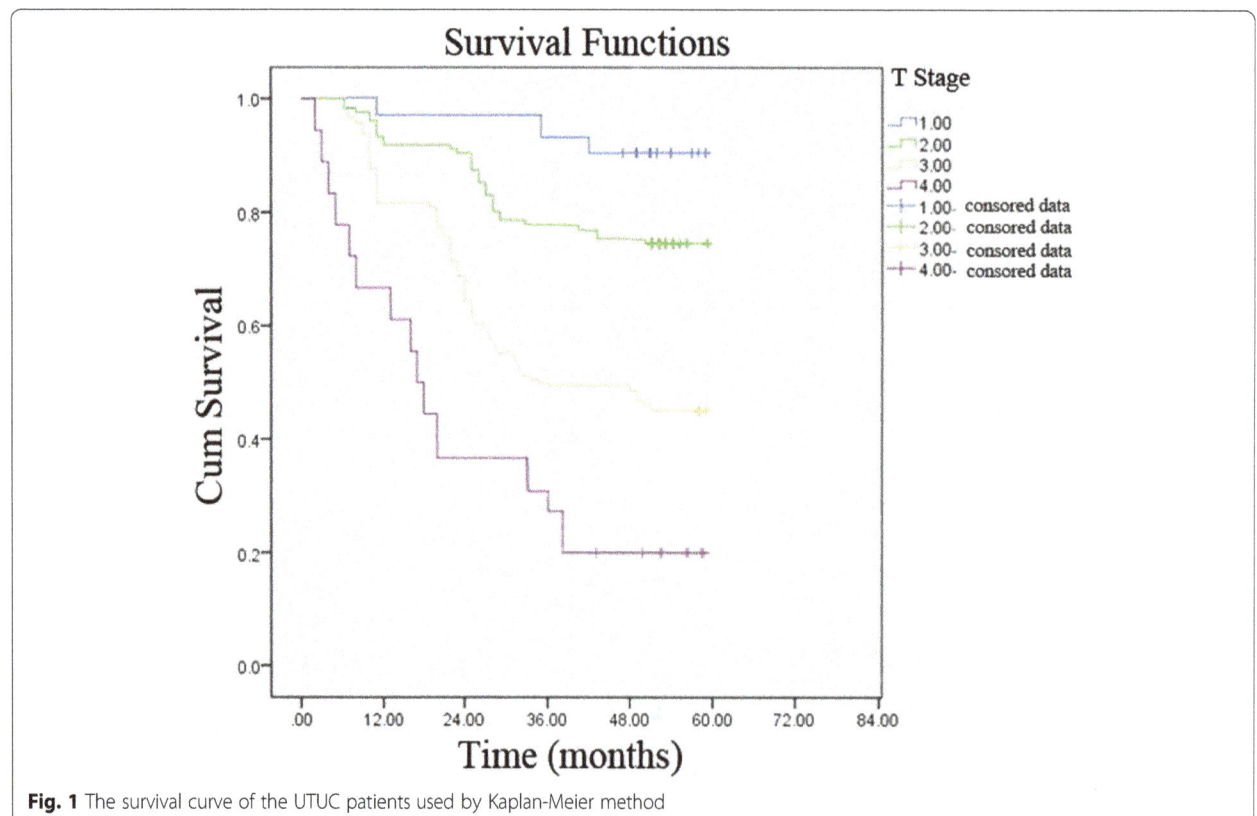

Fig. 1 The survival curve of the UTUC patients used by Kaplan-Meier method

Table 2 The outcomes of multiple COX regression analysis in the prognosis of UTUC

Variable	B	SE	Wald	Exp(B)	P
Smoking	0.964	0.214	20.207	2.381	< 0.01
THCAA	0.633	0.214	6.870	1.883	0.009
Age	0.357	0.169	4.468	0.700	0.035
Sex	0.002	0.145	0.000	1.002	0.991
Number of tumors	0.061	0.159	0.149	1.063	0.700
History of BC	0.698	0.228	9.356	2.010	0.002
LNM	1.994	0.353	31.915	7.343	< 0.01
Tumor size	0.449	0.158	8.086	0.638	< 0.01
Tumor location	0.162	0.260	0.390	0.850	0.532
Tumor stage	1.304	0.157	69.163	3.683	< 0.01
Tumor grade	2.157	0.298	52.291	8.646	< 0.01
Operation mode	0.472	0.378	1.559	1.603	0.212
DM	0.742	0.357	3.458	2.204	0.076

THCAA taking Chinese herbs containing aristolochic acid, *LNM* lymph node metastasis, *DM* diabetes mellitus

developed into invasive tumors at diagnosis compared with 15–25% of bladder tumors [1, 13]. UTUCs have a peak incidence in individuals aged 70–90 years and are three times more common in men in Western countries [1, 14]; these findings differed from those of our study in which the male-to-female ratio was 1:1.16. Previous studies showed that the survival rate of UTUC patients was related to the tumor stage and grade [4]. A multifactorial analysis of 252 UTUC cases by Hall et al. [15] revealed that tumor stage was the only indicator of postoperative survival. A study of 434 patients with UTUCs by Munoz and Ellison [16] showed that the 5-year survival rate of patients with Tis tumors was 95.1% and that of patients with local tumors was 88.9%; however, the 5-year survival rate of patients with distant metastasis was only 16.5%. In our study, tumor stage and grade were risk factors influencing the survival of

postoperative UTUC patients. A significant difference in 5-year survival rate occurred between low tumor staging (T1–T2) and high tumor staging (T3–T4), as well as between different tumor grades (G1–G2 and G3–G4). This suggests that early diagnosis and treatment with periodic follow-up are crucial for improving the survival rate.

UTUCs are prone to relapse and have a recurrence rate of 16–58% after surgery; thus, the current standard treatment of UTUCs is nephroureterectomy with bladder cuff resection [16]. The study also showed that the surgical approach (laparoscopic or open surgery) is not an influencing factor of postoperative survival. Mufti [17] also proposed that the surgical method (laparoscopy or open surgery) was not a prognostic factor, which is consistent with our results.

For most people, age is a risk factor of UTUC [18]. Raman et al. [19] investigated 13,800 patients with upper urinary tract tumors and showed that mortality owing to UTUCs increased with age. Similarly, we showed that compared with patients aged < 50 years, the relative risk of postoperative mortality increased among patients aged > 50 years. It is hypothesized that as the patient's age increases, the biological behavior of the tumor changes, with a decline in immune system function. LNM can be used to predict prognosis, especially for patients without lymph node dissection. Multicenter studies confirmed that LNM is closely related to higher tumor invasiveness, such as higher stage, higher grade, and distant metastasis. LNM can independently affect tumor recurrence and survival rate; hence, it is an independent risk factor for UTUC prognosis [20]. Our study also suggested that LNM was significantly associated with poor prognosis, which is consistent with the result of previous research. Tumor size has been also confirmed as a prognostic factor in some malignant tumors. The results of Simone's study [21] on UTUCs revealed that metastasis-free survival was closely related with tumor size: when the tumor diameter was < 3 cm, there

Table 3 The results of multiple logistic regression analysis of recurrent BC after RNU in UTUC patients

Variable	B	SE	Wald	Exp(B)	P
Age	0.170	0.525	0.105	1.186	0.746
Operation mode Number of tumors	0.016 0.030	0.322 0.389	0.002 0.006	1.016 1.030	0.960 0.939
LNM	0.228	0.574	0.158	1.256	0.691
Advanced tumor stage	1.064	0.300	12.548	2.899	< 0.01
Tumor location (UUC)	2.835	0.627	20.440	16.949	< 0.01
High-grade tumor	2.576	0.590	19.048	13.140	< 0.01
PBPC	−1.065	0.299	5.564	2.025	0.018
Preoperative Ureteroscopy	1.010	0.290	7.920	11.292	0.003
DM without Metfoemin use	2.156	0.354	6.785	3.872	0.032

LNM lymph node metastasis, *PBPC* postoperative bladder perfusion chemotherapy, *RUN* radical nephroureterectomy, *UUC* ureteral urothelial carcinoma, *DM* diabetes mellitus

was no metastasis within 5 years, whereas when it was > 3 cm, the 5-year metastasis-free survival rate was 67%. Our study also revealed that tumor size was a risk factor of UTUC, wherein a larger tumor diameter indicated worse prognosis.

It is known that smoking is a prognostic factor of UTUC. A study [22] revealed that smoking is the main risk factor of UTUC and lower urinary tract urothelial cancer. The incidence of urothelial carcinoma in smokers is three times greater than that in nonsmokers, probably owing to a mutation in tumor protein p53, chromosomal changes, immune regulation, etc. Our study also confirmed that smoking was a risk factor of poor prognosis in UTUC patients. Moreover, we found that consumption of herbal medicines such as Longdanxiegan pills, Paishi granule, Paishi decoction, and caulis aristolochiae manshuriensis, which contain aristolochic acid, also affected the prognosis of UTUC patients. DNA compounds can be formed in vivo under the influence of aristolochic acid [23], leading to the A-T base-pair proto-oncogene mutation, activation of RAS, and dysfunction of the cancer suppressor gene P53. Thus, smoking may play an important role in the occurrence of UTUCs. Additionally, our study confirmed that BC was a prognostic factor for UTUC, which is consistent with the findings of Nuhn [24]. This may be due to the similar pathogenesis of UTUC and BC or a missed diagnosis of UTUC in some BC patients (especially for ureteral TCCs). For the latter reason, urologists who examine patients with hematuria may often be satisfied with a BC diagnosis and omit ureteral TCCs that could also lead to BC. This explains our finding that a prior history of muscle-invasive urothelial carcinoma of the bladder was significantly associated with an increased risk of disease recurrence and cancer-specific death in UTUC patients. Therefore, further adjuvant treatment, ureteroscopy, CT urography, and close follow-up should be performed after BC surgery.

It is generally believed that UTUC patients should be treated with radical RNU with the resection of bladder cuff resection [25]. However, the recurrence rate of BC is very high even after radical surgery. The incidence of BC relapse after operation in patients with TCC of the urinary tract is 30–70% [26], while the rate in our study was slightly lower at 20.3%. In the case of postoperative BC recurrence, a tumor located in the ureter, especially at the lower end of the duct, is considered a high-risk factor for BC recurrence. Zigeuner [27] suggested that a ureteral tumor is prone to spread into the bladder because of its close anatomical position. This could be due to the mechanical stress caused by a higher urinary flow rate and larger chamber pressure, facilitating tumor cell metastasis. Furthermore, in recent years, studies worldwide have found that the risk of BC relapse in ureteral carcinoma is significantly higher than that of a renal

pelvis carcinoma after RNU [28], which corresponds to the findings of our study. This, in some degree, supports the cancer cell implantation theory as the mechanism of BC recurrence. Fang et al. [28] analyzed the risk factors of BC recurrence after primary UTUC radical resection in 438 cases and found that high-grade ureteral cancer and multiple tumors were high-risk factors of BC recurrence. Therefore, a close follow-up with cystoscopy is necessary for patients with a high-grade, high-stage tumor and ureteral cancer (especially those with lower urinary tract ureteral cancer). These results indicate that tumor size and LNM are not independent risk factors of BC recurrence in UTUC patients after operation. However, there is limited research on whether tumor size and LNM affect bladder tumor recurrence; thus, more samples and multicenter studies are required.

Marchioni et al. [29] confirmed that preoperative ureteroscopy increases the risk of postoperative BC recurrence, which is consistent with the results our study. If the cancer cell implantation theory as the main mechanism of BC recurrence is accepted, there is greater risk of cancer cell exfoliation and implantation in the bladder after ureteroscopy examination. Thus, preoperative ureteroscopy should not be the primary and routine method for diagnosing UTUCs if imaging diagnosis is relatively clear; rather, a safer imaging method should be performed.

Because UTUC is closely related to BC and is associated with a higher BC recurrence rate, postoperative intravesical instillation chemotherapy has been widely used to prevent BC recurrence in postoperative UTUC patients. Many studies showed that postoperative bladder perfusion chemotherapy can effectively reduce the recurrence rate of BC after UTUC surgery [30]. Our study showed that postoperative bladder perfusion chemotherapy was a protective factor of BC recurrence after RNU. Therefore, UTUC patients could benefit from early diagnosis and regular postoperative intravesical instillation chemotherapy.

Recent studies have demonstrated that the incidence and mortality of tumor patients with DM were significantly higher than those of patients without DM. In this study, we found that UTUC patients with DM were more likely to experience BC recurrence. Among postoperative UTUC patients, the BC recurrence rate in those with DM was approximately four times that in patients without DM, and the result was significantly different. However, the specific mechanism remains unknown, which could be closely associated with DM itself and the associated hyperglycemia, hyperinsulinemia, and lipid metabolism disorder. In a study of 251 people with non-muscle-invasive bladder carcinoma, DM was an independent risk factor for disease recurrence [31]. Liu's in vitro experiments showed that high doses of insulin can promote the proliferation of urinary tract epithelial cells [32]. DM is often accompanied by insulin resistance and hyperinsulinemia; thus, Liu's study results may be a plausible explanation for easily recrudescent BC after surgery in UTUC patients with DM. Metformin is currently a first-line oral hypoglycemic drug for the treatment of type 2 DM. Currently, research has shown that metformin can reduce the risk of cancer by inhibiting the proliferation of tumor cells in vivo and in vitro [33, 34]. Our study found that after RNU, the BC recurrence rate in UTUC patients with DM who did not take metformin was significantly higher than that in UTUC patients with DM who took metformin. Our study supported the fact that metformin can reduce the recurrence rate of BC in patients with UTUC and DM, which has not been reported thus far. Metformin mainly activates the AMPK pathway, promotes the expression of the P53 gene, and inhibits the mTOR pathway, thereby inhibiting tumor cell proliferation and reducing insulin and insulin-like growth factor levels [35]. However, whether these mechanisms also apply to the occurrence and progression of UTUCs in DM patients remain under study.

This study has some limitations. First, the research data represent a retrospective review of findings at a single center. Second, patients who were not surgically treated were not included in the analysis. Finally, lack of information on molecular biomarkers may reduce the strength of the findings. Therefore, further studies are necessary to confirm the role of molecular biomarkers as predictors for worse pathological outcomes of UTUCs.

Conclusions
In this study, the 5-year survival rate of UTUC patients from central China was not high compared with that of UTUC patients from other regions. We found that advanced tumor stage and presence of a high-grade tumor were risk factors for not only poor UTUC prognosis but also BC recurrence. In addition, preoperative ureteroscopy and DM without metformin use were high risk factors for BC recurrence, whereas postoperative bladder perfusion chemotherapy was a protective factor. Therefore, we suggest that UTUC patients with the above risk factors for BC recurrence should compulsorily undergo regular bladder perfusion chemotherapy. In addition, we suggest that preoperative ureteroscopy should not be exercised except when preoperative imaging diagnosis is difficult.

Abbreviations
BC: bladder cancer; CT: computed tomography; DM: diabetes mellitus; EMR: electronic medical records; LNM: lymph node metastasis; RNU: radical nephroureterectomy; TCC: transitional cell carcinomas; TCCs: transitional cell carcinomas; UTUC: upper urinary tract urothelial carcinoma; UTUCs: upper urinary tract urothelial carcinomas; UUC: ureteral urothelial carcinoma; UUTT: upper urinary tract tumor

Acknowledgements
We thank statistician Xiaoping Shang, the member of medical records room in the First Affiliated Hospital of Zhengzhou University for offering the important help, and we thank Editage editing company for polishing the language as well.

Authors' contributions
WQ made substantial contributions to conception and design this study, revise it critically for important intellectual content, and give final approval of the version to be published. ZT and WJ1 (Junwei Wu) were involved in drafting the manuscript. WJ2 (Jianguo Wen) made substantial contributions to conception and design this study. TD, WT and ZW made substantial contributions to acquisition of data, analysis and interpretation of data. All authors have read the manuscript and approved its publication.

Author details
[1]Department of Urology, The First Affiliated Hospital of Zhengzhou University, Zhengzhou 450052, Henan, China. [2]Department of Pediatric Surgery, The First Affiliated Hospital of Xinxiang Medical University, Xinxiang 453100, Henan, China.

References
1. Roupret M, Babjuk M, Comperat E, et al. European association of urology guidelines on upper urinary tract urothelial cell carcinoma:2015 update. Eur Urol. 2015;68(5):868–79.
2. Siegel RL, Miller KD, Jemal A. Cancer statistics, 2017. CA Cancer J Clin. 2017; 67(1):7–30.
3. Chen XP, Xiong GY, Li XS, Matin SF, et al. Predictive factors for worse pathological outcomes of upper tract urothelial carcinoma: experience from a nationwide high-volume Centre in China. BJU Int. 2013;112(7):917–24.
4. Chou YH, Huang CH. Unusual clinical presentation of upper urothelial carcinoma in Taiwan. Cancer. 1999;85(6):1342–4.
5. Yang MH, Chen KK, Yen CC, et al. Unusually high incidence of upper tract urothelial carcinoma in Taiwan. Urology. 2002;59(5):681–7.
6. Li CC, Chang TH, Wu WJ, et al. Significant predictive factors for prognosis of primary upper urinary tract cancer after radical nephroureterectomy in Taiwanese patients. Eur Urol. 2008;54(5):1127–35.
7. Lughezzani G, Sun M, Perrotte P, et al. Gender-related differences in patients with stage I to III upper tract urothelial carcinoma: results from the surveillance, epidemiology, and end results database. Urology. 2010;75(2): 321–7.
8. Rouprêt M, Babjuk M, Compérat E, et al. European Association of Urology guidelines on upper urinary tract urothelial carcinoma: 2017 update. Eur Urol. 2018;73(1):111–22.
9. Iborra I, Solsona E, Casanova J, Ricos JV, Rubio J, Climent MA. Conservative elective treatment of upper urinary tract tumors: a multivariate analysis of prognostic factors for recurrence and progression. J Urol. 2003;169(1):82–5.
10. Keeley FJ, Bibbo M, Bagley DH. Ureteroscopic treatment and surveillance of upper urinary tract transitional cell carcinoma. J Urol. 1997;157(5):1560–5.
11. Ku JH, Choi WS, Kwak C, Kim HH. Bladder cancer after nephroureterectomy in patients with urothelial carcinoma of the upper urinary tract. Urol Oncol. 2011;29(4):383–7.
12. Wu YP, Lin YZ, Lin MY, et al. Risk factors for bladder Cancer recurrence survival in patients with upper-tract urothelial carcinoma. Tumori. 2017: tj5000705.
13. Margulis V, Shariat SF, Matin SF, et al. Outcomes of radical nephroureterectomy: a series from the upper tract urothelial carcinoma collaboration. Cancer. 2009;115(6):1224–33.
14. Shariat SF, Favaretto RL, Gupta A, et al. Gender differences in radical nephroureterectomy for upper tract urothelial carcinoma. World J Urol. 2011;29(4):481–6.
15. Hall MC, Womack S, Sagalowsky AI, Carmody T, Erickstad MD, Roehrborn CG. Prognostic factors, recurrence, and survival in transitional cell carcinoma of the upper urinary tract: a 30-year experience in 252 patients. Urology. 1998;52(4):594–601.
16. Brown GA, Busby JE, Wood CG, et al. Nephroureterectomy for treating upper urinary tract transitional cell carcinoma: time to change the treatment paradigm? BJU Int. 2006;98(6):1176–80.
17. Matsui Y, Utsunomiya N, Ichioka K, et al. Risk factors for subsequent development of bladder cancer after primary transitional cell carcinoma of the upper urinary tract. Urology. 2005;65(2):279–83.
18. Liu JY, Li YH, Zhang ZL, et al. Age-specific effect of gender on upper tract urothelial carcinoma outcomes. Med Oncol. 2013;30(3):640.

19. Raman JD, Messer J, Sielatycki JA, Hollenbeak CS. Incidence and survival of patients with carcinoma of the ureter and renal pelvis in the USA, 1973-2005. BJU Int. 2011;107(7):1059–64.

20. Simone G, Papalia R, Loreto A. Et al. independent prognostic value of tumour diameter and tumour necrosis in upper urinary tract urothelial carcinoma. BJU Int. 2009;103(8):1052–7.

21. Novara G, Matsumoto K, Kassouf W. Et al. prognostic role of lymphovascular invasion in patients with urothelial carcinoma of the upper urinary tract:an international validation study. Eur Urol. 2010;57(6):1064–71.

22. Hartge P, Silverman D, Hoover R, et al. Changing cigarette habits and bladder cancer risk: a case-control study. J Natl Cancer Inst. 1987;78(6):1119–25.

23. Lord GM, Hollstein M, Arlt VM, et al. DNA adducts and p53 mutations in a patient with aristolochic acid-associated nephropathy. Am J Kidney Dis. 2004;43(4):e11–7.

24. Nuhn P, Novara G, Seitz C, et al. Prognostic value of prior history of urothelial carcinoma of the bladder in patients with upper urinary tract urothelial carcinoma: resulrs from a retrospective multicenter study. World J Urol. 2015;33(7):1005–13.

25. Rongyao L, Peng Z, Xuesong L, et al. Transperitoneal laparoscopic complete nephrectomy for upper urinary tract urothelial carcinoma. Beijing Da Xue Xue Bao. 2011;43(4):531–4.

26. Hisataki T, Miyao N, Masumori N, et al. Risk factors for the development of bladder cancer after upper tract urothelial cancer. Urology. 2000;55(5):663–7.

27. Zigeuner RE, Hutterer G, Chromecki T, Rehak P, Langner C. Bladder tumour development after urothelial carcinoma of the upper urinary tract is related to primary tumour location. BJU Int. 2006;98(6):1181–6.

28. Fang D, Xiong GY, Li XS, et al. Pattern and risk factors of intravesical recurrence after nephroureterectomy for upper tract urothelial carcinoma: a large Chinese center experience. J Formos Med Assoc. 2014;113(11):820–7.

29. Marchioni M, Giulia P, Luca C, et al. Impact of diagnostic ureteroscopy on intravesical recurrence in patients undergoing radical nephroureterectomy for upper tract urothelial cancer: a systematic review and meta-analysis. BJU Int. 2017;120(3):313–9.

30. Raman JD, Ng CK, Boorjian SA, Vaughan EJ, Sosa RE, Scherr DS. Bladder cancer after managing upper urinary tract transitional cell carcinoma: predictive factors and pathology. BJU Int. 2005;96(7):1031–5.

31. Hwang EC, Kim YJ, Hwang IS, et al. Impact of diabetes mellitus on recurrence and progression in patients with non-muscle invasive bladder carcinoma:a retrospective cohort study. Int J Urol. 2011;18(11):769–76.

32. Liu S, Li Y, Lin T, Fan X, Liang Y, Heemann U. High dose human insulin and insulin glargine promote T24 bladder cancer cell proliferation via P13K—independent activation of Akt. Diabetes Res Clin Praet. 2011;91(2):177–82.

33. Rattan R, Graham RP, Maguire JL, Giri S, Shridhar V. Mefformin suppresses ovarian cancer growth and metastasis with enhancement of cisplatin cytotoxicity in vivo. Neoplasia. 2011;13(5):483–91.

34. Gotlieb WH, Saumet J, Beauchamp MC, et al. In vitro metforminanti—neoplastic activity in epithelial ovarian cancer. Gynecol Oncol. 2008;110(2):246–50.

35. Jalving M, Gietema JA, Lefrandt JD, et al. Metformin:taking away the candyfor cancer. EurJ Cancer. 2010;46(13):2369–80.

4

Let-7i inhibits proliferation and migration of bladder cancer cells by targeting HMGA1

M-M Qin[1†], X. Chai[2†], H-B Huang[2], G. Feng[1], X-N Li[1], J. Zhang[1], R. Zheng[1], X-C Liu[1] and C. Pu[1*]

Abstract

Background: Let-7 is one of the earliest discovered microRNAs(miRNAs) and has been reported to be down-regulated in multiple malignant tumors. The effects and molecular mechanisms of let-7i in bladder cancer are still unclear. This study was to investigate the effects and potential mechanisms of let-7i on bladder cancer cells.

Methods: Total RNA was extracted from bladder cancer cell lines. The expression levels of let-7i and HMGA1 were examined by quantitative real-time PCR. Cell viability was detected using the CCK-8 and colony formation assays, while transwell and wound healing assays were used to evaluate migration ability. Luciferase reporter assay and western blot were used to confirm the target gene of let-7i.

Results: Compared with the SV-40 immortalized human uroepithelial cell line (SV-HUC-1), bladder cancer cell lines T24 and 5637 had low levels of let-7i expression, but high levels of high mobility group protein A1 (HMGA1) expression. Transfection of cell lines T24 and 5637 with let-7i mimic suppressed cell proliferation and migration. Luciferase reporter assay confirmed HMGA1 may be one of the target genes of let-7i-5p. Protein and mRNA expression of HMGA1 was significantly downregulated in let-7i mimic transfected cell lines T24 and 5637.

Conclusions: Up-regulation of let-7i suppressed proliferation and migration of the human bladder cancer cell lines T24 and 5637 by targeting HMGA1. These findings suggest that let-7i might be considered as a novel therapeutic target for bladder cancer.

Keywords: Let-7i, High mobility group protein A1, Bladder cancer, Proliferation, Migration

Background

Bladder cancer represents a common malignancy in urinary system, and its morbidity tends to yearly grow. Over 400,000 new cases of bladder cancer are reported worldwide every year [1]. The statistics of National Cancer Institute of China estimated that new cases of bladder cancer were 80,500, and death of bladder cancer were 32,900 in 2015 in China [2]. Approximately 70–75% of newly diagnosed bladder cancers are non-muscle invasive (NMIBC) [3]. NMIBC is typically treated with endoscopic transurethral resection (TUR). However, most patients have high risk of recurrence and disease progression. The median survival of patients with bladder cancer was 15 months, and the 5-year survival rate of bladder cancer was only 15% [4]. Therefore, the molecular mechanism that regulates the progression of bladder cancer is of great significance for treatment of bladder cancer.

MicroRNAs (miRNAs) are endogenous, non-coding RNAs and they play an important regulatory role through complimentary binding of the 3′ untranslated regions (3′UTRs) of target genes in RNA silencing and post-transcriptional regulation of gene expression [5]. Since the discovery of miRNAs [6], a variety of abnormal expressions of miRNAs have been found in many human cancers, including gastric cancer [7], breast cancer [8] and bladder cancer [9]. Abnormal expression of miRNAs and the growth, metastasis and apoptosis of human tumor cells were closely related [10–12]. Let-7 family is the earliest discovered miRNAs. Let-7 family play a significant role in the development and progression of many cancers, including prostate cancer [13] and bladder cancer [14]. However, the effects of let-7i, a member of the let-7 family, in bladder cancer are still unclear.

* Correspondence: philipcpu@163.com
†M-M Qin and X. Chai contributed equally to this work.
¹Clinical Laboratory, The First Affiliated Hospital of Wannan Medical College, No.2, West Zheshan Road, Wuhu 241001, Anhui, China
Full list of author information is available at the end of the article

High mobility group protein A1(HMGA1), a member of the HMGA family, can form multi protein stereo complexes by binding to the DNA region containing rich AT basic group, and regulate gene transcription of many genes [15]. HMGA1 as a key regulator of the autophagic pathway in cancer cells could contribute to cancer progression [16]. Previous study reported that let-7i was a key factor in development of prostate cancer by regulate HMGA2 [17]. Liu [18] also found that down-regulation of let-7a could inhibits growth and migration of breast cancer cells by targeting HMGA1.

However, how let-7i affects HMGA1 gene expression in bladder cancer cells are still unclear. Therefore, the aim of this study was to investigate the effects of let-7i on human bladder cancer cells proliferation and metastasis. Furthermore, to explore how let-7i affects HMGA1 expression in bladder cancer cells.

Methods
Materials
SV-HUC-1 and human bladder cancer cell lines T24 and 5637 were purchased from the Chinese Academy of Sciences (Shanghai, China); The 5637 series of bladder cancer is a human origin, which is a situ bladder cancer cell derived from the upper skin, with a moderate degree of malignancy. Bladder cancer T24, derived from human bladder transitional cell carcinoma cells, is an epithelioid metastatic adenocarcinoma with a high degree of malignancy. RPMI-1640 medium and fetal bovine serum were purchased from GIBCO (USA); CCK-8 Cell Proliferation Detection Kit was purchased from KeyGEN Bio TECH (Nanjing, China); 24-well plates with a transwell chamber was purchased from Corning (NY, USA); let-7i mimic, let-7i mimic negative control, HMGA1 primers and let-7i primers were purchased from RiboBio (Guangzhou, China); Trizol Universal reagent, miRcute Plus miRNA First-Strand cDNA Synthesis Kit and miRcute Plus miRNA qPCR Detection Kit (SYBR Green) were purchased from TIANGEN (Beijing, China); RevertAid™ First Strand cDNA Synthesis Kit was purchased from Thermo (Shanghai, China); SYBR®Premix Ex TaqTM(Tli RNaseH Plus) was purchased from TaKaRa (Beijing, China); The rabbit polyclonal antibodies against HMGA1 was purchased from Abcam (Cambridge, UK); The rabbit polyclonal antibodies against β-Actin was purchased from Cell Signaling Technology (Danvers, MA, USA).

Cell culture and transfection
T24 and 5637 cells in this experiment were newly resuscitated cells, which underwent 7–8 biological replications and were tested after the cells were in a stable state. The cells were routinely cultured in the RPMI-1640 medium containing 10% fetal bovine serum, 100 U/mL of streptomycin, and 100 U/mL of penicillin in a humidified cell incubator. Cell lines T24 and 5637 were plated at a density of 2×10^5 cells/well in 6-well plates. The let-7i mimic was cloned to Lipofectamine 3000, which was then transfected. Transient transfection was conducted using Lipofectamine 3000 (Invitrogen, USA) according to manufacturer's instructions. The let-7i mimic and negative control are designed by RiboBio(Guangzhou, China). Let-7i mimic was mature miRNA. Let-7i mimic and negative control were used at a concentration of 100 nmol.

Cell proliferation assay
Cell lines T24 and 5637 transfected with let-7i mimic or negative control were plated on 96-well plates at 2000 cells/well. After 24, 48 and 72 h of transfection, cells were incubated in 10% CCK-8 diluted in culture media at 37 °C until visual color conversion appeared. The absorbance was measured at 450 nm using a microplate reader according to the manufacturer's protocol.

Colony forming assay
Cell lines T24 and 5637 transfected with let-7i mimic or negative control were plated on 6-well plates at 500 cells/well and incubated in 5% CO_2 atmosphere at 37 °C for 14 days. Fresh medium is changed every 3 days during this period. Then cells were fixed and stained, followed by colony counting.

Wound healing and cell transwell assays
Wound healing and cell transwell assays were performed as previously described [18].

RNA extraction and RT-PCR
Total RNA was extracted from the bladder cancer cell lines using Trizol Universal reagent according to the manufacturer's instructions. Then, cDNA was obtained using the corresponding reverse transcriber reagent according to the manufacturer's instructions in United States labnet PCR instrument (BIO-RAD, USA). Quantitative polymerase chain reaction (PCR) was performed in ABI 7500 Sequence Detection System (Life Technologies, USA) using the corresponding PCR reagent according to the manufacturer's instructions. miRNA quantification with Bulge -loopTM miRNA RT-qPCR Primer Sets (one RT primer and a pair of qPCR primers for each set) specific U6 and let-7i are designed by RiboBio (Guangzhou, China). HMGA1 forward primer sequences: 5′-TCCATTCTTCGACATCCGTCA-3′ HMGA1 reverse primer sequences: 5′-GATCGTGGGCAGAACAGGAG-3′; GAPDH forward primer sequences: 5′-CATCAAGAAGGTGGTGAAGCAG-3′; GAPDH reverse primer sequences: 5′-GTGTCGCTGTTGAA.

GTCAGAG-3′. The relative quantification was performed by normalizing against the levels of GAPDH for mRNA or U6 for miRNA. Relative quantification of mRNA and miRNA expression was calculated using the $2^{-\Delta\Delta Ct}$ method.

Protein extraction and western blot

Total protein was collected and lysed in $1 \times$ Laemmli sample buffer (Sigma, USA) on ice; After the lysate boiled, protein samples (5 µl) were fractionated in 10% SDS-polyacrylamide gel and then transferred to nitrocellulose (NC) membrane (GE Healthcare, Piscataway, NJ, USA). Membranes were blocked with 10% non-fat milk and washed with TBST, and then incubated with primary antibody (dilution at 1:1000) at 4 °C for 12 h. The NC membranes were extensively washed three times, and then incubated with anti-rabbit horseradish peroxidase-conjugated secondary antibody. Following removal of the secondary antibody, the membranes were scanned by Fluor Chem FC3 (Protein Simple, San Jose, CA, USA). β-Actin was used as an internal control.

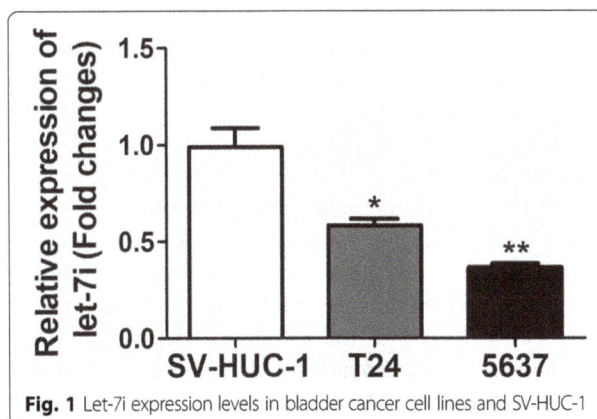

Fig. 1 Let-7i expression levels in bladder cancer cell lines and SV-HUC-1

Fluorescent reporter assay

Cells were cultured in 24-well plates and then co-transfected with 100 ng of HMGA1-UTR-WT or -MUT psi-CHECK2 vectors plus 100 nM let-7i-5p mimic or scrambled sequences using Lipofectamine 3000. 48 h

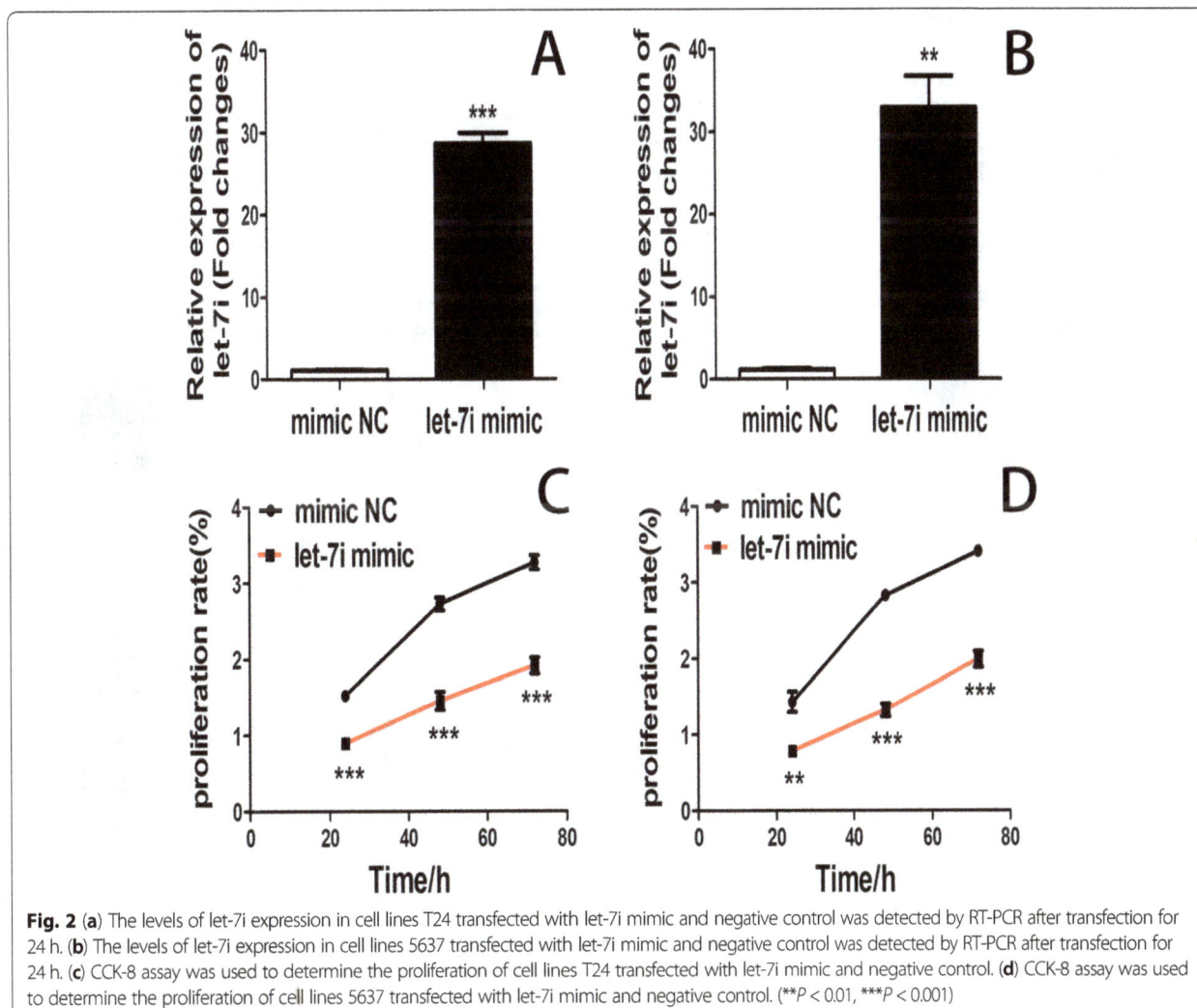

Fig. 2 (**a**) The levels of let-7i expression in cell lines T24 transfected with let-7i mimic and negative control was detected by RT-PCR after transfection for 24 h. (**b**) The levels of let-7i expression in cell lines 5637 transfected with let-7i mimic and negative control was detected by RT-PCR after transfection for 24 h. (**c**) CCK-8 assay was used to determine the proliferation of cell lines T24 transfected with let-7i mimic and negative control. (**d**) CCK-8 assay was used to determine the proliferation of cell lines 5637 transfected with let-7i mimic and negative control. (******$P < 0.01$, *******$P < 0.001$)

after transfection, luciferase activities were measured using Dual-Luciferase Reporter Assay System (Promega, USA). Firefly luciferase activity was used as an internal reference standard.

Statistical analysis

All statistical analyses were performed using the SPSS 19.0 version (SPSS Inc., Chicago, IL, USA) and GraphPad 5.0 software. Each experiment was performed in triplicate. All values for experimental results are expressed as the mean ± SEM. The statistical significance of differences between independent groups was determined by one-way analysis of variance (ANOVA) or t-test. A two-sided P value < 0.05 was considered statistically significant.

Results

Let-7i was down-regulated in bladder cancer cell lines

As shown in Fig. 1. Low expression of let-7i was found in bladder cancer cell lines T24 (0.58 ± 0.03) and 5637 (0.37 ± 0.02) as compared to SV-HUC-1 (0.99 ± 0.10, $P < 0.05$).

Overexpression of let-7i inhibited bladder cancer cells proliferation

Let-7i expression was effectively up-regulated in bladder cancer cell lines T24 and 5637 after transfected with let-7i mimic (Fig. 2a and b). CCK-8 assay was performed to detect the proliferation of cell lines T24 and 5637 after transfection

with let-7i mimic for 24, 48, and 72 h. Overexpression of let-7i significantly inhibited cell proliferation compared with the negative control cells. (Fig. 2c and d).

Overexpression of let-7i inhibited bladder cancer cells colony formation

Clone formation experiment was performed to detect the proliferation of cell lines T24 and 5637 after transfection with let-7i mimic and negative control for 14 days. Colonies formed from T24 cells transfected with let-7i mimic were significantly less than that of negative control transfected cells (Fig. 3a and b). While colonies formed from 5637 cells transfected with let-7i mimic were also significantly less than that of negative control transfected cells (Fig. 3c and d).

Overexpression of let-7i suppressed T24 and 5637 cells migration

Compared with the cells transfected with negative control, the cell healing rate in cell lines T24 with let-7i mimic was downregulated, and the ability to lateral migration in cell lines 5637 with let-7i mimic was also downregulated (Fig. 4).

Compared with the cells transfected with negative control, the migrated cells number in bladder cancer cell lines T24 with let-7i mimic was decreased, and the

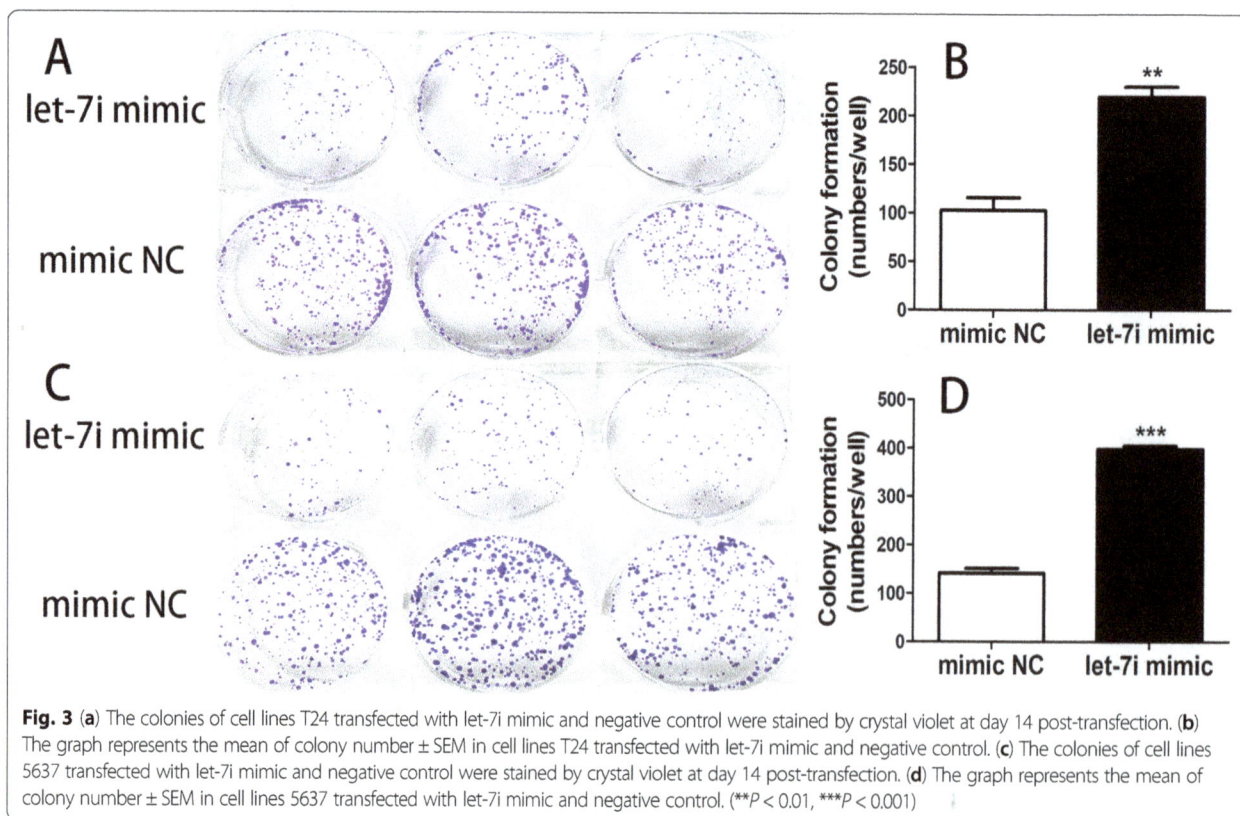

Fig. 3 (a) The colonies of cell lines T24 transfected with let-7i mimic and negative control were stained by crystal violet at day 14 post-transfection. (b) The graph represents the mean of colony number ± SEM in cell lines T24 transfected with let-7i mimic and negative control. (c) The colonies of cell lines 5637 transfected with let-7i mimic and negative control were stained by crystal violet at day 14 post-transfection. (d) The graph represents the mean of colony number ± SEM in cell lines 5637 transfected with let-7i mimic and negative control. (**$P < 0.01$, ***$P < 0.001$)

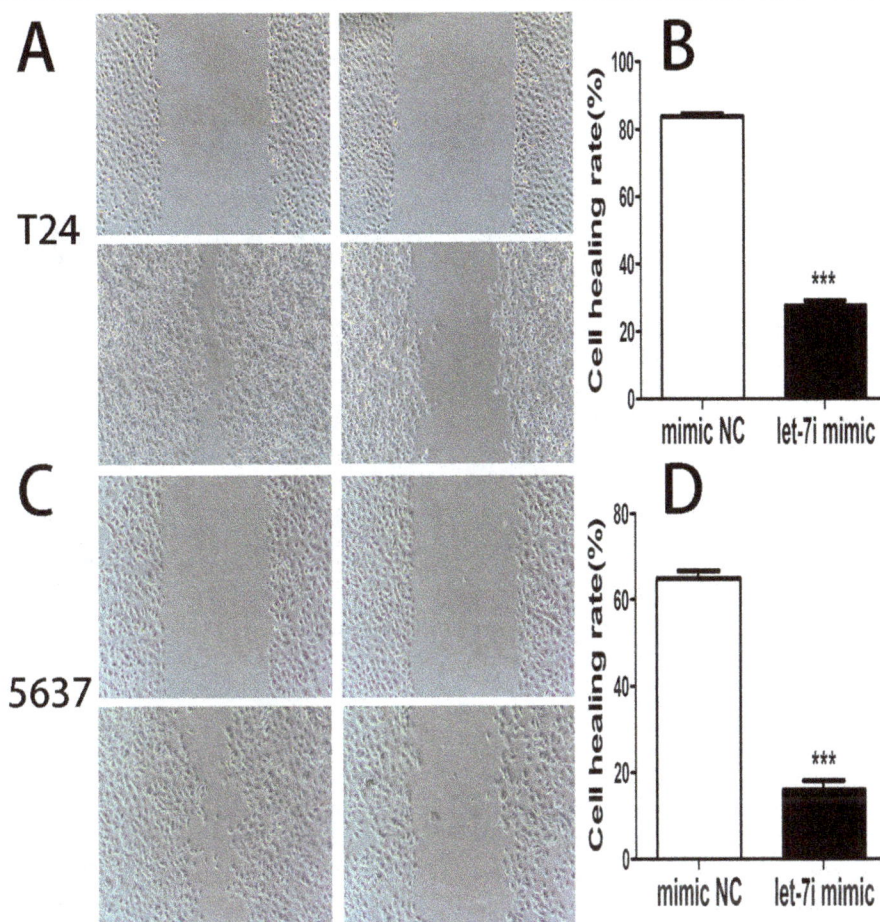

Fig. 4 (**a**) and (**b**) The lateral migration of cell lines T24 and 5637 transfected with let-7i mimic and negative control was examined by the cell scratch assay. (**c**) and (**d**) The graph represents the mean of wound closure rates ± SEM in cell lines T24 and 5637 transfected with let-7i mimic and negative control. (***$P < 0.001$)

ability to vertical migration in bladder cancer cell lines 5637 with let-7i mimic was also downregulated (Fig. 5).

HMGA1 was up-regulated in bladder cancer cell lines

High expression of HMGA1 mRNA was found in bladder cancer cell lines T24 ($3.65 ± 0.04$) and 5637 ($6.22 ± 0.38$) as compared to SV-HUC-1 ($0.99 ± 0.01$, $P < 0.001$). (Fig. 6a). Compared to SV-HUC-1, HMGA1 protein was also up-regulated in bladder cancer cell lines T24 and 5637. (Fig. 6 b and c).

HMGA1 was a target gene of let-7i

Let-7i targets were analyzed by using the bioinformatics software prediction (http://www.targetscan.com). Software analysis revealed that HMGA1 might be a potential target of let-7i based on putative target sequences of the HMGA1 3′ UTR (Fig. 7a). Luciferase assay showed that let-7i decreased the luciferase activity of the HMGA1 3′ UTR (Fig. 7b). Over-expression of let-7i obviously downregulated the

mRNA level of HMGA1. (Fig. 7c). Over-expression of let-7i also obviously downregulated the protein level of HMGA1. (Fig. 7d, e and f).

Discussion

In recent years, various studies support a role for miRNA in the origination and progression of human cancers [19, 20]. Dysregulation of miRNA activity to control both cell growth and cell metastasis may play important future roles in preventing and treating human various malignancies. Many members of let-7 family are abnormally expressed in many human tumors, such as prostate cancer [13], pancreatic cancer [21] and breast cancer [22]. Studies also showed that abnormal expression of let-7i in a variety of human tumors [23, 24], including bladder cancer [25]. However, the functions of let-7i in bladder cancer cells are unclear.

In the present study, let-7i was downregulated in bladder cancer cell lines. The results suggested that the decrease of let-7i level was correlated with the occurrence

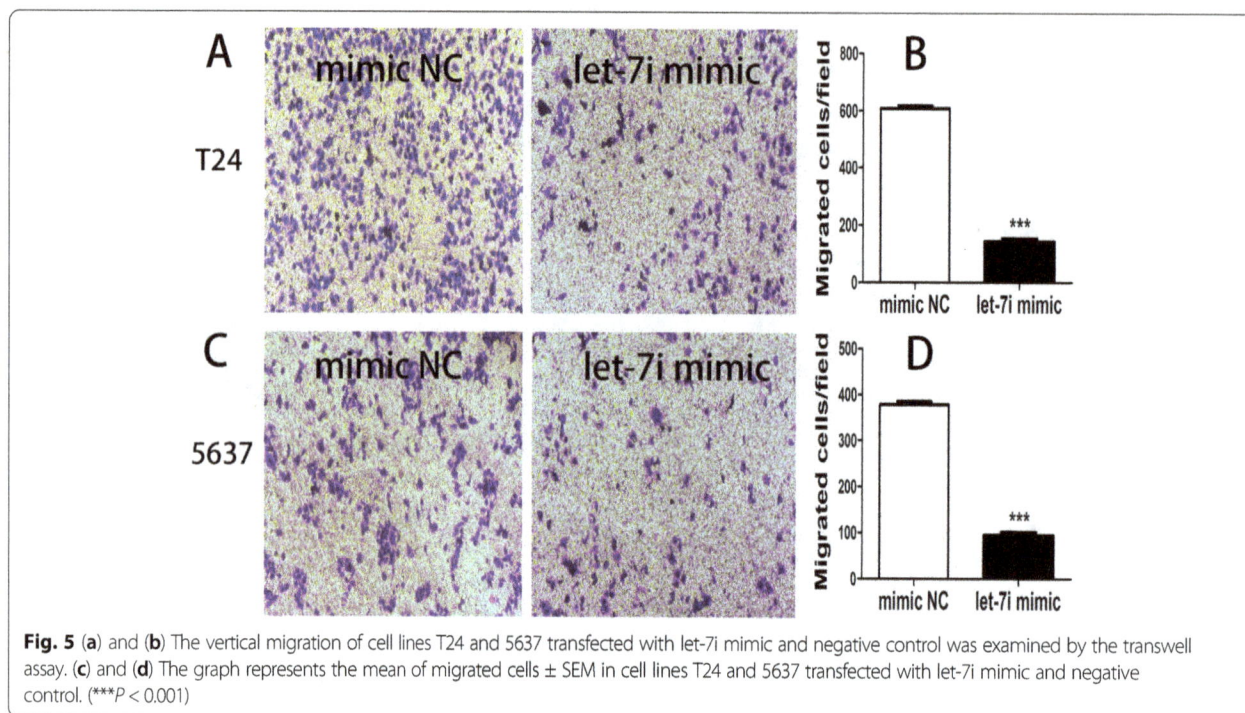

Fig. 5 (**a**) and (**b**) The vertical migration of cell lines T24 and 5637 transfected with let-7i mimic and negative control was examined by the transwell assay. (**c**) and (**d**) The graph represents the mean of migrated cells ± SEM in cell lines T24 and 5637 transfected with let-7i mimic and negative control. (***$P < 0.001$)

of bladder cancer. Our study was consistent with previous research [25]. Additionally, over-expression of let-7i suppressed bladder cell proliferation and migration. Song et al. found that down-regulation of the let-7i-5p inhibited the proliferation and metastasis of colon cancer cells [23, 26]. However, other study indicated that down-regulation of the let-7i facilitates gastric cancer invasion and metastasis [27]. In our study, CCK-8 and plate cloning assays showed that low level let-7i could promote the proliferation and colony formation of bladder cancer cells. Scratch and Transwell assays also indicated that the migration of bladder cancer cells was significantly inhibited after over-

expression of let-7i. These results revealed that down-regulation of the let-7i could inhibit breast cancer cells proliferation and migration.

High expression levels of HMGA1 were reported in a variety of human cancers. The expression of HMGA1 is upregulate in malignant tumor derived from the prostate, breast [28, 29]. Previous reports showed that HMGA1 could affect tumor metastasis through a variety of ways [30]. In addition, Studies have shown that HMGA1 can regulate proliferation and motility of bladder cancer cells [31]. Luciferase reporter assay showed that let-7i-5p mimic could downregulate the luciferase activity of the HMGA1

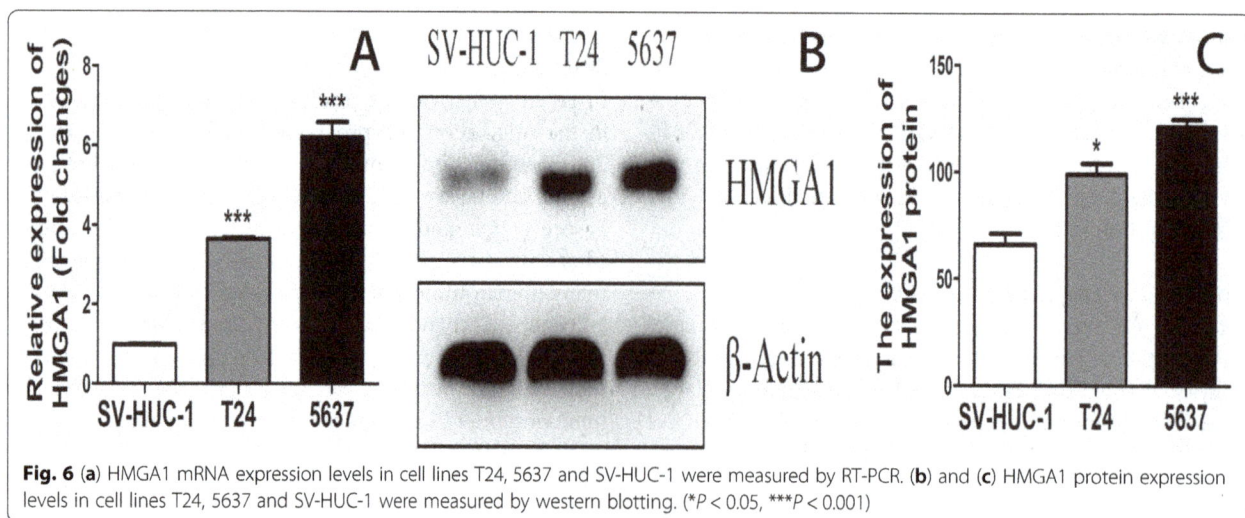

Fig. 6 (**a**) HMGA1 mRNA expression levels in cell lines T24, 5637 and SV-HUC-1 were measured by RT-PCR. (**b**) and (**c**) HMGA1 protein expression levels in cell lines T24, 5637 and SV-HUC-1 were measured by western blotting. (*$P < 0.05$, ***$P < 0.001$)

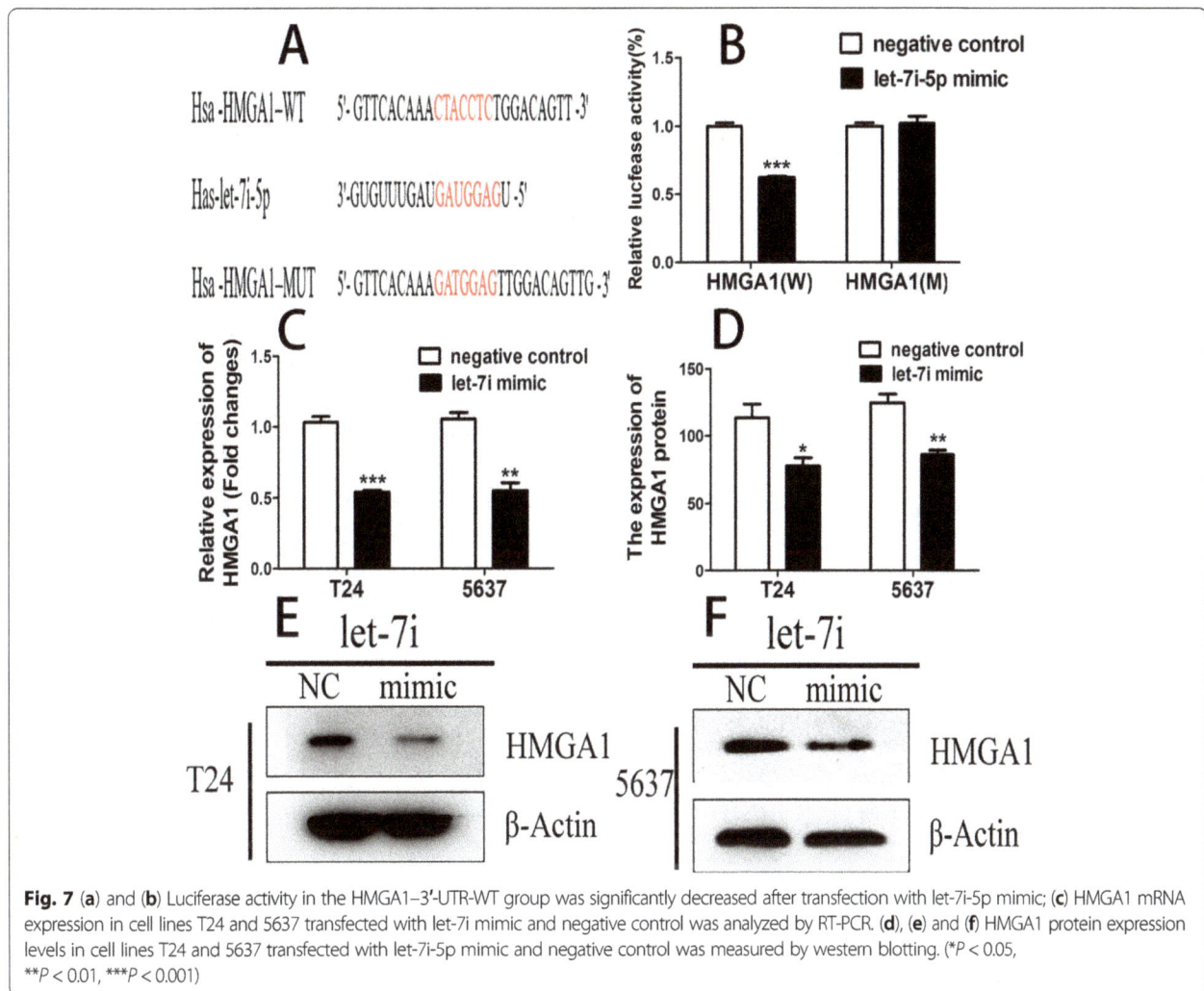

Fig. 7 (**a**) and (**b**) Luciferase activity in the HMGA1–3′-UTR-WT group was significantly decreased after transfection with let-7i-5p mimic; (**c**) HMGA1 mRNA expression in cell lines T24 and 5637 transfected with let-7i mimic and negative control was analyzed by RT-PCR. (**d**), (**e**) and (**f**) HMGA1 protein expression levels in cell lines T24 and 5637 transfected with let-7i-5p mimic and negative control was measured by western blotting. (*$P < 0.05$, **$P < 0.01$, ***$P < 0.001$)

WT 3′-UTR construct but not MUT 3′-UTR construct. Transfection of let-7i-5p mimic reduced HMGA1 mRNA and protein expression in bladder cancer cell lines, suggested that HMGA1 as a target gene for let-7i-5p. These results further confirmed let-7i regulated HMGA1 in bladder cancer. Increasing studies showed that the expression of let-7 in the tumor was downregulated and can inhibit the gene expression of HMGA2 and MYC at the transcriptional level [32]. Some study also showed that miR-625 and let-7i could suppresses cell proliferation and migration by targeting HMGA1 in breast cancer [18, 33]. Our study was consistent with previous reports.

However, there were also some limitations for our study. First, because levels are non-physiologic, the interpretation of the fluorescent reporter assay using co-transfection of let-7i and HMGA1 should be interpreted with caution. Second, there is no manipulating HMGA1 and reversing the effects of let-7i involved in this study. In addition, this study also lacks animal in vivo experiments, so more convincing experiments need to be further discussed in the future.

Conclusions

In conclusion, let-7i was down-regulated in bladder cancer cells and these in vitro studies showed that up-regulation of let-7i suppressed human bladder cancer cell proliferation and migration by targeting HMGA1. Our findings justify further studying let-7i as a potential clinical diagnostic or predictive biomarker and new target for molecular therapy for human bladder cancer.

Abbreviations
3′UTRs: 3′ untranslated regions; CCK8: Cell Counting Kit-8; HMGA1: High mobility group protein A1; NMIBC: non-muscle invasive; SV-HUC-1: SV-40 immortalized human uroepithelial cell line; T24 and 5637: bladder cancer cell lines; TUR: endoscopic transurethral resection

Acknowledgements
Not applicable.

Authors' contributions
CP and H-B H conceived and designed the experiments; M-M Q and XC performed the experiments; CP and X-N L contributed reagents/materials/analysis tools; X-N L and JZ, RZ, X-C L, analyzed the data; M-M Q, GF and XC wrote the paper. All authors read and approved the final manuscript.

Author details
[1]Clinical Laboratory, The First Affiliated Hospital of Wannan Medical College, No.2, West Zheshan Road, Wuhu 241001, Anhui, China. [2]Department of Urology, The First Affiliated Hospital of Wannan Medical College, Wuhu 241001, Anhui, China.

References

1. Ferlay J, Soerjomataram I, Dikshit R, et al. Cancer incidence and mortality worldwide: sources, methods and major patterns in GLOBOCAN 2012. Int J Cancer. 2015;136(5):E359–86.

2. Chen W, Zheng R, Baade PD, et al. Cancer statistics in China, 2015. CA Cancer J Clin. 2016;66(2):115–32.

3. Witjes JA, Compérat E, Cowan NC, De Santis M, Gakis G, Lebret T, Ribal MJ, Van der Heijden AG, Sherif A. EAU guidelines on muscle-invasive and metastatic bladder cancer: summary of the 2013 guidelines. Eur Urol. 2014; 65:778–92.

4. H v d M, Sengelov L, Roberts JT, et al. Long-term survival results of a randomized trial comparing gemcitabine plus cisplatin, with methotrexate, vinblastine, doxorubicin, plus cisplatin in patients with bladder cancer. J Clin Oncol. 2005;23(21):4602–8.

5. Jewell JL, Flores F, Guan KL. Micro(RNA) managing by mTORC1. Mol Cell. 2015;57(4):575–6.

6. Lee RC, Feinbaum RL, Ambros V. The C. elegans heterochronic gene lin-4 encodes small RNAs with antisense complementarity to lin-14. Cell. 1993; 75(5):843.

7. You W, Zhang X, Ji M, et al. MiR-152-5p as a microRNA passenger strand special functions in human gastric cancer cells. Int J Biol Sci. 2018;14(6):644–53.

8. Rohan T, Ye K, Wang Y, Glass AG, Ginsberg M, Loudig O. MicroRNA expression in benign breast tissue and risk of subsequent invasive breast cancer. PLoS One. 2018;13(2):e0191814.

9. Blanca A, Cheng L, Montironi R, et al. Mirna expression in bladder Cancer and their potential role in clinical practice. Curr Drug Metab. 2017;18(8):712.

10. Kim J, Yao F, Xiao Z, Sun Y, Ma L. MicroRNAs and metastasis: small RNAs play big roles. Cancer Metastasis Rev. 2018;37(1):5–15.

11. Akkafa F, Koyuncu İ, Temiz E, Dagli H, Dilmec F, Akbas H. miRNA-mediated apoptosis activation through TMEM 48 inhibition in A549 cell line. Biochem Biophys Res Commun. 2018;503(1):323–9.

12. Chivukula RR, Shi G, Acharya A, et al. An essential mesenchymal function for miR-143/145 in intestinal epithelial regeneration. Cell. 2014;157(5):1104–16.

13. Guelfi G, Cochetti G, Stefanetti V, et al. Next generation sequencing of urine exfoliated cells: an approach of prostate cancer microRNAs research. Sci Rep. 2018;8(1):7111.

14. Lu Y, Liu P, Van den Bergh F, et al. Modulation of gene expression and cell-cycle signaling pathways by the EGFR inhibitor gefitinib (Iressa) in rat urinary bladder cancer. Cancer Prev Res (Phila). 2012;5(2):248–59.

15. Arnoldo L, Sgarra R, Chiefari E, et al. A novel mechanism of post-translational modulation of HMGA functions by the histone chaperone nucleophosmin. Sci Rep. 2015;5:8552.

16. Conte A, Paladino S, Bianco G, et al. High mobility group A1 protein modulates autophagy in cancer cells. Cell Death Differ. 2017;24(11):1948–62.

17. Paz EA, LaFleur B, Gerner EW. Polyamines are oncometabolites that regulate the LIN28/let-7 pathway in colorectal cancer cells. Mol Carcinog. 2014; 53(Suppl 1):E96–106.

18. Liu K, Zhang C, Li T, et al. Let-7a inhibits growth and migration of breast cancer cells by targeting HMGA1. Int J Oncol. 2015;46(6):2526–34.

19. Zhang X, Wu M, Chong QY, et al. Amplification of Hsa-miR-191/425 locus promotes breast Cancer proliferation and metastasis by targeting DICER1. Carcinogenesis. 2018;39(12):1506-16.

20. Eminaga O, Fries J, Neiß S, et al. The upregulation of hypoxia-related miRNA 210 in primary tumor of lymphogenic metastatic prostate cancer. Epigenomics. 2018;10(10):1347-59.

21. Karmakar S, Kaushik G, Nimmakayala R, Rachagani S, Ponnusamy MP, Batra SK. MicroRNA regulation of K-Ras in pancreatic cancer and opportunities for therapeutic intervention. Semin Cancer Biol. 2019;54:63-71.

22. Tvingsholm SA, Hansen MB, KKB C, et al. Let-7 microRNA controls invasion-promoting lysosomal changes via the oncogenic transcription factor myeloid zinc finger-1. Oncogenesis. 2018;7(2):14.

23. Song J, Wang L, Ma Q, et al. Let-7i-5p inhibits the proliferation and metastasis of colon cancer cells by targeting kallikrein-related peptidase 6. Oncol Rep. 2018;40(3):1459-66.

24. Ottley EC, Nicholson HD, Gold EJ. Activin a regulates microRNAs and gene expression in LNCaP cells. Prostate. 2016;76(11):951–63.

25. Kozinn SI, Harty NJ, Delong JM, et al. MicroRNA profile to predict gemcitabine resistance in bladder carcinoma cell lines. Genes Cancer. 2013; 4(1–2):61–9.

26. Tian Y, Hao S, Ye M, et al. MicroRNAs let-7b/i suppress human glioma cell invasion and migration by targeting IKBKE directly. Biochem Biophys Res Commun. 2015;458(2):307–12.

27. Shi Y, Duan Z, Zhang X, Zhang X, Wang G, Li F. Down-regulation of the let-7i facilitates gastric cancer invasion and metastasis by targeting COL1A1. Protein Cell. 2019:10(2):143-8.

28. Sepe R, Piscuoglio S, Quintavalle C, et al. HMGA1 overexpression is associated with a particular subset of human breast carcinomas. J Clin Pathol. 2016;69(2):117–21.

29. Hillion J, Roy S, Heydarian M, et al. The high mobility group A1 (HMGA1) gene is highly overexpressed in human uterine serous carcinomas and carcinosarcomas and drives matrix Metalloproteinase-2 (MMP-2) in a subset of tumors. Gynecol Oncol. 2016;141(3):580–7.

30. Pegoraro S, Ros G, Piazza S, et al. HMGA1 promotes metastatic processes in basal-like breast cancer regulating EMT and stemness. Oncotarget. 2013;4(8): 1293–308.

31. Lin Y, Chen H, Hu Z, Mao Y, Xu X, Zhu Y, Xu X, Wu J, Li S, Mao Q, Zheng X, Xie L. miR-26a inhibits proliferation and motility in bladder cancer by targeting HMGA1. FEBS Lett. 2013;587:2467–73.

32. Cinkornpumin J, Roos M, Nguyen L, et al. A small molecule screen to identify regulators of let-7 targets. Sci Rep. 2017;7(1):15973.

33. Zhou WB, Zhong CN, Luo XP, et al. miR-625 suppresses cell proliferation and migration by targeting HMGA1 in breast cancer. Biochem Biophys Res Commun. 2016;470(4):838–44.

5

Follicular dendritic cell sarcoma (FDCS) of urinary bladder with coexisting urothelial carcinoma

Jing Sun[1,2], Cheng Wang[4], Dandan Wang[1], Jiangtao Wu[3], Leiming Wang[1], Lan Zhao[1] and Lianghong Teng[1*] ⓘ

Abstract

Background: Follicular dendritic cell sarcoma is a very rare bladder tumor with very few cases that have been reported in the English literature.

Case presentation: We report an unusual case of follicular dendritic cell sarcoma that is coexistent with urothelial carcinoma (UC) in the urinary bladder of a 73-year-old man, who first presented with lower abdominal pain. Microscopic examination of the first transurethral resection of bladder tumor (TURBT) sample showed a neoplasm containing spindle or ovoid-shaped cells that were arranged in storiform, nested or swirling patterns. Abundant mitotic Figs. (30 mitoses/10 high-power fields) and apoptotic bodies were present. The tumor cells were positive for CD21 and vimentin, partly positive for CD23, D2–40 and CD35. After 6 weeks, the tumor recurred lately, which surprisingly contained a component of urothelial carcinoma. The first TURBT sample was then reviewed and a coexisting UC mixed with FDCS was identified by examining the deeper levels of the tumor blocks.

Conclusions: This case is, to our knowledge, the first time to report the coexistence of FDCS and UC in the urinary bladder of an elderly patient. And these two tumors may share a similar molecular mechanism.

Keywords: Follicular dendritic cell sarcoma, Urothelial carcinoma, Urinary bladder, Transurethral resection of bladder tumor, Coexisting

Background

Follicular dendritic cell sarcoma (FDCS) is a rare neoplasm involving the proliferation of neoplastic dendritic cells [1, 2]. When it occurs in extra nodal sites, it is well known to be a diagnostic challenge [3, 4]. To our knowledge, up till now only one case of FDCS has been reported in urinary bladder [5]. There are only rare reports that FDCS can occur concurrently with other types of tumors such as Castleman disease [3]. Here we report a challenging case of FDCS in the urinary bladder, particularly coexisted with urothelial carcinoma (UC).

Case presentation

In August 2016, a cystoscopically visible protuberant neoplasm of the urinary bladder was found in a 73-year-old man, with clinical manifestation of lower abdominal

pain, frequency, urgency and dysuria during urination. Pelvic computed tomography (CT) examination showed a 1.5 cm nodular soft tissue shadow at the left anterior wall of the bladder (Fig. 1). The patient then underwent the procedure of transurethral resection of bladder tumor (TURBT). Resected sample was formalin fixed, paraffin embedded. The tissue blocks were cut into 3-μm sections, which were stained with hematoxylin and eosin. Microscopic examination showed the neoplasm was composed of spindle or ovoid-shaped cells that formed storiform, nested or swirling patterns. It involved mucosa and submucosa layers. The neoplastic spindle cells had indistinct cytoplasmic borders, a moderate amount of lightly acidophilic cytoplasm, round or ovoid nuclei with a thin nuclear membrane and small nucleoli. Abundant mitotic Figs. (30 mitoses/10 high-power fields) and apoptotic bodies were present, with no necrosis and hemorrhage. Multinucleated cells and pleomorphic cells were also seen. Some mature lymphocytes infiltrated between tumor cells and in perivascular

* Correspondence: tenglh2012@163.com
[1]Department of Pathology, Xuan Wu Hospital, Capital Medical University, Beijing, China
Full list of author information is available at the end of the article

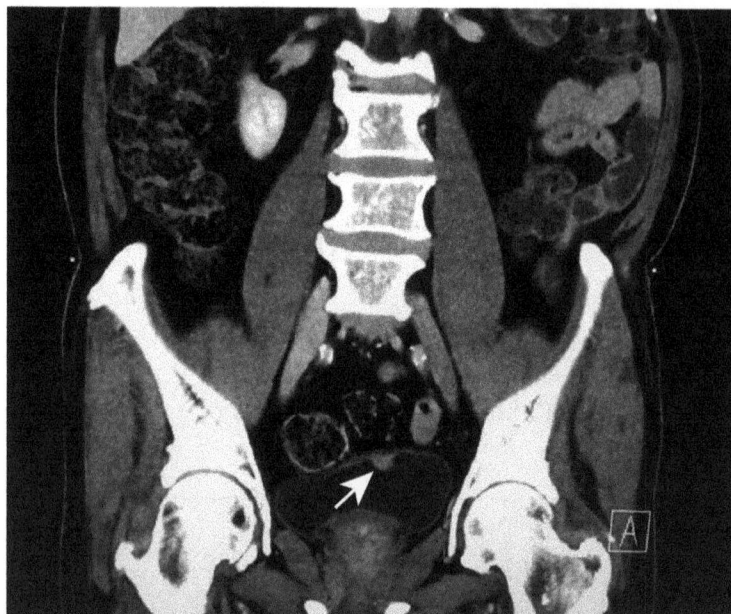

Fig. 1 Pelvic computed tomography examination shows a nodular soft tissue shadow (arrow) at the left anterior wall of the bladder

spaces (Fig. 2a, b). The residual lymphoid tissue was limited to small follicles.

Immunohistochemical stains were performed in our laboratory, utilizing an avidin biotin peroxidase complex method. Heat-induced antigen retrieval was performed and then the tissue was incubated with antibodies. Mouse monoclonal anti-human antibodies against CD3, CD5, CD20, CD21, CD23, CD30, CD56, CK, CK7, EMA, HMB45, Melan A, SMA, Vimentin, rabbit polyclonal anti-human antibodies against S-100, were purchased from Leica company. Mouse monoclonal anti-human antibodies CD35, D2–40, Desmin, Ki-67, MPO, P63, GATA-3, P16, P53, EGFR, ALK, CK5/6, rabbit polyclonal anti-human antibodies against CK20, P40, TFE-3, Uroplakin, were purchased from ZS company. Mouse monoclonal anti-human antibody BRAF V600E (VE1) was purchased from Roche company.

The tumor cells were positive for CD21 and vimentin, partly positive for CD23, D2–40 and CD35. The tumor cells were negative for CK, CK5/6, EMA, CK7, CK20, P63, P40, Uroplakin, Desmin, SMA, S100, TFE-3, HMB45, MelanA, MPO, ALK, CD3, CD5, CD20 and CD30. Ki-67 was expressed in about 30% of the tumor cell nuclei (Fig. 2c, d). Silver staining demonstrated abundant fibers circumfused each tumor cell. The pathological diagnosis of follicular dendritic cell sarcoma was given based on the morphology and immunohistochemistry.

Six weeks later, the tumor recurred, which appeared widely based, deeper than the primary surgical scar and was about 1.5 × 2 cm in size. A second transurethral resection was performed and microscopically the FDCS still could be seen in

bladder mucosa and submucosa. FDCS tumor cells were similar to those seen in the previous sample, which were spindle-shaped with round or ovoid nuclei with small nucleoli. But the number of mitotic Figs. (10 mitoses/10 high-power fields) was lower than that of the first sample. However, the tumor cells were found to infiltrate in muscularis propria. It was surprising that there was also an invasive urothelial carcinoma that was mixed with the FDCS. The UC of bladder infiltrated in mucosa and submucosa. The tumor cells of UC were arranged in nest or cord pattern, the cytoplasm was acidophilic and the nuclear were irregular. (Fig. 2e, f). Using immunohischemistry, UC were positive for CK, CK20, P63, GATA-3, negative for CD21, CD23, CD35 and D2–40. Otherwise, FDCS were positive for Vimentin, CD21, CD23, CD35 and D2–40, negative for CK and CK20. (Fig. 2g). UC and FDCS were both positive for P16, P53 and EGFR, and both negative for BRAF.

Because the second resection site was closed to the first one, we suspected the first sample might have been associated with urothelial carcinoma that was undetected in the first sample. We then obtained deeper levels of the initially resected tumor. Indeed, we identified the urothelial carcinoma in the deeper levels, which was coexisting with FDCS (Fig. 2h). After the second surgery the patient was treated with chemotherapy. At the time of writing this report, the patient had haven another relapse of urothelial carcinoma and one relapse of follicular dendritic cell sarcoma.

Discussion and conclusions

Follicular dendritic cell sarcoma is a proliferation of spindled to ovoid-shaped neoplastic cells. There is a

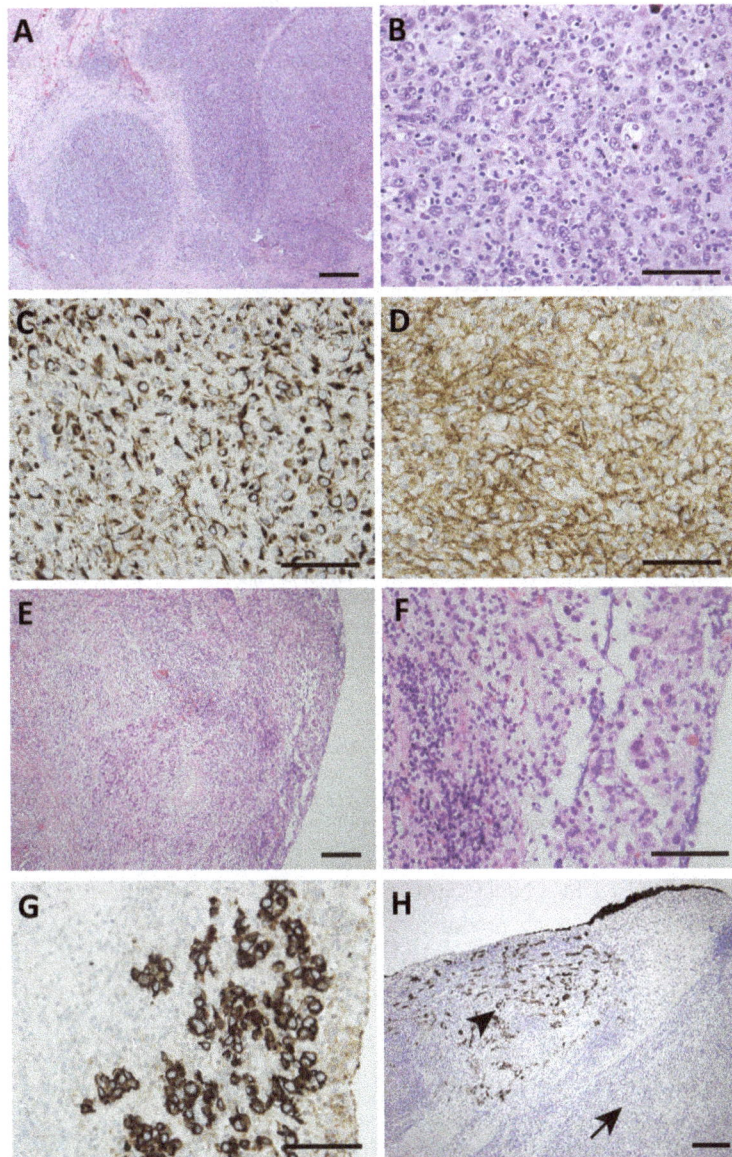

Fig. 2 HE and immunohistochemistry staining of the bladder tumor. HE staining **a-b**) showed FDCS tumor cells arranged in a storiform or nesting pattern, tumor cells had indistinct cytoplasmic borders, round or ovoid nuclei; Immunohistochemistry staining showed FDCS tumor cells were positive for vimentin (**c**) and CD21 (**d**); HE staining (**e-f**) showed UC tumor cells arranged in nest or cord pattern, tumor cells had acidophilic cytoplasm and irregular nuclear; Immunohistochemistry staining showed UC tumor cells were positive for CK (**g**); Immunohistochemistry staining of CK (**h**) showed infiltrated UC (arrow head) mixed with FDCS (arrow), UC were positive for CK, FDCS were negative for CK. Bar = 200 μm

wide age range from 9 to 82 years associated with FDCS, with an average age of 44 years in both sexes. Men and women have similar morbidity [4]. The patient in our report was 73 years old when he first presented with urinary symptoms.

Majority of FDCS occur in cervical lymph nodes, while approximately one-third of FDCS cases occur in extra-nodal sites. In most cases, the patients are asymptomatic and the neoplasms usually grow slowly and painlessly. Since FDCS is rare in the bladder and has morphologic features similar to other tumors, it may create a

diagnostic pitfall. FDCS may be confused with spindle cell carcinoma, malignant melanoma, lymphoma, inter-digitating dendritic cell sarcoma, thymoma, and meta-static undifferentiated carcinomas, et al. But FDCS immunophenotypic profile is quite specific and useful in its diagnosis. In this case, the morphologic features and immunophenotypes (CD21, CD23, CD35, D2–40 posi-tivity) were in keeping with follicular dendritic cell sarcoma. Majority of FDCS are considered low-grade sarcoma, while tumors with larger sizes and more mitotic figures tend to have relapses. In our case, the number of mitosis was high, which might explain the tumor recurrence 6 weeks later and the tumor cells were found to infiltrate into the muscular layer. So far only one case of FDCS was reported in urinary bladder [5]. In that case of bladder FDCS, cystitis glandularis and low-grade urothelial atypia were also found in the bladder mucosa adjacent to the tumor, which suggested that FDCS might be associated with metaplasia or even possible dysplasia in the nearby bladder mucosa. Our case is probably the first report on FDCS that occurred with UC at the same time. The UC was not present in the initial level of the first TURBT sample, which might be a useful lesson for our future practice, i.e., if there is FDCS detected in the urinary bladder, the possibility of a co-existing UC should be considered and the specimen should be examined thoroughly by examining additional tissue levels.

The etiology of FDCS is not clear. Approximately 10 to 20% of FDCS cases are associated with Castleman disease. Wang et al. reported some cases of Castleman disease contained areas of follicular dendritic cell proliferation, so FDCS was hypothesized to arise from such areas [6]. Additionally, Sun et al. stated that a similar feature of Castleman disease and FDCS was the expression of epidermal growth factor receptor (EGFR) [7]. It has also been found that, based on the study completed by Cheuk et al., Epstein-Barr virus was associated with the inflammatory pseudotumor-like variant of FDCS, which can selectively involve spleen and liver, characterized by frequent presence of systemic symptoms and marked female predominance [8]. Also FDCS is associated with complex cytogenetic abnormalities. Cell cycle regulatory gene such as P16 showed alteration [9] and tumor suppressor gene P53 mutation were also found in FDCS [10]. Recently Go et al. [11] found that the BRAF pathway was contributed to the pathogenesis of histiocytic and dendritic cell neoplasms, the BRAFV600E mutation was positive in 18.5% (5 of 27) of FDCS cases.

These cytogenetic abnormalities may share mechanisms of tumor genesis with a subset of other tumor types, such as urothelial carcinoma. P16 and P53 genes were altered more prominently in patients with high-grade tumors than low-grade tumors of urothelial carcinoma, which may play significant roles in the progression of bladder cancer [12]. There were many molecular risk factors, related to poor prognosis of UC, and one of these factors was the expression of EGFR [13]. Also, Boulalas et al. found that the involvement of BRAF mutations in the development of bladder UC was infrequent [14]. In our case, both P16 and P53 protein had shown positive stains in the FDCS and UC. Also, EGFR were over expressed, but no mutation was found about BRAF (V600E). These two tumors may share some same molecular mechanism, but the exact reason needs to be further studied.

In conclusion, follicular dendritic cell sarcoma can occur with urothelial carcinoma at the same time in the bladder, and these two tumors may share a similar molecular mechanism.

Abbreviations
ALK: Anaplastic lymphoma kinase; CD: Clusters of differentiation; CK: Cytokeratin; CT: Computed tomography; EGFR: Epidermal growth factor receptor; EMA: Epithelial membrane antigen; FDCS: Follicular dendritic cell sarcoma; Melan A: Melanoma marker A; MPO: Myeloperoxidase; SMA: Smooth muscle actin; TURBT: Transurethral resection of bladder tumor; UC: Urothelial carcinoma

Acknowledgements
Not applicable.

Authors' contributions
JS: wrote the pathological part of this manuscript; CW: contributed to writing and consulting; DDW: wrote the discussion; JTW: collected the clinical data; LMW: made the immunohistochemical diagnosis; LZ and LHT made the final diagnosis and helped revising the manuscript. All authors read and approved the final manuscript.

Author details
[1]Department of Pathology, Xuan Wu Hospital, Capital Medical University, Beijing, China. [2]Department of Pathology, Capital Medical University, Beijing, China. [3]Department of Urology, Xuan Wu Hospital, Capital Medical University, Beijing, China. [4]Department of Pathology and Laboratory Medicine, Dalhousie University, Nova Scotia, Canada.

References
1. Swerdlow SH, Campo E, Harris NL, Jaffe ES, Pileri SA, Stein H, Thiele J. WHO classification of Tumours of Haematopoietic and lymphoid tissues. Lyon, France: IARC Press. 2017:476–8.
2. Imal Y, Yamakawa M. Morphology, function and pathology of follicular dendritic cells. Pathol Int. 1996;46(11):807–33.
3. Wu A, Sheeja P. Follicular dendritic cell sarcoma. Arch Pathol Lab. Med. 2016;140(2):186–90.
4. Li L, Shi YH, Guo ZJ, Qiu T, Guo L, Yang HY, Zhang X, Zhao XM, Su Q. Clinicopathological features and prognosis assessment of extranodal follicular dendritic cell sarcoma. World J Gastroenterol. 2010;16(20):2504–19.
5. Duan GJ, Wu YL, Sun H, Lang L, Chen ZW, Yan XC. Primary follicular dendritic cellsarcoma of the urinary bladder: the first case report and potential diagnostic pitfalls. Diagn Pathol. 2017;12(1):35.
6. Wang RF, Han W, Qi L, Shan LH, Wang ZC, Wang LF. Extranodal follicular dendritic cell sarcoma: a clinicopathological report of four cases and a literature review. Oncol Lett. 2015;9(1):391–8.
7. Sun X, Chang KC, Abruzzo LV, Lai R, Younes A, Jones D. Epidermal growth factor receptor expression in follicular dendritic cells: a shared feature of follicular dendritic cell sarcoma and Castleman's disease. Hum Pathol. 2003; 34(9):835–40.
8. Cheuk W, Chan JK, Shek TW, Chang JH, Tsou MH, Yuen NW, Ng WF, Chan AC, Prat J. Inflammatory pseudotumor-like follicular dendriticcell tumor: a distinctive low-grade malignant intra-abdominal neoplasm with consistent Epstein-Barr virus association. Am J Surg Pathol. 2001;25(6):721–31.
9. Griffin GK, Sholl LM, Lindeman NIFletcher CD, Hornick JL. Targeted genomic sequencing of follicular dendritic cell sarcoma reveals recurrent alterations in NF-κB regulatory genes. Mod Pathol. 2016;29(1):67–74.
10. Li L, Shi YH, Guo ZJ, Qiu T, Guo L, Yang HY, Zhang X, Zhao XM. Su Q. Clinicopathological features and prognosis assessment of extranodal follicular dendritic cell sarcoma. World J Gastroenterol. 2010;16(20):2504–19.
11. Go H, Jeon YK, Huh J, Choi SJ, Choi YD, Cha HJ, Kim HJ, Park G, Min S, Kim JE. Frequent detection of BRAF(V) (600E) mutations in histiocytic and dendritic cell neoplasms. Histopathology. 2014;65(2):261–72.
12. Abat D, Demirhan O, Inandiklioglu N, Tunc E, Erdogan S, Tastemir D, Uslu IN, TansugZ. Genetic alterations of chromosomes, p53 and p16 genes in low-and high-grade bladder cancer. Oncol Lett 2014 ;8(1):25–32.
13. Parvin M, Sabet-Rasekh P, Hajian P, Mohammadi Torbati P, Sabet-Rasekh P, Mirzaei H. Evaluating the prevalence of the epidermal growth factor receptor in transitional cell carcinoma of bladder and its relationship with other prognostic factors. Iran J Cancer Prev. 2016;9(1):e4022.

6

Patient-reported outcomes in randomised clinical trials of bladder cancer

Mieke Van Hemelrijck[1][*] [iD], Francesco Sparano[2], Debra Josephs[1,3], Mirjam Sprangers[4], Francesco Cottone[2] and Fabio Efficace[2]

Abstract

Background: Despite international recommendations of including patient-reported outcomes (PROs) in randomised clinical trials (RCTs), a 2014 review concluded that few RCTs of bladder cancer (BC) report PRO as an outcome. We therefore aimed to update the 2014 review to synthesise current evidence-based knowledge of PROs from RCTs in BC. A secondary objective was to examine whether quality of PRO reporting has improved over time and to provide evidence-based recommendations for future studies in this area.

Methods: We conducted a systematic literature search using PubMed/Medline, from April 2014 until June 2018. We included the RCTs identified in the previous review as well as newly published RCTs. Studies were evaluated using a predefined electronic-data extraction form that included information on basic trial demographics, clinical and PRO characteristics and standards of PRO reporting based on recommendation from the International Society of Quality of Life Research.

Results: Since April 2014 only eight new RCTs for BC included PROs as a secondary outcome. In terms of methodology, only the proportion of RCTs documenting the extent of missing PRO data (75% vs 11.1%, $p = 0.03$) and the identification of PROs in trial protocols (50% vs 0%, $p = 0.015$) improved. Statistical approaches for dealing with missing data were not reported in most new studies (75%).

Conclusion: Little improvement into the uptake and assessment of PRO as an outcome in RCTs for BC has been made during recent years. Given the increase in (immunotherapy) drug trials with a potential for severe adverse events, there is urgent need to adopt the recommendations and standards available for PRO use in bladder cancer RCTs.

Keywords: PROs, Quality of life, Outcome measurement, RCT, Bladder cancer

Background

With an estimated 549,000 new cases and 200,000 deaths in 2018 worldwide, bladder cancer is the 10th most common form of cancer [1]. All groups of bladder cancer patients are, not surprisingly, subjected to significant treatment burdens that are emotionally and psychologically taxing. Several symptoms, such as blood in the urine, pain and nausea, associated with different treatments may result in increased prevalence of depression, anxiety and stress and, consequently, decreased quality of life (QoL) [2]. Given this disease burden, there is a need to further evaluate how patient-reported outcomes (PROs) are incorporated in clinical bladder cancer research. Inclusion of QoL or other PROs in clinical trials and methodological rigor already at the stage of protocol writing are essential to eventually generate data that can robustly inform patient care [3].

Randomized controlled trials (RCTs), across a wide range of cancer malignancies, increasingly include PROs in an effort to better understand overall treatment effectiveness of newer drugs [4]. Inclusion of PROs in cancer research is not only valued by oncologists and patients, but also by regulatory stakeholders. To illustrate, the US Food and Drug Administration (FDA) included PROs as

* Correspondence: Mieke.vanhemelrijck@kcl.ac.uk
[1]King's College London, School of Cancer and Pharmaceutical Sciences, Translational Oncology and Urology Research (TOUR), London SE1 9RT, UK
Full list of author information is available at the end of the article

one of the clinical outcomes assessments (COAs) that can be used to determine whether or not a drug has demonstrated treatment benefit [5]. Similarly, the European Medicines Agency (EMA) has issued recent guidelines on the use of PRO endpoints in cancer research [6].

In the context of bladder cancer, a systematic review encompassing the years 2004–2014 examined the quality of PRO reporting and methodological strengths and weaknesses of RCTs. It concluded that few RCTs report PRO as an outcome and improvement in methodology was required [7]. Another more recent systematic review using the COnsensus-based Standards for the selection of health Measurement INstruments (COSMIN) [8] specifically evaluated the psychometric properties of PRO measurements in bladder cancer (1990–2017) [9]. No existing PRO stood out as the most appropriate to measure QoL in bladder cancer patients due to heterogeneity of the disease and its treatments and due to lack of validation studies [9]. Moreover, a recent systematic review highlighted the mental health implications in bladder cancer patients [10] – and hence the potential effects the disease and its treatments can have on QoL.

This study therefore aimed to update the review by Feuerstein et al. [7], by including all the RCTs of that review as well as newly published RCTs in order to synthesise current evidence-based knowledge of PROs from RCTs in bladder cancer. A secondary objective was to examine whether quality of PRO reporting improved over time and to provide evidence-based recommendations for future studies in this area.

Methods
Search strategy and identification of studies
We conducted a systematic literature search using PubMed/Medline, from April 2014 until June 2018. Methodology for study identification and evaluation followed standardised criteria used in the PROMOTION Registry (http://promotion.gimema.it) and was previously described in similar systematic reviews [7, 11, 12]. For the purpose of this updated review on bladder cancer RCTs, the following script was used to identify a PRO component: (*"quality of life" OR "health related quality of life" OR "health status" OR "health outcomes" OR "patient outcomes" OR "depression" OR "anxiety" OR "emotional" OR "social" OR "psychosocial" OR "psychological" OR "distress" OR "social functioning" OR "social wellbeing" OR "emotional" OR "patient reported symptom" OR "patient reported outcomes" OR pain OR fatigue OR "patient reported outcome" OR "PRO" OR "PROs" OR "HRQL" OR "QOL" OR "HRQOL" OR "symptom distress" OR "symptom burden" OR "symptom assessment" OR "functional status" OR sexual OR functioning) AND bladder*. The search strategy was restricted to RCTs. In case of multiple publications from the same RCT, all

relevant data possibly published in secondary articles were combined.

Selection criteria
Only English-language reports of RCTs comparing conventional treatments and involving adult patients with bladder cancer were included – irrespective of disease stage. The minimum, overall sample size was set at 50 patients. Screening studies or those involving patients with benign disease were excluded. We did not consider conference abstracts as these did not contain sufficient information. RCTs of interventions that were psychological, behavioural, complementary or alternative were also excluded.

We included all studies evaluating a PRO either as a primary or secondary outcome – either as a multidimensional QoL outcome or any other type of PRO. Those studies evaluating only treatment adherence or satisfaction were also excluded. For comparability purposes, selection criteria of eligible articles were the same as of the previous systematic review [7]. Details on the search strategy and selection process were documented according to the PRISMA guidelines [13].

Methods of evaluation of studies
Two reviewers (MVH, FS) extracted information from the identified studies and a third reviewer (FE) was consulted in case of disagreement. All data were entered by the reviewers into a password protected online database (REDCap) [14] by completing a predefined electronic-data extraction form (eDEF). Full details on information contained in the eDEF have been previously reported [11]. A double-blind data entry procedure was performed as each reviewer completed the eDEF independently. Discrepancies in evaluations were electronically recorded and when disagreements occurred in the evaluation of any item included in the eDEF, the reviewers revisited the paper to reconcile any differences until consensus was achieved.

Type of data extraction and data analysis
For the purpose of this review, the following types of information were considered: 1) basic trial demographics; 2) clinical and PRO characteristics and 3) elements of PRO reporting based on recommendation from the International Society of Quality of Life Research (ISOQOL) [15]. Quality of PRO reporting was therefore evaluated with the ISOQOL checklist, which comprises a common set of 17 key issues regardless of PRO being primary or secondary outcome. Eleven additional issues were considered when a PRO is a primary outcome of the study. Each item of the ISOQOL checklist was rated as 'yes' if documented in the publication (scored as 1) or 'no' if not documented (scored 0). To further refine the

investigation of the accuracy of reporting, we divided the ISOQOL item addressing the problem of missing data into two (i.e., reporting the extent of missing data and reporting statistical approaches for dealing with missing data). We thus rated each RCT with a score ranging from 0 to a maximum of 18 (RCT with PRO as a secondary outcome) or 29 (PRO as primary outcome). In both cases, a higher score indicates better quality of the PRO reporting. Our rule of thumb for this analysis was to consider RCTs addressing less than 50% of items included in the ISOQOL recommendations [15] as having "suboptimal quality". That is, 9 items out of 18 for RCTs which included PRO as secondary outcome and 15 items out of 29 for RCTs which included PRO as primary outcome.

Main characteristics of eligible studies were reported by proportions, means and standard deviation, according to the type of variable. Differences between studies were assessed by Fisher exact test or Wilcoxon-Mann-Whitney test. Based on the ISOQOL checklist score, comparisons of reporting quality were performed. To ensure comparability between studies with PRO as primary or secondary outcome, for each study the raw score was standardised dividing it by the number of applicable items (18 for secondary or 29 for primary), then multiplied by 100. This way, we obtained an adjusted checklist score ranging from 0 (worst quality) to 100 (best quality). Based on such score, we compared studies with PRO as secondary outcome (studies until March 2014 vs those from April 2014), studies with PRO as primary vs. studies with PRO as secondary outcome and studies using a validated PRO measure or not. In addition, we computed the proportion of studies that had a checklist score below or equal to the cut-off value of 50. All tests were two-sided and statistical significance was set at $\alpha = 0.05$. Analyses were performed by SAS software v. 9.4 (SAS Institute Inc., Cary, NC).

Results

Overview of RCT characteristics

The search identified 586 abstracts published in the period 2014–2018. Eight studies fulfilled the eligibility criteria (Fig. 1). In all the newly identified RCTs [16–23], PROs were secondary outcome, whereas of the nine old studies [24–33] five RCTs (55.6%) employed PROs as

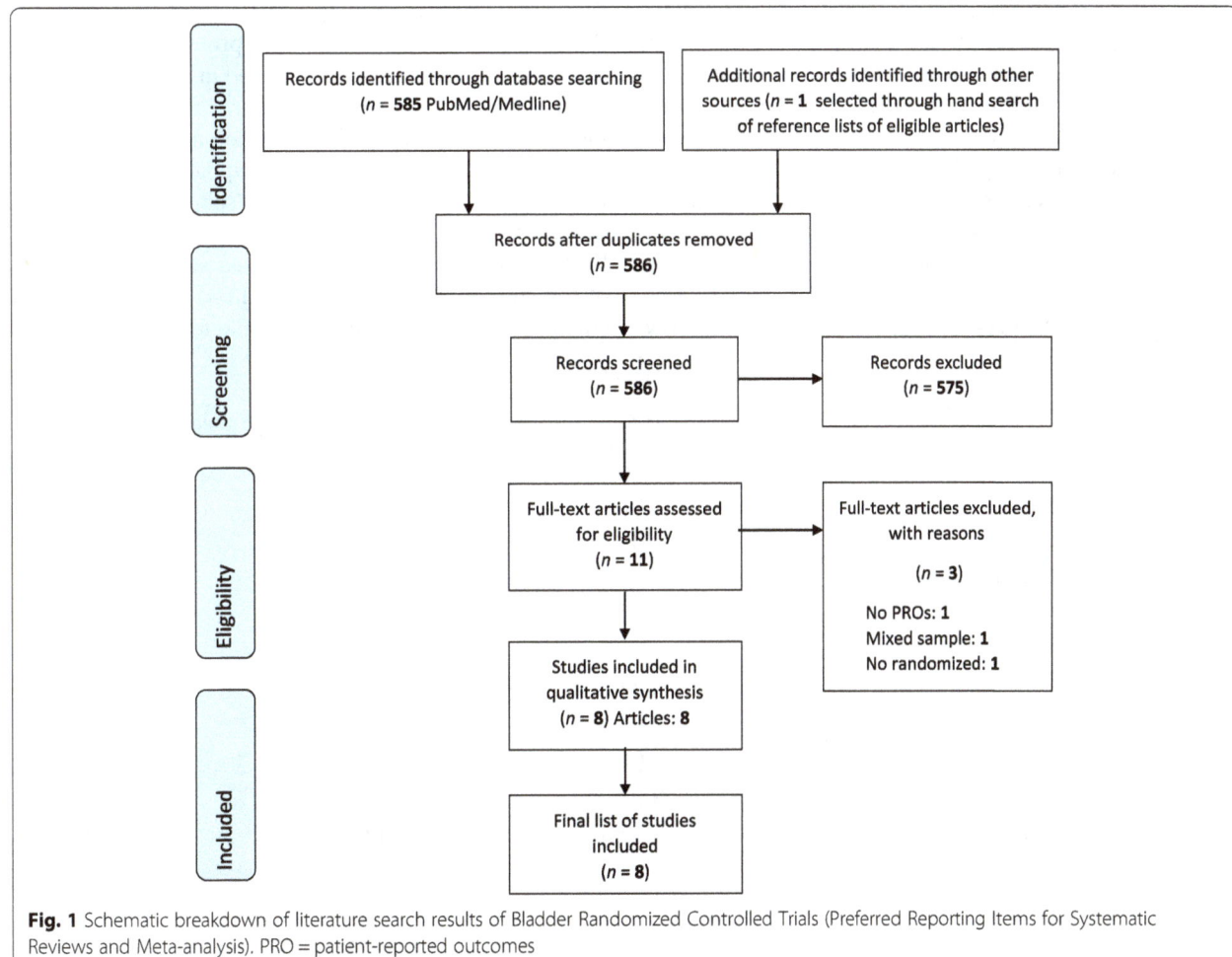

Fig. 1 Schematic breakdown of literature search results of Bladder Randomized Controlled Trials (Preferred Reporting Items for Systematic Reviews and Meta-analysis). PRO = patient-reported outcomes

primary outcome [27–30, 33]. All but one of the newly identified RCTs were not supported by industry (87.5%) and none of the RCTs was carried out in a multinational context. The majority of new trials (5, 62.5%) enrolled patients with non-metastatic disease. Compared to the old studies, where two RCTs (22.2%) enrolled more than 200 patients, only one of the newly identified RCTs (12.5%) enrolled more than 200 patients overall. Six new RTCs (75%) assessed PROs over a time period of 6 months, one study (12.5%) up to 1 year and in one study (12.5%) the length of assessment was more than 1 year. Details are reported in Table 1.

Most recent (2014–2018) evidence of bladder cancer RCTs with PROs

Among the eight newly identified RCTs, only three [18, 19, 23] used a multidimensional PRO instrument (e.g. the European Organization for Research and Treatment of Cancer Quality of Life Questionnaire-Core 30 (EORTC QLQ-C30) [34]) and of these, two used a bladder cancer-specific questionnaire (the Functional Assessment of Cancer Therapy-Bladder (FACT-Bl) and the FACT-Vanderbilt Cystectomy Index (VCI) questionnaires) (Table 2). In three studies [16, 17, 20], no differences in pain scores were detected between the experimental treatment arms (solifenacin, sevoflurane and glycopyrrolate, respectively) and the control arms (standard care, desflurane and atropine, respectively). In the study conducted by Huang et al. [21], VAS scores for bladder pain were significantly lower at the end of the induction cycle in the group treated with pirarubicin combined with hyaluronic acid compared to pirarubicin alone, while dexmedetomidine was associated with lower postoperative pain scores compared to placebo [22]. Low

dose of Bacillus Calmette-Guerin (BCG) was associated with better outcomes in terms of global QoL, role functioning and financial problems, as assessed by the EORTC QLQ-C30, compared to standard dose [18]. No differences in QoL, as assessed with the FACT-BI, were found between laparoscopic and robot-assisted radical cystectomy [19]. Finally, no difference in QoL, as assessed by the FACT-VCI, was detected between robot-assisted radical cystectomy and open radical cystectomy [23].

Comparison of PRO quality reporting between 2004 and 2014 and 2014–2018

Only one (12.5%) of the eight new RCTs reported a PRO hypothesis [18] and two (25%) reported the statistical approach for dealing with missing data [19, 23]. Three RCTs (37.5%) documented the mode of PRO administration [16, 17, 21], four (50%) documented the rationale for the choice of PRO instrument [16, 19, 21, 23], whereas two RCTs (25%) reported generalisability issues [17, 21] or interpretation in terms of clinical significance [21, 22].

Compared to previous studies, only two statistically significant improvements were noted: there was an increase in proportion of RCTs documenting the extent of missing PRO data (75% vs 11.1%, $p = 0.015$) and an increase of RCTs documenting PROs in trial protocols (50% vs 0%, $p = 0.03$). Further details are reported in Table 3.

We compared the ISOQOL scores for studies with a PRO as secondary outcome identified in the previous review with those identified in this update. The quality of PRO reporting was considered as "suboptimal" for all of the old studies, while this was not the case for the new RCTs, whose quality was considered suboptimal in 50% of the studies. The mean standardized score for the old studies was 30.5 (median 33.3), while for the new studies

Table 1 Overview of RCT characteristics

Characteristic	Category	RCT published between Jan.2004 –Mar. 2014 (n. 9), N. (%)	RCTs published between Apr.2014 – Jun.2018 (n. 8), N. (%)	Total (n. 17), N. (%)
International (if more than one country)	No	8 (88.9)	8 (100)	16 (94.1)
	Yes	1 (11.1)	0 (0)	1 (5.9)
Industry supported (fully or in part)	No	6 (66.7)	7 (87.5)	13 (76.5)
	Yes	3 (33.3)	1 (12.5)	4 (23.5)
PRO endpoint	Primary	5 (55.6)	0 (0)	5 (29.4)
	Secondary	4 (44.4)	8 (100)	12 (70.6)
Secondary paper on PRO	No	8 (88.9)	8 (100)	16 (94.1)
	Yes	1 (11.1)	0 (0)	1 (5.9)
Length of PRO assessment during RCT	Up to 6 months	4 (44.5)	6 (75)	10 (58.8)
	Up to 1 year	2 (22.2)	1 (12.5)	3 (17.7)
	More than 1 year	3 (33.3)	1 (12.5)	4 (23.5)
Overall study sample size	<=200	7 (77.8)	7 (87.5)	14 (82.3)
	> 200	2 (22.2)	1 (12.5)	3 (17.7)

Table 2 Overview of bladder cancer RCTs with a PRO evaluation published between 2004 and 2018

Author	Intervention	Type of bladder cancer	Sample size[a]	Main Clinical Outcome	PRO instrument used	Summary findings for main clinical outcome and PRO[b]
PRO primary endpoint						
Marandola et al. 2005 [27]	Spinal anaesthesia with 10 mg of 0.5% hyperbaric bupivacine vs. 15 µg of sufentanil	Scheduled for TURBT	62	Motor and sensory blockages (primary)	Verbal analogue pain scale	• Bupivacine patients experienced more intense motor blockade • Statistical significance on PRO outcomes not reported
Ozyuvaci et al. 2005 [28]	General anaesthesia vs combined epidural and general anaesthesia for radical cystectomy	Scheduled for radical cystectomy	50	Intraoperative outcomes	Visual analogue scale	• Significant reduction of intraoperative blood loss for those in the combined group • Lower post-operative pain scores for the combined group
Gontero et al. 2013 [29]	Intravesical gemcitabine vs 1/3 dose BCG instillation	NMIBC	120	Recurrence and progression	EORT QLQ-C30	• No difference in recurrence and progression • On univariate analysis, at T1, gemcitabine had better cognitive and emotional functioning and urinary symptom distress. At T2, gemcitabine had better cognitive functioning and less nausea and vomiting symptom distress
Johnson et al. 2013 [33]	10 mg extended release oxybutynin daily or placebo 6 weeks prior to BCG treatment	BCG Naïve NMIBC	50	Adverse reactions and systemic symptoms	Self-reported urinary symptoms	• More urinary frequency and burning, fever and flu-like symptoms when receiving treatment • Worse urinary symptoms when receiving treatment
Karl et al. 2014 [30]	Early recovery vs conservative regimen after radical cystectomy	Scheduled for radical cystectomy	101	Postoperative morbidity, adverse events, mobility	EORTC QLQ-C30	• Early recovery associated with lower rates of wound healing disorders, DVT and fever • Early recovery associated with improvements in most QLQ-C30 scales
PRO secondary endpoint						
Skinner et al. 2009 [31] Ahmadi et al. 2013 [32]	T pouch vs Studer pouch diversion after radical cystoprostatectomy	Scheduled for cystoprostatectomy	295	Renal function and anatomy at 3 years following surgery (primary)	Modified version of the Bladder Cancer Index	• No differences • Not reported
Koga et al. 2010 [26]	Maintenance vs observation following complete response after BCG	NMIBC	53	Efficacy of duration (primary)	EORTC QLQ-C30	• Maintenance BCG associated with lower recurrence rate on univariate, but not multivariate, analyses • No difference in QoL
Sabichi et al. 2011 [25]	Celecoxib vs. placebo	NMIBC	146	Time to recurrence (primary)	EORTC QLQ-C30	• No effect on time to recurrence. • No difference in QoL
James et al. 2012 [24]	Radiotherapy with or without chemotherapy	MIBC	360	Survival free of locoregional disease (primary)	Not reported	• Locoregional disease-free survival was significantly better in the chemoradiotherapy group than in the radiotherapy group • PRO not reported
Kim et al. 2015 [20]	Glycopyrrolate vs atropine in combination with neostigmine after TURBT	Scheduled for TURBT	74	Incidence of catheter-related bladder discomfort postoperatively (primary)	Numerical rating scale	• Incidence of CRBD was significantly lower in the glycopyrrolate group than in the atropine group postoperatively • No difference in pain scores
Huang et al. 2015 [21]	Pirarubicin combined with hyaluronic acid vs pirarubicin alone after TURBT	Scheduled for TURBT	127	Recurrence (efficacy) (primary)	Visual analogue scale	• No difference in treatment efficacy • The VAS for bladder pain was significantly lower, at the end of the induction cycle, in the experimental group
Kim et al. 2015 [22]	Dexmedetomidine vs placebo during TURBT	Scheduled for TURBT	109	Incidence of catheter-related bladder	Numerical rating scale	• Incidence of CRBD was significantly higher in the control group • The postoperative pain score was higher in the control group

Table 2 Overview of bladder cancer RCTs with a PRO evaluation published between 2004 and 2018 (*Continued*)

Author	Intervention	Type of bladder cancer	Sample size[a]	Main Clinical Outcome	PRO instrument used	Summary findings for main clinical outcome and PRO[b]
				discomfort postoperatively (primary)		
Kim et al. 2016 [17]	Sevoflurane vs desflurane during TURBT	Scheduled for TURBT	89	Incidence of catheter-related bladder discomfort 24 h postoperatively (primary)	Numerical rating scale	• Sevoflurane was associated with less frequent postoperative CRBD • No difference in postoperative pain scores
Yokomizo et al. 2016 [18]	80 mg BCG (standard) vs 40 mg BCG induction therapy	NMIBC or CIS	166	Non-inferiority with a null hypothesis of 15% decrease in complete response rate	EORT QLQ-C30	• Noninferiority not proven. • Low dose BCG associated with higher quality of life
Khan et al. 2016 [19]	Laparoscopic radical cystectomy vs. robot-assisted radical cystectomy	Scheduled for cystectomy	60	30- and 90-day complication rates	FACT-BI	• 30-d complication rate higher in the open radical prostatectomy arm; but no differences at 90-d • No difference in QoL between both arms
Chung et al. 2017 [16]	Solifenacin vs standard care prior, during, and after TURBT	NMIBC	134	Incidence of catheter-related bladder discomfort (CRBD) at 1 and 2 h post TURBT (primary)	Visual analogue scale	• No difference in incidence rates • No difference in postoperative pain scores
Parekh et al. 2018 [23]	Robot-assisted radical cystectomy vs. open radical cystectomy	Scheduled for cystectomy	302	Progression-free survival at 2 years after surgery	Short Form-8 FACT-VCI	• Robotic cystectomy was non-inferior to open cystectomy for 2 years progression-free survival • No difference in QoL between both arms

Abbreviations: BCG Bacillus Calmette-Guerin, *CIS* Carcinoma in situ, *CRBD* Catheter-related bladder discomfort, *DVT* Deep vein thrombosis, *EORTC* European Organization for Research and Treatment of Cancer, *FACT-BI* Functional Assessment of Cancer Therapy-Bladder, *FACT-VCI* Functional Assessment of Cancer Therapy-Vanderbilt Cystectomy Index, *MIBC* Muscle invasive bladder cancer, *NMIBC* Non-muscle invasive bladder cancer, *PRO* Patient-Reported Outcomes, *QLQ-C30* Quality of Life Questionnaire-Core30, *QoL* Quality of life, *RCT* Randomized controlled trial, *TURBT* Transurethral resection of bladder tumor
[a]The overall trial sample size refers to all the patients that agreed to participate to the study giving informed consent. We refer to the number of patients actually enrolled, not necessarily those who were randomized
[b]Differences in the main traditional clinical outcome were extracted based on reported statistical significance. Differences in PRO outcomes were based on statistical significance and/or clinically meaningful difference

Table 3 Comparison of PRO quality reporting over time in Bladder Cancer RCTs with PROs as a secondary outcome

Methodological issue	Category	RCT with PROs (Jan.2004 –Mar. 2014) (n. 9), N. (%)	RCTs with PROs (Apr.2014 – Jun.2018) (n. 8), N. (%)	P-value
Title and abstract				
The PRO should be identified as an outcome in the abstract	No	1 (11.1)	3 (37.5)	0.29
	Yes	8 (88.9)	5 (62.5)	
Introduction, background, and objectives				
The PRO hypothesis should be stated and specify the relevant PRO domain if applicable	No	5 (55.6)	5 (62.5)	1
	Yes	2 (22.2)	1 (12.5)	
	N/A (if explorative)	2 (22.2)	2 (25)	
Methods				
Outcomes				
The mode of administration of the PRO tool and the methods of collecting data should be described	No	7 (77.8)	5 (62.5)	0.62
	Yes	2 (22.2)	3 (37.5)	
Electronic mode of PRO administration[a]	No	1 (11.1)	2 (25)	1
	Yes	1 (11.1)	0 (0)	
	N/A	7 (77.8)	6 (75)	
The rationale for choice of the PRO instrument used should be provided	No	4 (44.4)	4 (50)	1
	Yes	5 (55.6)	4 (50)	
Evidence of PRO instrument validity and reliability should be provided or cited	No	4 (44.4)	3 (37.5)	0.44
	Yes, for all PRO instruments	5 (55.6)	3 (37.5)	
	Yes, only for some PRO instruments	0 (0)	2 (25)	
The intended PRO data collection schedule should be provided	No	2 (22.2)	1 (12.5)	1
	Yes	7 (77.8)	7 (87.5)	
PROs should be identified in the trial protocol post-hoc analyses	No	9 (100)	4 (50)	0.03[a]
	Yes	0 (0)	4 (50)	
The status of PRO as either a primary or secondary outcome should be stated	No	2 (22.2)	3 (37.5)	0.62
	Yes	7 (77.8)	5 (62.5)	
Statistical methods				
There should be evidence of appropriate statistical analysis and tests of statistical significance for each PRO hypothesis tested	No	0 (0)	2 (25)	0.223
	Yes	2 (22.2)	0 (0)	
	N/A	7 (77.8)	6 (75)	
The extent of missing data should be stated[b]	No	8 (88.9)	2 (25)	0.015[a]
	Yes	1 (11.1)	6 (75)	
Statistical approaches for dealing with missing data should be explicitly stated[b]	No	9 (100)	6 (75)	0.206
	Yes	0 (0)	2 (25)	
Results				
Participant flow				
A flow diagram or a description of the allocation of participants and those lost to follow-up should be provided for PROs specifically	No	7 (77.8)	5 (62.5)	0.62
	Yes	2 (22.2)	3 (37.5)	
The reasons for missing data should be explained	No	8 (88.9)	5 (62.5)	0.294
	Yes	1 (11.1)	3 (37.5)	

Table 3 Comparison of PRO quality reporting over time in Bladder Cancer RCTs with PROs as a secondary outcome *(Continued)*

Methodological issue	Category	RCT with PROs (Jan.2004 –Mar. 2014) (n. 9), N. (%)	RCTs with PROs (Apr.2014 – Jun.2018) (n. 8), N. (%)	P-value
Baseline data				
The study patients characteristics should be described including baseline PRO scores	No	6 (66.7)	3 (37.5)	0.347
	Yes	3 (33.3)	5 (62.5)	
Outcomes and estimation				
PRO outcomes also reported in a graphical format[a]	No	5 (55.6)	6 (75)	0.62
	Yes	4 (44.4)	2 (25)	
Discussion				
Limitations				
The limitations of the PRO components of the trial should be explicitly discussed	No	5 (55.6)	4 (50)	1
	Yes	4 (44.4)	4 (50)	
Generalizability				
Generalizability issues uniquely related to the PRO results should be discussed	No	5 (55.6)	6 (75)	0.62
	Yes	4 (44.4)	2 (25)	
Interpretation				
PROs are interpreted (Not only re-stated)[a]	No	2 (22.2)	5 (62.5)	0.153
	Yes	7 (77.8)	3 (37.5)	
The clinical significance of the PRO findings should be discussed	No	6 (66.7)	6 (75)	1
	Yes	3 (33.3)	2 (25)	
Methodology used to assess clinical significance is discussed[a]	Anchor based (e.g., minimal important difference)	1 (11.1)	0 (0)	1
	Distribution based (e.g. effect size)	1 (11.1)	2 (25)	
	Both	1 (11.1)	0 (0)	
	Missing	6 (66.7)	6 (75)	
The PRO results should be discussed in the context of the other clinical trial outcomes	No	2 (22.2)	1 (12.5)	1
	Yes	7 (77.8)	7 (87.5)	

For descriptive purposes, subheadings of this table reflect those reported in the ISOQOL recommended standards [15]; however, rating of items was independent of location of the information within the manuscript

[a]These items were not included in the ISOQOL recommended standards [15] and in the calculation of the ISOQOL score but have been evaluated in our study and reported in this table to have a wider outlook on the level of reporting

[b]These items were originally combined in the ISOQOL recommended standards [15] but have been split in this report to better investigate possible discrepancies between documentation of PRO missing data (ie, reporting how many patients did not complete a given questionnaire at any given time point) versus actual reporting of statistical methods to address this issue. Also, we wanted to be consistent with items reported in the CONSORT PRO Extension [35] (ie, statistical approaches for dealing with missing data is reported as a stand-alone issue)

the mean score was 48.6 (median 50). However, this positive trend was not statistically significant ($p = 0.072$).

The quality of PRO reporting among all of the studies published between 2004 and 2018 was found to be poor. Overall, only six studies (35.3%) addressed 50% or more of the issues recommended by the ISOQOL checklist (data not shown). The mean standardised ISOQOL score for all these studies was 44.7, below the cut-off value of 50. For three of the five RCTs with PRO as primary outcome (60%) the quality of PRO reporting was considered as "suboptimal". This percentage was higher for RCTs with a PRO as secondary outcomes, with eight of the twelve studies

(66.6%) considered as "suboptimal". The mean standardised ISOQOL score for the RCTs with PRO as primary outcome was 49.7, while for RCTs with PRO as secondary outcome was 42.6. No statistically significant differences in the ISOQOL score were found between RCTs with PRO as primary or secondary outcomes ($p = 0.459$).

It needs to be noted that only one of the seven (14.3%) studies using validated PRO instruments (e.g. EORTC QLQ-C30) had a high level of quality of PRO reporting, compared to those using non-validated instruments (5 RCTs, 50%). No differences were found in the mean standardised ISOQOL scores between the studies that used validated PRO instruments and those using non-validated instruments.

Discussion

Since April 2014 only eight new RCTs for bladder cancer that also included a PRO component, were identified and in all these studies PROs were considered as secondary outcomes. Also, during this time period little improvements were noted in the quality of PRO reporting. Indeed, when comparing the new studies identified in this update with previously published RCTs between January 2004 and March 2014 [7], we did not find significant improvement in the mean standardised ISOQOL checklist scores, possibly due to the small number of studies considered. When comparing each individual item of the ISOQOL checklist over time, we only observed two statistically significant improvements with respect to the reporting of missing data and the identification of PROs in trial protocols. Some of the key recommended issues (e.g. reporting of statistical approaches for dealing with missing data, PRO hypothesis statement and generalizability issues regarding the PRO results) are still poorly documented.

The number of newly conducted RCTs of bladder cancer with a PRO component published from 2014 is strikingly low when compared with the number of RCTs conducted in other cancer types, such as breast, lung and prostate cancer [4, 36, 37]. Nevertheless, in the current era of immunotherapy development, including monoclonal antibodies directed against inhibitory checkpoints receptors on T-cells (known as immune checkpoint inhibitors, ICIs), a vast number of trials for bladder cancer are under way – with several of them also assessing PROs. For instance, CHECKMATE 274 (ClinicalTrials.gov Identifier: NCT02632409) is an RCT of the ICI nivolumab versus placebo in patients who have undergone radical cystectomy for muscle-invasive bladder cancer (MIBC). In this study PROs are evaluated as an exploratory outcome using a multidimensional QoL measure. Another study of an ICI, avelumab, in the maintenance setting following first line chemotherapy (JAVELIN; ClinicalTrials.gov Identifier: NCT02603432) also evaluates PRO as a secondary outcome. POTOMAC (ClinicalTrials.gov Identifier: NCT03528694), a trial of the ICI durvalumab plus Bacillus Calmette-Guerin (BCG) versus BCG alone in patients with high risk non-muscle invasive bladder cancer (NMIBC) assesses several PROs as secondary outcome measures. Of note however, many currently ongoing studies in bladder cancer, including those evaluating PARP-inhibitors, FGFR-inhibitors and tyrosine kinase inhibitors do not include PRO assessments [38, 39].

Important International PRO initiatives are ongoing, for example, the standardisation of statistical analyses of PRO data in clinical trials [40]. Also, an international,

consensus-based, PRO-specific guidance, the Standard Protocol Items: Recommendations for Interventional Trials (SPIRIT)-PRO Extension, was recently made available [3]. This guidance aims to support investigators with protocol writing and to ensure that all methodological issues are appropriately considered. Finally, the CONSORT PRO Extension has been published in 2013 and this is particularly helpful to investigators at the time of publishing final results of RCTs with a PRO component [35]. Taken together these recommendations will hopefully help investigators improving the design of clinical trials and the assessment of PROs, thus ensuring high-quality data that may inform patient-centred care. Furthermore, it is worth highlighting that the European Organisation for Research and Treatment of Cancer (EORTC) Quality of Life Group has developed various tumour and treatment-specific QoL Modules – with several currently in development, including specific ones for non-muscle invasive BC, muscle invasive BC, and metastatic bladder cancer [41]. Finally, it is important to note, however, that word limits in journal guidelines may sometimes limit authors in the opportunity to report on secondary outcomes (i.e. PROs) for their trials [42] – especially if the results for the primary outcome are negative.

This study has limitations. First, despite our comprehensive search strategy, it is possible that some RCTs with a PRO component might have been missed. Another limitation is the exclusion of non–English language papers. However, it is unlikely that such omission would have significantly altered the conclusion of this review [43]. In addition, we did not compare the published RCT results with their respective protocols, although this might have provided further information. Finally, our results cannot be generalised to RCTs investigating non-conventional medical interventions. A strength of the current review is that we used a formal, objective approach to evaluate PRO reporting in the bladder cancer literature. Since all studies use different reporting criteria and methods, the information was extracted and assessed by two independent researchers. In case of inconsistencies, a third arbiter helped achieving consensus.

Conclusion

The current systematic review identified little improvement in the uptake and assessment of PROs in RCTs for bladder cancer during the last 4 years. Therefore, given the scarcity of rigorous PRO data, it is difficult to draw meaningful conclusions that can robustly inform patient care and support clinical decision-making. Given the increase in (immunotherapy) drug trials with a potential for severe adverse events in bladder cancer patients, there is urgent need to adopt the recommendations and standards available for PRO use in bladder cancer RCTs.

Acknowledgements
We would like to thank the Dianne and Graham Roberts Charitable Settlement for their support.

Authors' contributions
Data collection and analysis: FS, FC, MVH, FE. Draft of manuscript: MVH. Final editing of manuscript: FS, DJ, MJ, FC, FE. All authors read and approved the final manuscript.

Author details
[1]King's College London, School of Cancer and Pharmaceutical Sciences, Translational Oncology and Urology Research (TOUR), London SE1 9RT, UK. [2]Data Center and Health Outcomes Research Unit, Italian Group for Adult Hematologic Disease (GIMEMA), Rome, Italy. [3]Guy's and St Thomas' NHS Foundation Trust, Medical Oncology, London, UK. [4]Department of Medical Psychology, Location AMC, Amsterdam University Medical Centers, Amsterdam, The Netherlands.

References

1. Bray F, Ferlay J, Soerjomataram I, Siegel RL, Torre LA, Jemal A. Global cancer statistics 2018: GLOBOCAN estimates of incidence and mortality worldwide for 36 cancers in 185 countries. CA Cancer J Clin. 2018;68(6):394–424.
2. Rutherford C, Costa DSJ, King MT, Smith DP, Patel MI. A conceptual framework for patient-reported outcomes in non-muscle invasive bladder cancer. Support Care Cancer. 2017;25(10):3095–102.
3. Calvert M, Kyte D, Mercieca-Bebber R, Slade A, Chan AW, King MT, et al. Guidelines for inclusion of patient-reported outcomes in clinical trial protocols: the SPIRIT-PRO extension. JAMA. 2018;319(5):483–94.
4. Efficace F, Fayers P, Pusic A, Cemal Y, Yanagawa J, Jacobs M, et al. Quality of patient-reported outcome reporting across cancer randomized controlled trials according to the CONSORT patient-reported outcome extension: a pooled analysis of 557 trials. Cancer. 2015;121(18):3335–42.
5. U.S. Food and Drug Administration: Guidance for Industry and FDA Staff Qualification Process for Drug Development Tools, 2014. https://www.fda.gov/downloads/drugs/guidances/ucm230597.pdf. Accessed 14 June 2017.
6. European Medicine Agency. The use of patient-reported outcome (PRO) measures in oncology studies. Appendix 2 to the guideline on the evaluation of anticancer medicinal products in man. 2016. http://www.ema.europa.eu/docs/en_GB/document_library/Other/2016/04/WC500205159.pdf Accessed 9 July 2017.
7. Feuerstein MA, Jacobs M, Piciocchi A, Bochner B, Pusic A, Fayers P, et al. Quality of life and symptom assessment in randomized clinical trials of bladder cancer: A systematic review. Urol Oncol. 2015;33(7):331 e17–23.
8. Prinsen CAC, Mokkink LB, Bouter LM, Alonso J, Patrick DL, de Vet HCW, et al. COSMIN guideline for systematic reviews of patient-reported outcome measures. Qual Life Res. 2018;27(5):1147–57.
9. Mason SJ, Catto JWF, Downing A, Bottomley SE, Glaser AW, Wright P. Evaluating patient-reported outcome measures (PROMs) for bladder cancer: a systematic review using the COnsensus-based standards for the selection of health measurement INstruments (COSMIN) checklist. BJU Int. 2018; 122(5):760–73.
10. Pham H, Torres H, Sharma P. Mental health implications in bladder cancer patients: a review. Urol Oncol. 2019;37(2):97–107.
11. Efficace F, Feuerstein M, Fayers P, Cafaro V, Eastham J, Pusic A, et al. Patient-reported outcomes in randomised controlled trials of prostate cancer: methodological quality and impact on clinical decision making. Eur Urol. 2014;66(3):416–27.
12. Mercieca-Bebber RL, Perreca A, King M, Macann A, Whale K, Soldati S, et al. Patient-reported outcomes in head and neck and thyroid cancer randomised controlled trials: a systematic review of completeness of reporting and impact on interpretation. Eur J Cancer. 2016;56:144–61.
13. Moher D, Liberati A, Tetzlaff J, Altman DG, Group P. Preferred reporting items for systematic reviews and meta-analyses: the PRISMA statement. J Clin Epidemiol. 2009;62(10):1006–12.
14. Harris PA, Taylor R, Thielke R, Payne J, Gonzalez N, Conde JG. Research electronic data capture (REDCap)--a metadata-driven methodology and workflow process for providing translational research informatics support. J Biomed Inform. 2009;42(2):377–81.
15. Brundage M, Blazeby J, Revicki D, Bass B, de Vet H, Duffy H, et al. Patient-reported outcomes in randomized clinical trials: development of ISOQOL reporting standards. Qual Life Res. 2013;22(6):1161–75.
16. Chung JM, Ha HK, Kim DH, Joo J, Kim S, Sohn DW, et al. Evaluation of the efficacy of Solifenacin for preventing catheter-related bladder discomfort after transurethral resection of bladder tumors in patients with non-muscle invasive bladder Cancer: a prospective, randomized, Multicenter Study. Clin Genitourin Cancer. 2017;15(1):157–62.
17. Kim HC, Hong WP, Lim YJ, Park HP. The effect of sevoflurane versus desflurane on postoperative catheter-related bladder discomfort in patients undergoing transurethral excision of a bladder tumour: a randomized controlled trial. Can J Anaesth. 2016;63(5):596–602.
18. Yokomizo A, Kanimoto Y, Okamura T, Ozono S, Koga H, Iwamura M, et al. Randomized controlled study of the efficacy, safety and quality of life with low dose bacillus Calmette-Guerin instillation therapy for nonmuscle invasive bladder Cancer. J Urol. 2016;195(1):41–6.
19. Khan MS, Gan C, Ahmed K, Ismail AF, Watkins J, Summers JA, et al. A single-Centre early phase randomised controlled three-arm trial of open, robotic, and laparoscopic radical cystectomy (CORAL). Eur Urol. 2016;69(4):613–21.
20. Kim HC, Lim SM, Seo H, Park HP. Effect of glycopyrrolate versus atropine coadministered with neostigmine for reversal of rocuronium on postoperative catheter-related bladder discomfort in patients undergoing transurethral resection of bladder tumor: a prospective randomized study. J Anesth. 2015;29(6):831–5.
21. Huang W, Wang F, Wu C, Hu W. Efficacy and safety of pirarubicin combined with hyaluronic acid for non-muscle invasive bladder cancer after transurethral resection: a prospective, randomized study. Int Urol Nephrol. 2015;47(4):631–6.
22. Kim HC, Lee YH, Jeon YT, Hwang JW, Lim YJ, Park JE, et al. The effect of intraoperative dexmedetomidine on postoperative catheter-related bladder discomfort in patients undergoing transurethral bladder tumour resection: a double-blind randomised study. Eur J Anaesthesiol. 2015;32(9):596–601.
23. Parekh DJ, Reis IM, Castle EP, Gonzalgo ML, Woods ME, Svatek RS, et al. Robot-assisted radical cystectomy versus open radical cystectomy in patients with bladder cancer (RAZOR): an open-label, randomised, phase 3, non-inferiority trial. Lancet. 2018;391(10139):2525–36.
24. James ND, Hussain SA, Hall E, Jenkins P, Tremlett J, Rawlings C, et al. Radiotherapy with or without chemotherapy in muscle-invasive bladder cancer. N Engl J Med. 2012;366(16):1477–88.
25. Sabichi AL, Lee JJ, Grossman HB, Liu S, Richmond E, Czerniak BA, et al. A randomized controlled trial of celecoxib to prevent recurrence of nonmuscle-invasive bladder cancer. Cancer Prev Res (Phila). 2011;4(10):1580–9.
26. Koga H, Ozono S, Tsushima T, Tomita K, Horiguchi Y, Usami M, et al. Maintenance intravesical bacillus Calmette-Guerin instillation for ta, T1 cancer and carcinoma in situ of the bladder: randomized controlled trial by the BCG Tokyo strain study group. Int J Urol. 2010;17(9):759–66.
27. Marandola M, Antonucci A, Tellan G, Fegiz A, Fazio R, Scicchitano S, et al. Subarachnoid sufentanil as sole agent vs standard spinal bupivacaine in transurethral resection of the bladder. Minerva Anestesiol. 2005;71(3):83–91.
28. Ozyuvaci E, Altan A, Karadeniz T, Topsakal M, Besisik A, Yucel M. General anesthesia versus epidural and general anesthesia in radical cystectomy. Urol Int. 2005;74(1):62–7.
29. Gontero P, Oderda M, Mehnert A, Gurioli A, Marson F, Lucca I, et al. The impact of intravesical gemcitabine and 1/3 dose Bacillus Calmette-Guerin instillation therapy on the quality of life in patients with nonmuscle invasive bladder cancer: results of a prospective, randomized, phase II trial. J Urol. 2013;190(3):857–62.
30. Karl A, Buchner A, Becker A, Staehler M, Seitz M, Khoder W, et al. A new concept for early recovery after surgery for patients undergoing radical cystectomy for bladder cancer: results of a prospective randomized study. J Urol. 2014;191(2):335–40.
31. Skinner EC, Skinner DG. Does reflux in orthotopic diversion matter? A randomized prospective comparison of the Studer and T-pouch ileal neobladders. World J Urol. 2009;27(1):51–5.
32. Ahmadi H, Skinner EC, Simma-Chiang V, Miranda G, Cai J, Penson DF, et al. Urinary functional outcome following radical cystoprostatectomy and ileal neobladder reconstruction in male patients. J Urol. 2013;189(5):1782–8.
33. Johnson MH, Nepple KG, Peck V, Trinkaus K, Klim A, Sandhu GS, et al. Randomized controlled trial of oxybutynin extended release versus placebo for urinary symptoms during intravesical Bacillus Calmette-Guerin treatment. J Urol. 2013;189(4):1268–74.

34. Aaronson NK, Ahmedzai S, Bergman B, Bullinger M, Cull A, Duez NJ, et al. The European Organization for Research and Treatment of Cancer QLQ-C30: a quality-of-life instrument for use in international clinical trials in oncology. J Natl Cancer Inst. 1993;85(5):365–76.

35. Calvert M, Blazeby J, Altman DG, Revicki DA, Moher D, Brundage MD. Reporting of patient-reported outcomes in randomized trials: the CONSORT PRO extension. JAMA. 2013;309(8):814–22.

36. Fiteni F, Anota A, Westeel V, Bonnetain F. Methodology of health-related quality of life analysis in phase III advanced non-small-cell lung cancer clinical trials: a critical review. BMC Cancer. 2016;16:122.

37. Efficace F, Aaronson NK, Sparano F, Sprangers M, Fayers P, Pusic AL, et al. Quality of Patient-Reported Outcome (PRO) reporting in Randomized Controlled Trials (RCTs) over time. Evidence from 480 RCTs from 2004 to 2016. 24th Annual Conference of the International Society for Quality of Life Research (ISOQOL), Philadelphia, USA. Qual Life Res. 2017;26(1):139 (abs.3056).

38. Rimar KJ, Tran PT, Matulewicz RS, Hussain M, Meeks JJ. The emerging role of homologous recombination repair and PARP inhibitors in genitourinary malignancies. Cancer. 2017;123(11):1912–24.

39. Nogova L, Sequist LV, Perez Garcia JM, Andre F, Delord JP, Hidalgo M, et al. Evaluation of BGJ398, a fibroblast growth factor receptor 1-3 kinase inhibitor, in patients with advanced solid tumors harboring genetic alterations in fibroblast growth factor receptors: results of a global phase I, dose-escalation and dose-expansion study. J Clin Oncol. 2017;35(2):157–65.

40. Pe M, Dorme L, Coens C, Basch E, Calvert M, Campbell A, et al. Statistical analysis of patient-reported outcome data in randomised controlled trials of locally advanced and metastatic breast cancer: a systematic review. Lancet Oncol. 2018;19(9):e459–e69.

41. EORTC Quality of Life Group. EORTC Quality of Life 2019 Available from: https://www.eortc.org/research_field/quality-of-life/.

42. Marandino L, La Salvia A, Sonetto C, De Luca E, Pignataro D, Zichi C, et al. Deficiencies in health-related quality-of-life assessment and reporting: a systematic review of oncology randomized phase III trials published between 2012 and 2016. Ann Oncol. 2018;29(12):2288–95.

43. Morrison A, Polisena J, Husereau D, Moulton K, Clark M, Fiander M, et al. The effect of English-language restriction on systematic review-based meta-analyses: a systematic review of empirical studies. Int J Technol Assess Health Care. 2012;28(2):138–44.

7

Comparison of gemcitabine and anthracycline antibiotics in prevention of superficial bladder cancer recurrence

Tian-Wei Wang[1], Hui Yuan[2], Wen-Li Diao[2], Rong Yang[2], Xiao-Zhi Zhao[2] and Hong-Qian Guo[2]* (iD)

Abstract

Background: Because of the failure, shortage and related toxicities of Bacillus Calmette-Guérin (BCG), the other intravesical chemotherapy drugs are also widely used in clinical application. Gemcitabine and anthracycline antibiotics (epirubicin and pirarubicin) are widely used as first-line or salvage therapy, but which drug is better is less discussed.

Methods: A total of 124 primary NMIBC patients administered intravesical therapy after transurethral resection of bladder tumor (TURBT) at Nanjing Drum Tower hospital from January 1996 to July 2018. After TURBT, all patients accepted standard intravesical chemotherapy. Recurrence was defined as the occurrence of a new tumor in the bladder. Progression was defined as confirmed tumor invading muscular layer. Treatment failure was defined as need for radical cystectomy (RC), systemic chemotherapy and radiation therapy.

Results: Of the 124 patients who underwent intravesical chemotherapy, 84 patients were given gemcitabine, 40 patients were given epirubicin or pirarubicin, with mean follow-up times (mean ± SD) of (34.8 ± 17.9) and (35.9 ± 22.1) months respectively. The clinical and pathological features of patients show no difference between two groups. Recurrence rate of patients given gemcitabine was 8.33% (7 out of 84), the recurrence rate was 45% (18 out of 40) for epirubicin or pirarubicin ($P < 0.0001$). The progression rates of gemcitabine, anthracycline antibiotics groups were 2.38% (2 out of 84) and 20% (8 out of 40), respectively ($P < 0.001$). The rate of treatment failure is 8.33% (7 out of 84) and 25% (10 out of 40), respectively ($P = 0.012$). Gemcitabine intravesical chemotherapy group was significantly related to a lower rate of recurrence (HR = 0.165, 95% CI 0.069–0.397, $P = 0.000$), progression (HR = 0.160, 95% CI 0.032–0.799, $P = 0.026$) and treatment failure (HR = 0.260, 95% CI 0.078–0.867, $P = 0.028$).

Conclusion: In conclusion, gemcitabine intravesical chemotherapy group was significantly related to a lower rate of recurrence, progression and treatment failure. Gemcitabine could be considered as a choice for these patients who are not suitable for BCG.

Keywords: Gemcitabine, Anthracycline antibiotics, NMIBC, Intravesical therapy

Background

According to EAU Guidelines, bladder cancer (BCa) is the 11th mostly diagnosed cancer in the population. About 75% of bladder cancers are NMIBC at initial diagnosis [1], 60% of these patients experience recurrence and 10% experience progression in 5 years [2].T1 tumor, HG/G3tumor, CIS, multifocal, recurrent before and tumor size is larger than 3 cm are regarded as high-risk

tumors. Micropapillary, plasmocytoid, nested, sarcomatoid, microcystic, squamous, and adeno variants of urothelial carcinoma have a poor prognosis [1]. In order to control disease recurrence and progression, intravesical therapy is conventional used after TURBT.

Intravesical BCG therapy is a standard treatment for NMIBC after TURBT [3]. Although BCG has been regarded as the most effective intravesical therapy, it also has disadvantages in clinical use. Firstly, intravesical BCG therapy is associated with adverse effects such as reactive arthritis [4] and Poncet's disease [5]. Secondly, the production of BCG can't meet the market demand,

* Correspondence: dr.ghq@nju.edu.cn
[2]Department of Urology, Nanjing Drum Tower Hospital, Medical School of Nanjing University, 321 Zhongshan Rd., Nanjing 210008, China
Full list of author information is available at the end of the article

which leads to a world-wide shortage of BCG [6]. Thirdly, up to 40% patients do not respond to intravesical BCG therapy [7]. For all these reasons and more, gemcitabine and anthracycline antibiotics are also widely used clinically as first-line therapy or salvage therapy. However, whether gemcitabine is superior to other intravesical chemotherapy drugs is rarely discussed.

In the present study, we aimed to assess the impact of different intravesical chemotherapy drugs on recurrence, progression and treatment failure in patients with NMIBC.

Methods

A total of 124 primary NMIBC patients administered intravesical therapy after TURBT at Nanjing Drum Tower hospital from January 1996 to July 2018 were retrospectively analyzed. Inclusion criteria: The patients were primary diagnosed with NMIBC and all of them accepted TURBT followed by intravesical therapy; The demographic, clinical and pathological information was accurate. Histology was affirmed by experienced pathologists at the department of pathology. The grade classification of urothelium carcinomas was according to 2004 WHO classifications and the TNM classification was based on 2002 TNM classification approved by the Union Internationale Contre le Cancer. All patients were stratified according to AUA risk strata. The surgeons evaluated the location, size and numbers of tumors during the operations. All of these patients accepted the immediate chemotherapy after operation. The intravesical therapeutic regimen is shown below: Perfusion once a week for 6 weeks; then once every 2 weeks for 12 weeks; next once a month for 6 months; following once every 2 months until a full year. The respectively per dosage of gemcitabine, pirarubicin and epirubicin is 1000 mg, 40 mg and 40 mg. Treatment plan was timely adjusted according to the review results.

Follow up

Patients were followed up every 3 months with urine cytology and cystoscopy during the first year, every 6 months for the next 2 years, and then yearly thereafter. Ultrasonography, CT scanning, cystoscopy and urinary cytology were used to evaluate recurrence. Recurrence was defined as the occurrence of a new tumor in the bladder. Progression was defined as confirmed tumor invading muscular layer. Treatment failure was defined as need for radical cystectomy (RC), systemic chemotherapy and radiation therapy.

Statistical analysis

Statistical analysis was performed using SPSS version 22.0. The categorized data was presented as count value, the continuous variables were reported as mean ± SD. The continuous and categorized data were compared using the t test and Chi square test. Meier method was used to generate the survival curves. The log-rank test was used to verify statistical significance between curves. The multivariable proportional hazards model was used to test prognostic factors with $P < 0.2$ in univariate analysis. Multivariate analyses of data were performed using the Cox proportional hazards model. Figures drawing were performing with GraphPad Prism 7. For all statistical comparisons, a value of $p < 0.05$ was considered statistically significant.

Results

Of the 124 patients who underwent intravesical chemotherapy at Nanjing drum tower hospital, 84 patients were given gemcitabine, 40 patients were given epirubicin or pirarubicin, with mean follow-up times (mean ± SD) of (34.8 ± 17.9) and (35.9 ± 22.1) months respectively. The clinical and pathological features of patients show no difference between two groups. The baseline characteristics of patients according to treatments are shown in Table 1.

Clinical outcome of the two groups is shown in Table 2. Recurrence rate of patients who was given

Table 1 Characteristics of patients

Patient data	Intravesical chemotherapy drug		P
	Gemcitabine ($n = 84$) n(%)	Epirubicin or Pirarubicin ($n = 40$) n(%)	
Gender			
Male	61 (72.62%)	30 (75%)	0.779
Female	23 (27.38%)	10 (25%)	
Age (years)			
< 65	39 (46.43%)	14 (35%)	0.229
≥ 65	45 (53.57%)	26 (65%)	
Multifocality			
Single	41 (53.25%)	20 (57.14%)	0.701
Multiple	36 (46.75%)	15 (42.86%)	
Size (cm)			
< 3	57 (67.86%)	25 (62.5%)	0.427
≥ 3	27 (32.14%)	15 (37.5%)	
Grade			
Low	42 (57.53%)	19 (51.35%)	0.538
High	31 (42.47%)	18 (48.65%)	
Risk			
Low	19 (22.62%)	13 (32.50%)	0.452
Immediate	25 (29.76%)	9 (22.50%)	
High	40 (47.62%)	18 (45.00%)	
reTURBT			
Yes	33 (39.29%)	17 (42.50%)	0.733
No	51 (60.71%)	23 (57.50%)	
Follow up months			
(mean ± SD)	34.8 (17.9)	35.9 (22.1)	0.772

Table 2 Recurrence, progression and treatment failure rates of the two groups

	Gemcitabine	Epirubicin or Pirarubicin	P
Recurrence			
Yes	7 (8.33%)	18 (45%)	0.000
No	77 (91.67%)	22 (55%)	
Progression			
Yes	2 (2.38%)	8 (20%)	0.001
No	82 (97.62%)	32 (80%)	
Treatment failure			
Yes	7 (8.33%)	10 (25%)	0.012
No	77 (91.67%)	30 (75%)	

gemcitabine was 8.33% (7 out of 84), the recurrence rates were 45% (18 out of 40) for epirubicin or pirarubicin ($P < 0.001$). The progression rates of gemcitabine, epirubicin or pirarubicin groups were 2.38% (2 out of 84) and 20% (8 out of 40), respectively ($P < 0.01$). The rate of treatment failure was 8.33% (7 out of 84) and 25% (10 out of 40), respectively ($P < 0.05$), as shown in Table 2. Taken together, intravesical chemotherapy with different drugs showed an obvious statistically difference, the epirubicin or pirarubicin group had a higher recurrence free survival, progression free survival and treatment failure free survival rate than gemcitabine group.

The log-rank tests show obvious differences between the two groups in recurrence free survival rates, progression free survival rates and treatment failure free survival rates. The Kaplan-Meier estimates of two groups are graphically presented in Fig. 1a–c. Tumor recurrence, progression and treatment failure differ significantly between these groups. Comparing with epirubin or pirarubicin group, gemcitabine group showed obvious advantage in inhibiting tumor recurrence, progression and treatment failure. After univariate analysis, variables with $p < 0.2$ were enrolled into multivariate analysis (Table 3). Gemcitabine intravesical chemotherapy group was significantly related to a lower rate of recurrence (HR = 0.165, 95% CI 0.069–0.397, $P = 0.000$), lower rate of progression (HR = 0.160, 95% CI 0.032–0.799, $P = 0.026$) and treatment failure (HR = 0.260, 95% CI 0.078–0.867, $P = 0.028$).

Toxicity evaluation

Common side effects in both groups included chemical cystitis, urinary frequency, hematuria and suprapubic discomfort. Overall 4% of patients experienced side effects and no patients stopped chemotherapy because of side effects. None of the toxicities were fatal.

Discussion

Although BCG is used as first-line intravesical therapy for NMIBC patients after TURBT, its shortcomings also poses a management dilemma in clinical application, which force clinicians to search for better therapeutic strategies. As some patients do not respond to BCG or cannot tolerate its side effects, Yang et al. used Gemcitabine and cisplatin (GC) adjuvant chemotherapy instead of BCG intravesical therapy, which showed favorable results [8]. Some researches tried to

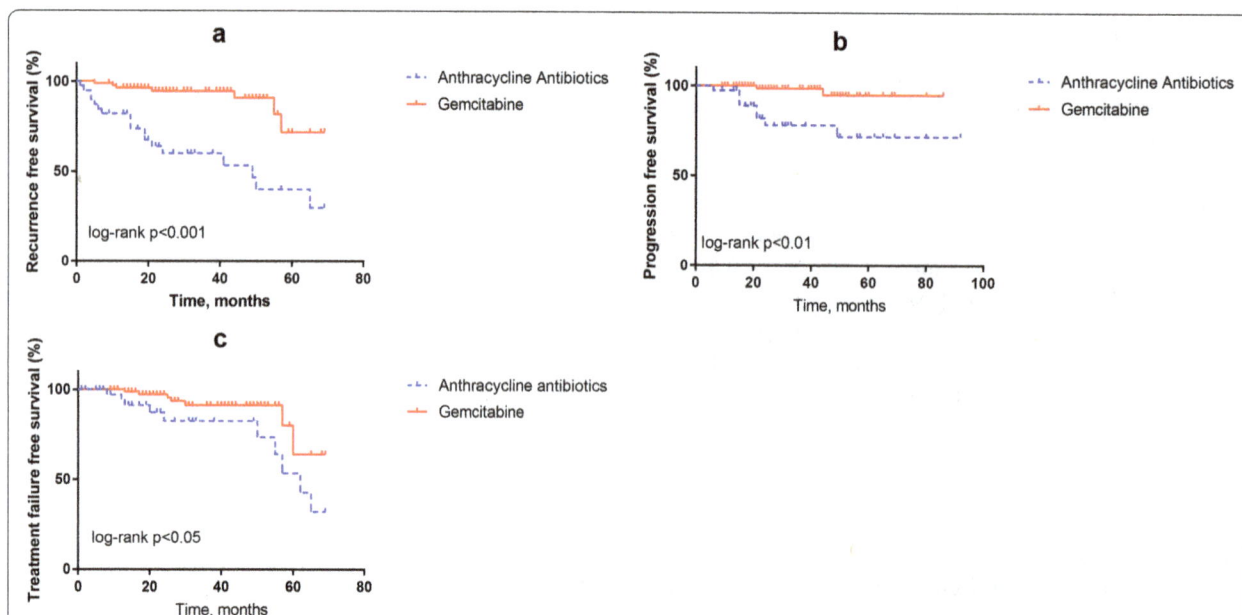

Fig. 1 a–c Kaplan–Meier curves for all patients. **a** Recurrence free survival; **b** progression free survival; **c** Treatment failure free survival. Tumor recurrence, progression and treatment failure differ significantly between these groups. Comparing with epirubin or pirarubicin group, gemcitabine group showed obvious advantage in inhibiting tumor recurrence, progression and treatment failure

Table 3 Univariate and multivariate standard Cox proportional hazards analysis of variables associated with tumor recurrence, progression and treatment failure in all patients

Variable	Univariate HR (95% CI)	P	Multivariate HR (95% CI)	p
Recurrence				
Gender	1.338 (0.817–2.191)	0.247		
Age	1.497 (0.658–3.403)	0.336		
Multifocality	1.526 (0.642–3.629)	0.339		
Size	1.869 (0.850–4.108)	0.120	2.668 (1.146–6.215)	0.023
Grade	0.443 (0.190–1.033)	0.060	1.243 (0.232–6.664)	0.800
Risk				
Low[a]				
Immediate	1.934 (0.696–5.371)	0.206	2.762 (0.461–16.543)	0.266
High	3.019 (1.186–7.685)	0.020	3.632 (0.535–24.633)	0.187
reTURBT	0.441 (0.182–1.068)	0.070	0.667 (0.134–3.313)	0.620
Gemcitabine vs Epirubicin or Pirarubicin	0.159 (0.066–0.382)	0.000	0.179 (0.072–0.447)	< 0.001
Progression				
Gender	1.266 (0.583–2.747)	0.552		
Age	0.765 (0.221–2.644)	0.672		
Multifocality	4.063 (0.819–20.143)	0.086	4.168 (0.827–21.000)	0.084
Size	2.188 (0.195–24.519)	0.525		
Grade	1.333 (0.376–4.727)	0.657		
Risk				
Low[a]				
Immediate	0.993 (0.181–5.432)	0.993		
High	1.945 (0.486–7.780)	0.347		
reTURBT	0.323 (0.068–1.521)	0.153	0.278 (0.055–1.394)	0.120
Gemcitabine vs Epirubicin or Pirarubicin	0.110 (0.023–0.518)	0.005	0.155 (0.031–0.781)	0.024
Treatment failure				
Gender	0.447 (0.128–1.561)	0.207		
Age	2.094 (0.736–5.960)	0.166	2.244 (0.591–8.527)	0.235
Multifocality	2.156 (0.739–6.290)	0.160	1.447 (0.479–4.368)	0.512
Size	0.897 (0.314–2.562)	0.840		
Grade	1.485 (0.491–4.485)	0.484		
Risk				
Low[a]				
Immediate	1.315 (0.443–3.906)	0.622		
High	0.455 (0.099–2.080)	0.310		
reTURBT	1.429 (0.537–3.804)	0.475		
Gemcitabine vs Epirubicin or Pirarubicin	0.377 (0.140–1.018)	0.054	0.248 (0.074–0.830)	0.024

[a]Referenced category. reTURBT, repeated transurethral resection of bladder tumor

reduce the standard dose of BCG to lessen the shortage of BCG. However, there is no consensus suggesting that intravesical BCG standard dose can be replaced by now [9]. Kyla N. Velaer et al. reported their experience on sequential intravesical gemcitabine and docetaxel as salvage therapy after BCG failure [10]. With the growth demand of BCG and the increasing number of patients, the contradiction will become more and more prominent.

Due to various reasons, gemcitabine is widely used in bladder cancer. In Australia, gemcitabine was setted as first-line intravesical therapy since 2010 [11]. Thiru Prasanna et al. deemed that intravesical gemcitabine had better DFS and lower toxicity when compared with BCG [11]. Pirarubicin and epirubicin has been widely used in intravesical chemotherapy since 1980s and has been proved to be effective. However, William B. Tabayoyong et al. collected seven trials about epirubicin and reported that six trials showed no improvement in recurrence with the maintenance treatment to induction [12]. What's more, most researchers think pirarubicin and epirubicin have been only able to reduce recurrence but not progression [13]. Gemcitabine, Pirarubicin and epirubicin are widely used in China, but seldom assessed the efficiency between these therapeutic choices.

In our research, we found a trend toward better recurrence free survival, progression free survival and treatment failure free survival in gemcitabine group. It is also important that gemcitabine intravesical chemotherapy is an independent protective factor not only for recurrence, but also for progression and treatment failure. Through multivariate analysis, we noted that the size of tumor larger than 3 cm is more likely to recurrent, which is in accord with EAU Guidelines.

There are potential limitations in our analysis. First, it is a retrospective analysis, and our material have limited data. Second, the current study never includes BCG treatment because of limited data. Third, there were other variables never bring into consideration such as molecular subtype of urothelial carcinoma, which may have influenced on results. Most importantly, the limited data may makes the estimate of the treatment effect less robust. Furthermore, a large randomized controlled trial is required to clarify the importance of gemcitabine therapy.

Conclusion

In conclusion, gemcitabine intravesical chemotherapy group was significantly related to a lower rate of recurrence, progression and treatment failure compared to anthracycline antibiotics group. Gemcitabine is superior to epirubicin or pirarubicin in inhibiting tumor recurrence and progression. We deduce that gemcitabine is also better than epirubicin or pirarubicin in salvage therapy and we will further discuss it. BCG is still the first-line intravesical therapy, but gemcitabine could be considered as a choice for those patients who are not suitable for BCG.

Abbreviations

AUA: American urological association; BCa: Bladder cancer; BCG: Bacillus Calmette-Guérin; DFS: Disease free survival; EAU: European Association of Urology; GC: Gemcitabine and cisplatin adjuvant chemotherapy; NMIBC: Non-muscle invasive bladder cancer; RC: Radical cystectomy; TURBT: Transurethral resection of bladder tumor

Acknowledgements

The authors thanks to all the staff in the urology department of Nanjing Drum Tower Hospital for their assistance.

Authors' contributions

W-TW: data collection or management, data analysis and manuscript writing. HY: data collection or management and data analysis. W-LD: data collection or management and data analysis. RY: data collection or management and data analysis. Z-XZ: protocol development. H-QG: protocol development and manuscript editing. All authors have read and approved the final manuscript.

Author details

[1]Nanjing Medical University, 101 Longmian Rd, Nanjing 211166, China. [2]Department of Urology, Nanjing Drum Tower Hospital, Medical School of Nanjing University, 321 Zhongshan Rd., Nanjing 210008, China.

References

1. Babjuk M, et al. EAU guidelines on non–muscle-invasive Urothelial carcinoma of the bladder: update 2016. Eur Urol. 2017;71(3):447–61.
2. Ferro M, et al. An increased body mass index is associated with a worse prognosis in patients administered BCG immunotherapy for T1 bladder cancer. World J Urol. 2019;37(3):507-14.
3. Kawai K, et al. Bacillus Calmette-Guerin (BCG) immunotherapy for bladder cancer: current understanding and perspectives on engineered BCG vaccine. Cancer Sci. 2013;104(1):22–7.
4. Yoshimura H, et al. Ultrasonographic findings in a patient with reactive arthritis induced by intravesical BCG therapy for bladder cancer. J Med Ultrason. 2018. https://doi.org/10.1007/s10396-018-0889-7.
5. Sampaio et al. Poncet's disease after the intravesical instillation of Bacillus Calmette – Guérin (BCG):a case report. BMC Res Notes. 2017;10:416.
6. Bandari J, et al. Manufacturing and the market: rationalizing the shortage of Bacillus Calmette-Guérin. Eur Urol Focus. 2018;4(4):481-84.
7. Zlotta AR, Fleshner NE, Jewett MA. The management of BCG failure in non-muscle-invasive bladder cancer: an update. Can Urol Assoc J. 2009;3(6 Suppl 4):S199–205.
8. Yang GL, et al. Commentary on "A novel treatment strategy for newly diagnosed high-grade T1 bladder cancer:Gemcitabine and cisplatin adjuvant chemotherapy—A single-institution experience." Urol Oncol. 2017; 35(2):38.e9–38.e15.
9. Wu C, et al. Assessing the feasibility of replacing standard-dose Bacillus Calmette–Guérin immunotherapy with other intravesical instillation therapies in bladder cancer patients: a network meta-analysis. Cell Physiol Biochem. 2017;41(4):1298–312.
10. Velaer KN, et al. Experience with sequential intravesical gemcitabine and docetaxel as salvage therapy for non-muscle invasive bladder cancer. Curr Urol Rep. 2016;17(5):38.
11. Prasanna T, et al. Intravesical Gemcitabine versus Intravesical Bacillus Calmette-Guérin for the Treatment of Non-Muscle Invasive Bladder Cancer: An Evaluation of Efficacy and Toxicity. 2017;7(undefined):260.
12. Tabayoyong WB, et al. Systematic review on the utilization of maintenance intravesical chemotherapy in the management of non-muscle-invasive bladder cancer. Eur Urol Focus. 2018;4(4):512–21.
13. Huang B, et al. Efficacy of intra-arterial chemotherapy combined with intravesical chemotherapy in T1G3 bladder cancer when compared with intravesical chemotherapy alone after bladder-sparing surgery: a retrospective study. World J Urol. 2019;37(5):823–9.

8

CoQ10 ameliorates monosodium glutamate-induced alteration in detrusor activity and responsiveness in rats via anti-inflammatory, anti-oxidant and channel inhibiting mechanisms

Dalia F. El Agamy and Yahya M. Naguib* (iD)

Abstract

Background: Competent detrusor muscles with coordinated contraction and relaxation are crucial for normal urinary bladder storage and emptying functions. Hence, detrusor instability, and subsequently bladder overactivity, may lead to undesirable outcomes including incontinence. Multiple mechanisms may underlie the pathogenesis of detrusor overactivity including inflammation and oxidative stress. Herein, we tested the possibility that CoQ10 may have a potential therapeutic role in detrusor overactivity.

Methods: Forty adult male Wistar albino rats weighing 100-150 g were used in the present study. Rats were divided (10/group) into control (receiving vehicles), monosodium glutamate (MSG)-treated (receiving 5 mg/kg MSG daily for 15 consecutive days), MSG + OO-treated (receiving concomitantly 5 mg/kg MSG and olive oil for 15 consecutive days), MSG + CoQ10-treated (receiving concomitantly 5 mg/kg MSG and 100 mg/kg CoQ10 daily for 15 consecutive days) groups.

Results: MSG resulted in significant increase in bladder weight and sensitised the bladder smooth muscles to acetylcholine. MSG has also resulted in significant increase in bladder TNF-α, IL-6, malondialdehyde, nerve growth factor and connexion 43, with significant decrease in the antioxidant enzymes superoxide dismutase and catalase. Olive oil had no effect on MSG induced alterations of different parameters. Treatment with CoQ10 has resulted in a significant restoration of all the altered parameters.

Conclusion: Taken together, our results suggest that CoQ10 antagonizes the deleterious effects of MSG on detrusor activity. We propose that CoQ10 could be a therapeutic strategy targeting urinary bladder dysfunction.

Keywords: Detrusor overactivity, Monosodium glutamate, CoQ10, Connexin43, Nerve growth factor

Background

Normal lower urinary tract storage and voiding functions rely on a competent urinary bladder. Disturbance of the urinary bladder storage competence may result in embarrassing symptoms such as urgency, frequency, nocturia and even incontinence [1]. Most patients with symptoms such as urgency urge incontinence, frequency or nocturia are considered to be treated from overactive

detrusor even without a definitive diagnosis. This was rationale based on the reluctance to subject patients to invasive urodynamic studies unless it is absolutely necessary [2]. Detrusor smooth muscle (DSM) has spontaneous action potentials and spontaneous phasic activity. There is poor electrical coupling between DSM fibers that facilitates muscle bundles to adjust their length to achieve minimum surface area/volume ratio during filling phase with no contraction or increase in intravesical pressure. A disturbance in this mechanism may give rise to synchronous activation of muscle bundles resulting in

* Correspondence: yahya.naguib@med.menofia.edu.eg
Clinical Physiology Department, Faculty of Medicine, Menoufia University, Menoufia, Egypt

instability of the urinary bladder [3]. Several molecular mechanisms affecting bladder smooth muscle, urothelium, and nerves has been proposed to explain the complex pathophysiology. Those included altered channel activities and enhanced bladder response to chemical and mechanical stimuli [4].

Monosodium Glutamate (MSG), the sodium salt of glutamate, is one of the world's most extensively used food additive [5]. Although MSG is considered as a bladder irritant, few data are available on the effect of MSG on the renal system and even fewer is known about the effects of MSG on the urinary bladder. MSG was found to be associated with urolithiasis and urinary tract obstruction in experimental setting [6]. MSG was capable to induce bladder epithelial hyperplasia in rats [7]. MSG increases the level of glutamate; a major excitatory neurotransmitter that plays an important role in the reflex pathways controlling the lower urinary tract functions [8]. Tonic activation of glutamate receptors contributes to the bladder overactivity [9].

Connexins (Cxs) are a family of specific proteins with plethora of functions. They may act as intercellular ion channels (gap junctions, GJs), second messengers, small signalling molecules, and conductors for electrical signals [10]. Connexins play an important role in the coordinated contraction and relaxation responses required for bladder emptying and filling [11]. Gap junction proteins are dynamic membrane proteins that have short half-lives of only few hours. The mechanisms regulating connexins turnover are complex. Various protein kinases phosphorylate connexins and phosphorylation may trigger its internalization and degradation [12]. There is a close relationship between elevated detrusor muscle Cx43 expression and detrusor muscle overactivity [13].

Coenzyme Q10, CoQ10 or ubiquinone-10, is an endogenous compound that acts as a powerful antioxidant, a crucial cofactor in the mitochondrial electron transport system, as well as a modulator of gene expression [14, 15]. CoQ10 tends to decrease both pro-inflammatory and oxidative stress markers in experimental animals [16, 17]. Interestingly, CoQ10 was shown to regulate adenosine monophosphate-activated protein kinase (AMPK) phosphorylation in a dose and time dependent manners [18, 19]. (AMPK) is an intracellular energy sensor which is activated under low cellular energy status. AMPK maintains cellular energy homeostasis and has regulatory effects on the cellular metabolism [20]. AMPK has anti-inflammatory, anti-oxidative and channel-inhibiting properties. It counteracts the biological actions of several inflammatory mediators and growth factors including those implicated in the up-regulation of Cx43 expression in the detrusor muscle and bladder overactivity. In addition, AMPK was reported to suppress Cx43 in a mouse model of cystitis [21].

Herein, we hypothesised that CoQ10 could ameliorate the deleterious effects of MSG on detrusor muscle activity. We also tested the possibility that the anti-inflammatory, antioxidant and channel inhibiting properties of CoQ10 may underlie its actions.

Methods
Animals and

Forty male Wistar rats weighing approximately 100–150 g were obtained from a local animal providing facility. Rats were kept under controlled temperature, humidity, and 12 h light/dark cycles. Rats were given access to standard rodent chow and water ad libitum. To allow proper acclimatization, rats were kept for 10 days prior to experimentation. Animal care and use were approved by the Ethics Committee of the Faculty of Medicine-Menoufia University-Egypt.

Experimental design

All experiments were carried in accordance with the Guide for the Care and Use of Laboratory Animals published by the US National Institutes of Health (NIH Publication no. 85–23, revised in 1996). Rats were divided randomly (10 rats/group) following the acclimatization period into: (1) control group: rats received 0.9% saline orally via gavage, and olive oil via intra-peritoneal injection, (2) MSG-treated group: rats received single daily dose (5 g/kg body weight dissolved in 0.9% saline via oral gavage) of monosodium glutamate (MSG, Sigma-Aldrich, UK) for 15 consecutive days, (3) MSG and olive oil (OO)-treated group: rats received MSG (5 g/kg body weight dissolved in 0.9% saline via oral gavage), and OO via intra-peritoneal injection (IP) for 15 consecutive days, and (4) MSG and CoQ10-treated group: rats received MSG (5 g/kg body weight dissolved in 0.9% saline via oral gavage), and CoQ10 (Sigma-Aldrich, UK, 10 mg/kg body weight dissolved in olive oil IP) daily for 15 consecutive days.

Blood sampling

Rats were fasted overnight after the last doses of MSG and CoQ10. Rats were then anaesthetised by injecting sodium thiopental (STP) (60 mg/kg IP). Blood samples were collected via cardiac puncture, left to clot for 10–15 min and then centrifuged at 4000 rpm for another 10 min. Serum samples were stored at − 20 °C for subsequent analysis of serum tumor necrosis factor alpha (TNF-α) and interleukin 6 (IL-6). All rats were then scarified by cervical dislocation.

Dissection of urinary bladder

Instantaneously after the rats were sacrificed the urinary bladder was dissected, weighed, and transferred to Kreb's solution. The bladder was incised longitudinally from the base to the dome. Then the bladder was opened up to form a flat sheet and the base and the top of the dome were cautiously excised. The sheet was then cut longitudinally into three equal parts; for tissue homogenization, Cx43 RT-PCR, and for the assessment of the in vitro bladder contractile activity.

Preparation of urinary bladder tissue homogenate

Bladder tissue was homogenized in ice cold phosphate buffer (pH 7.4). Using a surgical scalpel, bladder tissue was cross-chopped into fine slices, suspended in chilled 0.25 M sucrose solution and rapidly blotted on a filter paper. Mincing and homogenization of tissue were performed to release soluble proteins in ice-cold Tris hydrochloride buffer (10 mM, pH 7.4). Tissue homogenate was centrifuged at 7000 rpm for 20 min and the supernatant was collected and stored at $-20\,°C$ for subsequent estimation of malondialdehyde (MDA), superoxide dismutase (SOD), catalase (CAT), and nerve growth factor (NGF).

Assessment of the contractile activity of urinary bladder strips

One third of the urinary bladder was cut into 3–4 longitudinal strips measuring 2–4 * 6–12 mm depending on its size. The strips were transferred into a Petri-dish containing Krebs' solution aerated with carbogen (95% oxygen and 5% carbon dioxide) at room temperature. Each strip was then suspended in a 10 ml organ bath containing the freshly prepared Krebs' solution, maintained at $37\,°C$ and continuously bubbled with carbogen. The preparation was attached to a force transducer (Grass, USA), and isometric tension was recorded by physiograph (MKIII-S Universal Coupler, Narco Bio-System, USA). The strip was allowed to equilibrate for 60 min. A resting tension of 1 g was maintained throughout the experiment. Following equilibration, phasic activity of the tissues was recorded and the response of the tissue to $10^{-5}\,M$ acetylcholine (cholinergic receptor agonist) was recorded [22].

Biochemical assays

Serum levels of TNF-α and IL-6 (Quantikine® ELISA, R&D Systems Inc., MN, USA), and tissue homogenate level of NGF (MyBioSource, Inc., USA) were measured by enzyme linked immune sorbent assay (ELISA) technique according to the manufacturer's instructions. Measurement was performed with ELISA automatic optical reader and the absorbance was taken at 450 nm (SUNRISE Touchscreen, TECHAN, Salzburg, Austria). Tissue level of MDA (QuantiChrom™, BioAssay Systems, USA), CAT (EnzyChrom™, BioAssay Systems, USA), and SOD (EnzyChrom™, BioAssay Systems, USA) were determined by colorimetric method on a Jenway Genova autoanalyser (UK).

Quantification of Cx43 mRNA

Total RNA was extracted from rat bladders using TRI reagent (Sigma-Aldrich, UK). Extracted RNAs were reverse transcribed using the high capacity RNA-to-cDNA kit (Applied Biosystems, Foster City, CA, USA) according to the manufacturer's instructions. Real-time RT-PCR was performed using a Biosystem 7300 (Applied Biosystems, CA, USA). To quantify changes in gene expression, the comparative Ct method was used to calculate the relative-fold changes normalized relative to the housekeeping gene GAPDH. The gene specific primers for Cx43 were: sense TGGGGGAAAGGCGTGAG and antisense CTGCTG GCTCTGCTGGAAGGT, while primers for GAPDH were: sense TGAAGGTCGGTGTGAACGGATTTGGC, and antisense CATGTAGGCCATGAGGTCCACCAC. Results are shown as the mean of three samples, with each sample assayed in duplicate.

Statistical analysis

Results are expressed as mean ± standard deviation (SD). Kolmogorov-Smirnov test was performed on all data sets to ensure normal distribution ($p > 0.5$). Student t-test or repeated-measures Analysis of Variances (ANOVA) were used for statistical analysis of the different groups whichever appropriate, using Origin® software and the probability of chance (p values). P values < 0.05 were considered significant.

Results

Urinary bladder weight and detrusor response to acetylcholine

Treatment with MSG resulted in significant increase in the weight of the urinary bladder when compared to the control group (113 ± 3.2 vs 73.9 ± 2.9 mg, $P < 0.001$). Insignificant difference was observed in bladder weight in the MSG + OO group (111.9 ± 2.8 mg) when compared to the corresponding value in the MSG treated group ($P = 0.926$), while urinary bladder weight was significantly higher ($P < 0.001$) if compared to the control group. The weight of the urinary bladder was significantly decreased in the MSG + CoQ10 group (79.8 ± 5.2 mg) when compared to the MSG or MSG + OO treated groups ($P < 0.001$), albeit it was still significantly higher when compared to the control group ($P = 0.016$). Detrusor smooth muscle contractility in response to acetylcholine (ACh) was significantly increased in MSG treated group when compared to the control group (1.9 ± 0.19 vs 0.5 ± 0.11 mg tension, $P < 0.001$). Detrusor muscle responsiveness was insignificantly changed in MSG + OO (1.8 ± 0.19 mg tension) when compared to the MSG treated group ($P = 0.992$), and significantly increased if compared to the control group ($P < 0.001$). Detrusor responsiveness was significantly decreased in the MSG + CoQ10 treated group (0.7 ± 0.21 mg tension) when compared to MSG or MSG +

OO treated groups ($P < 0.001$). There was insignificant difference between the MSG + CoQ10 treated group when compared to the control group ($P = 0.144$) (Fig. 1).

Serum level of TNF-α and IL-6

MSG treatment resulted in significant increase in serum level of TNF-α and IL-6 (101.8 ± 10.9 pg/ml and 199.5 ±

12.6 pg/ml respectively), when compared to the control group (43.5 ± 7.9 and 148.5 ± 8.78 respectively, $P < 0.001$). In the MSG + OO treated group, there was insignificant difference in TNF-α and IL-6 levels (99 ± 11.9 pg/ml and 195.9 ± 10.5 pg/ml respectively) when compared to the MSG treated group ($P = 0.938$ and $P = 0.873$ respectively), while they were significantly higher when

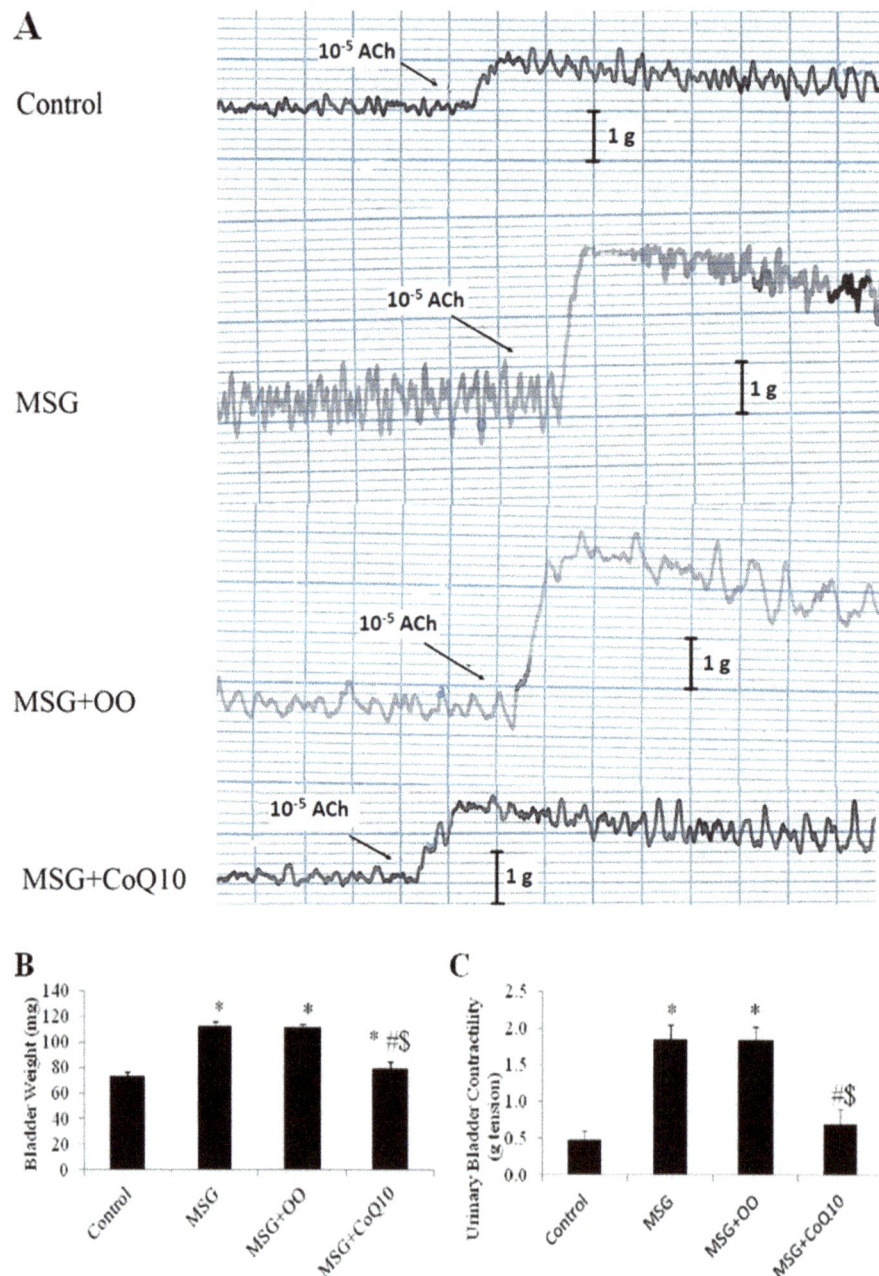

Fig. 1 CoQ10 restores detrusor smooth muscle contractile response and bladder weight in MSG treated rats. **a** Representative traces of detrusor muscle response to acetylcholine (Ach) in monosodium glutamate (MSG), MSG + OO, and MSG + CoQ10 treated rats. **b** Effect of CoQ10 treatment on urinary bladder strips contractility in control, monosodium glutamate (MSG), MSG + OO, and MSG + CoQ10 treated rats. **c** Effect of CoQ10 treatment on urinary bladder weight in control, monosodium glutamate (MSG), MSG + OO, and MSG + CoQ10 treated rats. * Significant when compared to control group. # Significant when compared to MSG group. $ Significant when compared to MSG + OO group ($n = 10$)

compared to the control group ($P < 0.001$). The MSG + CoQ10 treated group had significantly lower levels of TNF-α and IL-6 (51.9 ± 5.9 pg/ml and 161.4 ± 4.4 pg/ml respectively) when compared to the MSG or MSG + OO treated groups ($P < 0.001$), while there was insignificant difference if compared to the control group ($P = 0.313$ and $P = 0.054$ respectively) (Fig. 2).

Urinary bladder homogenate level of MDA, SOD, and CAT activities

Tissue level of MDA was significantly higher in the MSG treated group when compared to the control group (0.64 ± 0.03 vs 0.31 ± 0.03 nmol/mg tissue, $P < 0.001$). The MSG + OO treated group showed insignificant difference in tissue level of MDA (0.62 ± 0.02 nmol/mg tissue) when compared to the MSG treated group ($P = 0.6$), while MDA level was significantly higher when compared to the control group ($P < 0.001$). The MSG + CoQ10 group had significantly lower level of MDA (0.49 ± 0.04 nmol/mg tissue) when compared to the MSG or MSG + OO treated groups ($P < 0.001$), while it was still significantly higher than the corresponding value in the control group ($P < 0.001$). On the contrary, the enzyme activity of tissue SOD and CAT in the MSG treated group was significantly lower than the control group (10.6 ± 1.06 and 25.6 ± 1.06 vs 27.8 ± 2.66 and 50.9 ± 5.33 U/mg tissue respectively, $P < 0.001$). In the MSG + OO group, SOD and CAT enzymes activity levels were insignificantly different (11.1 ± 1.46 and 26.5 ± 1.93 U/mg tissue respectively) when compared to the MSG treated group ($P = 0.945$ and $P = 0.948$ respectively), while enzymes activity levels were significantly lower when compared to control group ($P < 0.001$). In the MSG + CoQ10 group, SOD and CAT activity levels were significantly higher when compared to the MSG or MSG + OO treated groups (21.6 ± 1.68 and 37.8 ± 2.9 U/mg tissue respectively, $P < 0.001$). SOD and CAT levels

were significantly lower in the MSG + CoQ10 group when compared to the control group ($P < 0.001$) (Fig. 3).

Urinary bladder homogenate level of NGF

The tissue level of NGF was significantly higher in the MSG treated group when compared to the control group (184.1 ± 21.6 vs 82.3 ± 11.9 pg/mg protein, $P < 0.001$). There was insignificant difference in NGF level MSG + OO group (185.6 ± 23.06 pg/mg protein) when compared to the MSG treated group ($P = 0.999$), while NGF level was significantly higher when compared to the control group ($P < 0.001$). NGF level was significantly lower in the MSG + CoQ10 treated group (103.9 ± 22.4 pg/mg protein) when compared to MSG or MSG + OO treated groups ($P < 0.001$), while there was insignificant difference if compared to the group control ($P = 0.167$) (Fig. 4a).

RT-PCR of Cx43 mRNA level in rat bladder

Urinary bladder Cx43 expression was significantly up-regulated in the MSG treated group when compared to the control group (1.45 ± 0.11 vs 1, $P < 0.001$). There was insignificant difference in Cx43 expression in the MSG + OO group (1.44 ± 0.11) when compared to MSG treated group ($P = 0.992$), while the expression was significantly higher when compared to control group ($P < 0.001$). Cx43 expression in the MSG + CoQ10 treated group was significantly down-regulated (1.12 ± 0.12) when compared to the MSG or MSG + OO treated groups ($P < 0.001$). There was insignificant difference in Cx43 expression between MSG + CoQ10 treated and the control group ($P = 0.112$) (Fig. 4b).

Discussion
Monosodium glutamate is a widely used flavour enhancer and food additive that may impact several physiological functions [23]. Although it has been reported earlier that MSG may induce urinary bladder endothelial

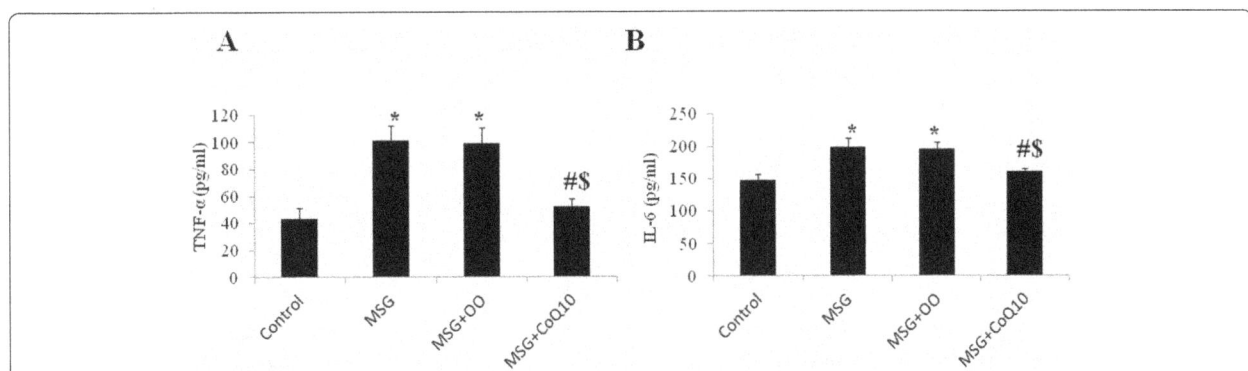

Fig. 2 CoQ10 attenuates MSG-induce inflammation. **a** Effect of CoQ10 treatment on serum level of TNF-α in control, monosodium glutamate (MSG), MSG + OO, and MSG + CoQ10 treated rats. **b** Effect of CoQ10 treatment on serum level of IL-6 in control, monosodium glutamate (MSG), MSG + OO, and MSG + CoQ10 treated rats. * Significant when compared to control group. # Significant when compared to MSG group. $ Significant when compared to MSG + OO group ($n = 10$)

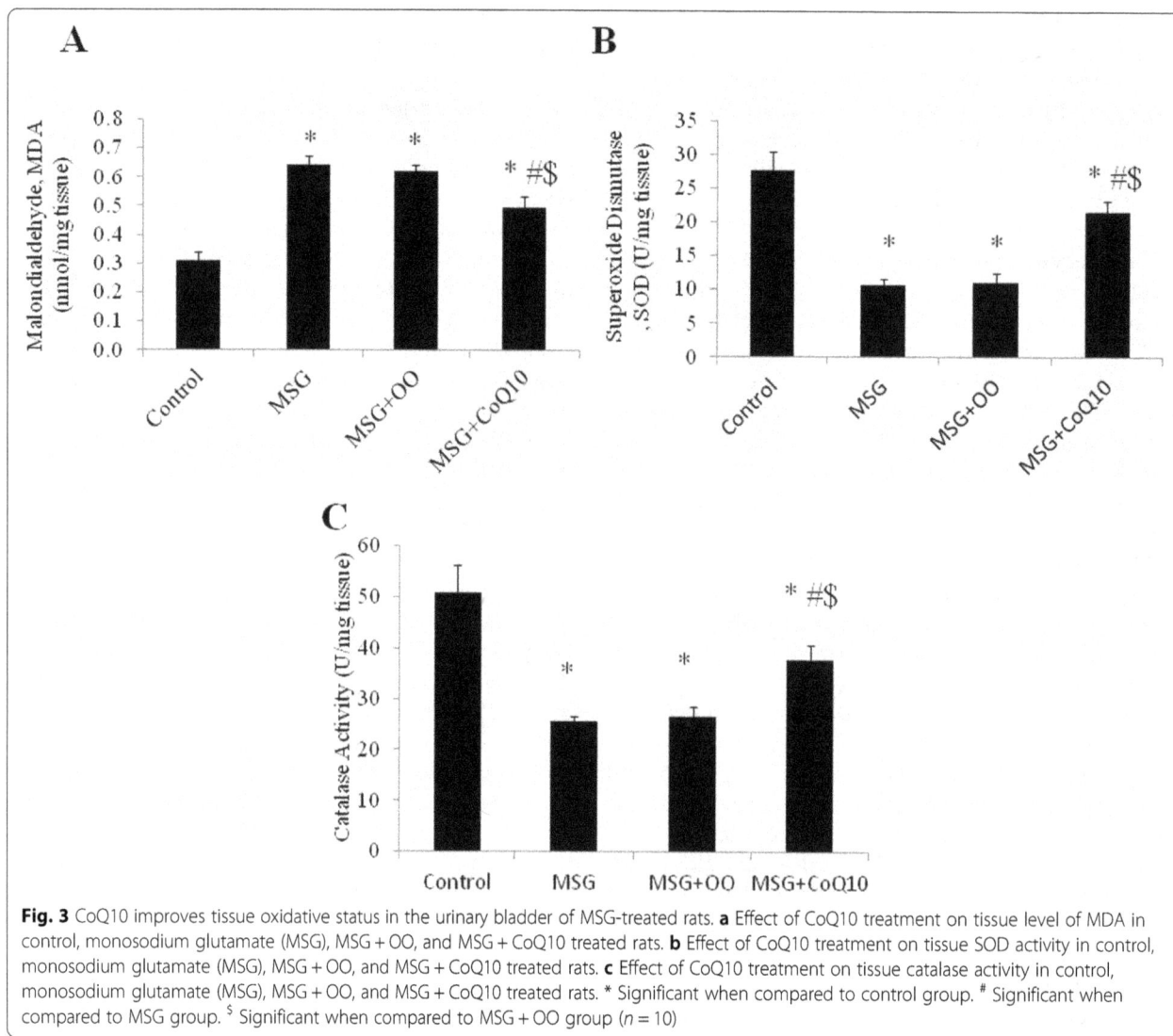

Fig. 3 CoQ10 improves tissue oxidative status in the urinary bladder of MSG-treated rats. **a** Effect of CoQ10 treatment on tissue level of MDA in control, monosodium glutamate (MSG), MSG + OO, and MSG + CoQ10 treated rats. **b** Effect of CoQ10 treatment on tissue SOD activity in control, monosodium glutamate (MSG), MSG + OO, and MSG + CoQ10 treated rats. **c** Effect of CoQ10 treatment on tissue catalase activity in control, monosodium glutamate (MSG), MSG + OO, and MSG + CoQ10 treated rats. * Significant when compared to control group. # Significant when compared to MSG group. $ Significant when compared to MSG + OO group ($n = 10$)

hyperplasia and altered motility [7, 24], the impact of MSG on the urinary bladder has not been properly studied. We show here that MSG may affect detrusor muscle contractility and responsiveness. We also show a potential role of the AMPK activator CoQ10 in ameliorating MSG-induced detrusor overactivity. We also show that CoQ10 exerts this action via modulating the expression of Cx43, decreasing NGF level, anti-inflammatory and anti-oxidative effects.

The present study shows that the MSG treated rats had increased urinary bladder sensitization to acetylcholine as well as increased bladder weight when compared to the control rats. Excitingly, these findings were minimized in the CoQ10 treated rats. The urinary bladder wall is lined by bundles of smooth muscle fibers; the detrusor muscle. There is poor electrical coupling between the smooth muscles bundles; a sensible property of the urinary bladder that

allows the detrusor to remain quiescent with little change in intravesical pressure as the bladder fills during the urine storage phase [25]. The expression of connexins in detrusor is lower than other tissues such as the myocardium. Therefore, it does not form an effective electrical functional syncitium, allowing bladder filling with no contraction or rise of intravesical pressure. However, if the electrical activity was well coupled, intravesical spontaneous pressure changes is expected with synchronous activation of the urinary bladder and bladder instability [3]. Oxidative stress impairs the contractile responses of tissue to different agents; oxidative stress impairs the contractile response of corpus cavernosum strips and aorta rings in response to phenylephrine. The effect was abolished by the use of the anti-oxidant L-carnitine [26]. Oxidative stress was found to be a key factor in the development of detrusor overactivity in

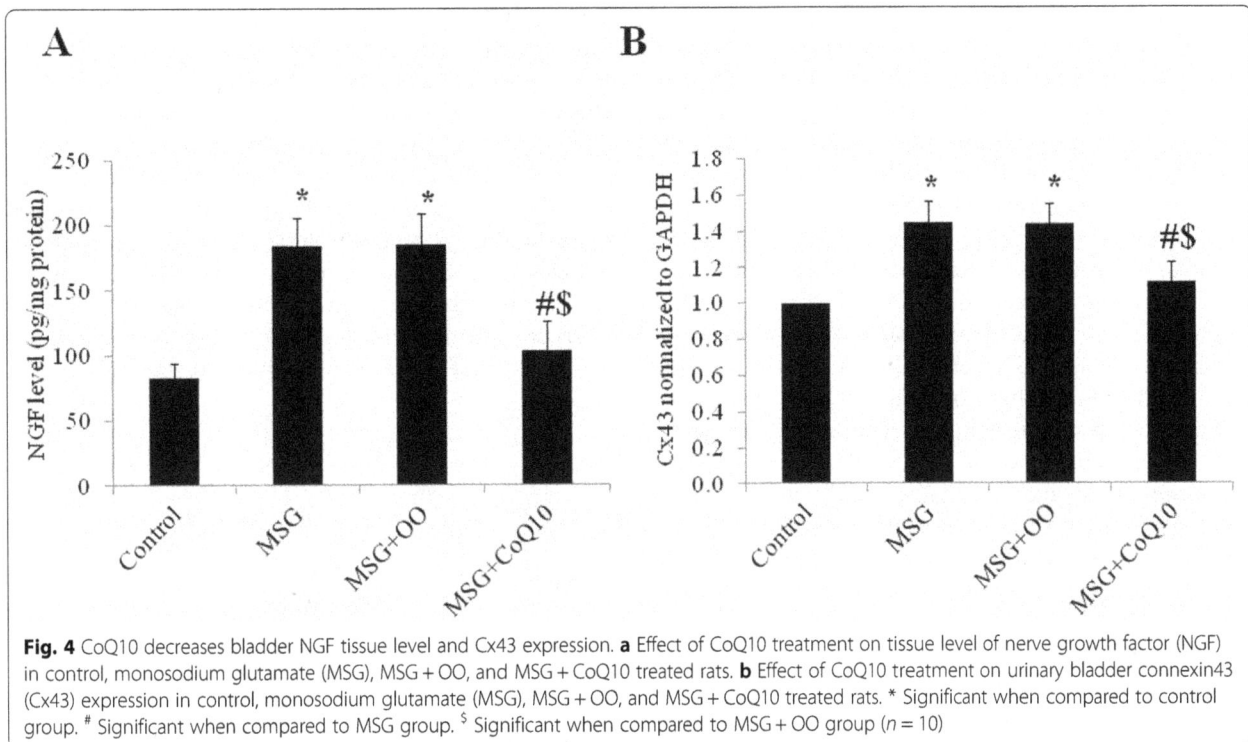

Fig. 4 CoQ10 decreases bladder NGF tissue level and Cx43 expression. **a** Effect of CoQ10 treatment on tissue level of nerve growth factor (NGF) in control, monosodium glutamate (MSG), MSG + OO, and MSG + CoQ10 treated rats. **b** Effect of CoQ10 treatment on urinary bladder connexin43 (Cx43) expression in control, monosodium glutamate (MSG), MSG + OO, and MSG + CoQ10 treated rats. * Significant when compared to control group. # Significant when compared to MSG group. $ Significant when compared to MSG + OO group (n = 10)

atherosclerosis-induced chronic bladder ischemia [27]. Bladder hyperactivity could be due to sensitization of afferent pathways, increased tissue damaging molecules such as NGF and prostaglandins, and up-regulation of Cx43 expression [28, 29]. Interestingly, CoQ10 has been shown to restore contractile responses to all form of stimulation in a rabbit model of obstructive bladder dysfunction [30]. Therefore, we expected that it may have a beneficial role in the restoration of normal bladder activity altered by MSG treatment. Tissue hypertrophy can be a resultant of increased inflammatory mediators, oxidative stress markers and growth factors. ROS activate a wide variety of hypertrophy signaling kinases and transcription factors [31], and is a causative factor for increased bladder weight in diabetic rats [32]. Inflammatory cytokines and growth factors have the potential to induce bladder hypertrophy and remodeling [33].

In the present study, the urinary bladder of MSG-treated rats had significantly higher levels of IL-6 and TNF-α when compared with the controls. IL-6 and TNF-α levels were significantly reduced following CoQ10 treatment. Several previous studies have shown that excess exposure to glutamate rises the level proinflammatory cytokines TNF-α and IL-6. Xu et al. reported that exogenous glutamate enhanced the inflammatory responses in brain and intestine at the transcriptional level [34]. MSG administration activates peroxisome proliferator-activated receptors that have a potential role in the control of

inflammation and the impairment of pro-inflammatory cytokine signalling pathways in the liver and fat tissue [35, 36]. Inflammatory cytokines play a key role in the modulation of connexins expression and the pathogenesis of urinary bladder dysfunction [37, 38]. CoQ10 has anti-inflammatory and immunomodulatory properties. CoQ10 has been shown to reduce TNF-α, IL-2 and IL-6 levels in different settings [39]. Therefore, treatment with CoQ10 could attenuate the MSG-induced rise in proinflammatory status. Increased bladder lipid peroxidation and decreased antioxidant enzymes activity in MSG-treated rats were observed in the present study. MSG increased bladder level of MDA, and decreased tissue activity of SOD and CAT enzymes. MSG induced lipid peroxidation and increased activities of CAT and SOD in the liver of MSG-treated animals [40, 41]. CoQ10 has been shown to decrease bladder MDA level with subsequent prolongation of micturition frequency and increase of bladder capacity in a rat model of chronic bladder ischemia [42].

In the present study the level of NGF in the bladder tissue homogenate was significantly increased in the MSG-treated rats. This was counteracted by the treatment with CoQ10. NGF is a small protein that plays physiological and pathophysiological roles in the lower urinary tract. It normally exits in the afferent nerves and ganglia of the bladder wall; and either plays an important role in normal sensation of bladder distension, or sensitizes the afferent nerves to induce bladder hyperactivity [43]. Elevation of several proinflammatory cytokines such as TNF-α was associated with increased NGF mRNA over-expression and elevated NGF production [44, 45]. Nevertheless, previously published data demonstrated that an increase in NGF expression even without associated inflammation sensitizes the visceral reflex pathways leading to bladder overactivity [46]. Overproduction of NGF is involved in urgency and bladder dysfunction [47]. Moreover, NGF induces detrusor overactivity, modulates urothelial response to inflammation and sensory threshold of urgency, and is involved in abnormal afferent signaling and bladder sensation [48]. Cushing et al. reported that NGF increases Cx43 phosphorylation and function and regulates intercellular communication between neurons during nervous system development and repair [49]. NGF also increased Cx43 expression in various other tissues such as pulmonary arteries [50], ovaries [51], and atrial myocytes [52].

In our hands, an increase in the expression of Cx43 mRNA was evident following MSG treatment. This was countered by treatment with CoQ10. Urinary bladder Cx43 is a gap junction protein that enhances intercellular electrical and chemical transmission and increases bladder response to cholinergic stimuli. Cx43 overexpression may lead to a decrease in the functional bladder capacity resulting in an increase in frequency of micturition and urgency [53]. Physiological circadian oscillation of detrusor muscle Cx43 participates in the diurnal variation in bladder capacity [21]. Multiple pathological factors have been identified to upregulate Cx43 expression such as inflammatory mediators, oxidative stress and growth factors in different cell types. Li et al. reported that proinflammatory cytokines potently increase Cx43 expression and function in bladder smooth muscle cells. Oxidative stress has been also shown to increase Cx43 in bladder smooth muscles [29]. Several growth factors including fibroblast growth factor (FGF) and NGF have been implicated in the increase of Cx43 level and function [49, 54]. Increased intercellular electrical coupling between adjacent detrusor cells allows easy spread of electrical activity and generate significant contractions, and involuntary intravesical pressure rises. When the condition is left untreated, irreversible changes in DSM occur with decreased bladder compliance, increased intravesical pressure during the bladder filling phase and dysfunction of the upper urinary tract [13]. Activation of A MPK has been shown to decrease Cx43 expression via the inhibition of CREB; a transcription factor that binds to cAMP response element sites and controls various cellular activities [21]. This may explain, at least in part, how the treatment with CoQ10 may have decreased CX43 expression levels in the current study. However, it does not point clearly whether this is a direct effect or secondarily to decreased inflammation and oxidative stress, or NGF level.

Conclusion

The current study demonstrates that MSG can alter detrusor smooth muscle activity with possible detrimental effects on bladder storage and voiding functions. The inflammatory and oxidative stress consequences of ingesting MSG led to increase in urinary bladder tissue level of NGF and Cx43 expression; resulting in increased sensitization and probably electrical coupling of detrusor muscles. The use of the multi-modal AMPK activator CoQ10 could be a potential adjuvant treatment. CoQ10 possesses anti-inflammatory and anti-oxidative properties, enabling it to play a possible therapeutic role.

Abbreviations

AMPK: Adenosine monophosphate-activated protein kinase; CAT: Catalase; CoQ10: Coenzyme Q10; DSM: Detrusor smooth muscle; FGF: Fibroblast growth factor; IL-6: Interleukin 6; MDA: Malondialdehyde; MSG: Monosodium glutamate; NGF: Nerve growth factor; SOD: Superoxide dismutase; STP: Sodium thiopental; TNF-α: Tumor necrosis factor alpha

Acknowledgments

Authors wish to thank the Faculty of Medicine - Menoufia University for providing most of the required facilities.
Authors would also like to acknowledge the assistance of Prof. Dr. Eman Badr and members of the Central Lab – Faculty of Medicine – Menoufia University.

Authors' contributions

DFE carried out the smooth muscle contractile experiments and biochemical assays, and participated in the study design. YMN carried out the PCR experiments, participated in the study design and coordination, performed the statistical analysis and drafted the manuscript. Both authors have read and approved the final version of the manuscript.

References

1. Tornic J, Panicker JN. The management of lower urinary tract dysfunction in multiple sclerosis. Curr Neurol Neurosci Rep. 2018;18(8):54.
2. Abrams P. Describing bladder storage function: overactive bladder syndrome and detrusor overactivity. Urology. 2003;62(5):28–37.
3. Meng E, Young JS, Brading AF. Spontaneous activity of mouse detrusor smooth muscle and the effects of the urothelium. Neurourol Urodyn. 2008; 27(1):79–87.
4. Sacco E. Physiopathology of overactive bladder syndrome. Urologia. 2012; 79(1):24–35.
5. He K, Du S, Xun P, Sharma S, Wang H, Zhai F, Popkin B. Consumption of monosodium glutamate in relation to incidence of overweight in Chinese adults: China Health and Nutrition Survey (CHNS). Am J Clin Nutr. 2011; 93(6):1328–36.
6. Sharma A, Prasongwattana V, Cha'on U, Selmi C, Hipkaeo W, Boonnate P, Pethlert S, Titipungul T, Intarawichian P, Waraasawapati S, et al. Monosodium glutamate (MSG) consumption is associated with urolithiasis and urinary tract obstruction in rats. PloS One. 2013;8(9):e75546.
7. de Groot AP, Feron VJ, Immel HR. Induction of hyperplasia in the bladder epithelium of rats by a dietary excess of acid or base: Implications for toxicity/carcinogenicity testing. Food Chem Toxicol. 1988;26(5):425–34.
8. Yoshiyama M. Glutamatergic mechanisms controlling lower urinary tract function. Low Urin Tract Symptoms. 2009;1(s1):S101–4.
9. Uy J, Yu M, Jiang X, Jones C, Shen B, Wang J, Roppolo JR, de Groat WC, Tai C. Glutamatergic Mechanisms Involved in Bladder Overactivity and Pudendal Neuromodulation in Cats. J Pharmacol Exp Ther. 2017;362(1):53–8.
10. Evans WH, Martin PEM. Gap junctions: structure and function (Review). Mol Membr Biol. 2002;19(2):121–36.
11. Neuhaus J, Weimann A, Stolzenburg J-U, Wolburg H, Horn L-C, Dorschner W. Smooth muscle cells from human urinary bladder express connexin 43 in vivo and in vitro. World J Urol. 2002;20:250–4.
12. Laird DW. Connexin phosphorylation as a regulatory event linked to gap junction internalization and degradation. Biochim Biophys Acta Biomembr. 2005;1711(2):172 82.

13. Haferkamp A, Mundhenk J, Bastian PJ, Reitz A, Dorsam J, Pannek J, Schumacher S, Schurch B, Buttner R, Muller SC. Increased expression of Connexin 43 in the overactive neurogenic detrusor. Eur Urol. 2004;46(6):799–805.

14. Crane FL. Biochemical functions of coenzyme Q10. J Am Coll Nutr. 2001; 20(6):591–8.

15. Groneberg DA, Kindermann B, Althammer M, Klapper M, Vormann J, Littarru GP, Doring F. Coenzyme Q10 affects expression of genes involved in cell signalling, metabolism and transport in human CaCo-2 cells. Int J Biochem Cell Biol. 2005;37(6):1208–18.

16. Kunitomo M, Yamaguchi Y, Kagota S, Otsubo K. Beneficial effect of Coenzyme Q10 on increased oxidative and nitrative stress and inflammation and individual metabolic components developing in a rat model of metabolic syndrome. J Pharmacol Sci. 2008;107(2):128–37.

17. Sohet FM, Neyrinck AM, Pachikian BD, de Backer FC, Bindels LB, Niklowitz P, Menke T, Cani PD, Delzenne NM. Coenzyme Q10 supplementation lowers hepatic oxidative stress and inflammation associated with diet-induced obesity in mice. Biochem Pharmacol. 2009;78(11):1391–400.

18. Lee SK, Lee JO, Kim JH, Kim N, You GY, Moon JW, Sha J, Kim SJ, Lee YW, Kang HJ, et al. Coenzyme Q10 increases the fatty acid oxidation through AMPK-mediated PPARÎ± induction in 3 T3-L1 preadipocytes. Cell Signal. 2012;24(12):2329–36.

19. Massimiliano G, Francesca G, Josè MAS, Luca M, Tamara YFH, Josè LQ, Bullon P, Maurizio B. AMPK as a new attractive therapeutic target for disease prevention: the role of dietary compounds ampk and disease prevention. Curr Drug Targets. 2016;17(8):865–89.

20. Hardie DG. AMP-activated protein kinase-an energy sensor that regulates all aspects of cell function. Genes Dev. 2011;25(18):1895–908.

21. Zhang X, Yao J, Gao K, Chi Y, Mitsui T, Ihara T, Sawada N, Kamiyama M, Fan J, Takeda M. AMPK Suppresses Connexin43 Expression in the Bladder and Ameliorates Voiding Dysfunction in Cyclophosphamide-induced Mouse Cystitis. Sci Rep. 2016;6:19708.

22. Ng YK, de Groat WC, Wu HY. Muscarinic regulation of neonatal rat bladder spontaneous contractions. Am J Physiol Regul Integr Comp Physiol. 2006; 291:R1049–59.

23. Okwudiri OO, Sylvanus AC, Peace IA. Monosodium Glutamate Induces Oxidative Stress and Affects Glucose Metabolism in the Kidney of Rats. Int J Biochem Res Rev. 2012;2(1):1–11.

24. Chen SY, Wang SD, Cheng CL, Kuo JS, Groat WCD, Chai CY. Glutamate activation of neurons in CV-reactive areas of cat brain stem affects urinary bladder motility. Am J Physiol. 1993;265:F520–9.

25. Yoshimura N, Chancellor MB. Differential diagnosis and treatment of impaired bladder emptying. Rev Urol. 2004;6(Suppl 1):S24–31.

26. Sener GK, Paskaloglu KB, Satiroglu H, Alican I, Kaçmaz A, Sakarcan A. L-carnitine ameliorates oxidative damage due to chronic renal failure in rats. J Cardiovasc Pharmacol. 2004;43:698–705.

27. Nomiya M, Sagawa K, Yazaki J, Takahashi N, Kushida N, Haga N, Aikawa K, Matsui T, Oka M, Fukui T, et al. Increased bladder activity is associated with elevated oxidative stress markers and proinflammatory cytokines in a rat model of atherosclerosis-induced chronic bladder ischemia. Neurourol Urodyn. 2012;31:185–9.

28. Masuda H, Kihara K, Saito K, Matsuoka Y, Yoshida S, Chancellor MB, de Groat WC, Yoshimura N. Reactive oxygen species mediate detrusor overactivity via sensitization of afferent pathway in the bladder of anaesthetized rats. BJU Int. 2008;101(6):775–80.

29. Li K, Yao J, Shi L, Sawada N, Chi Y, Yan Q, Matsue H, Kitamura M, Takeda M. Reciprocal Regulation between Proinflammatory Cytokine-induced Inducible NO Synthase (iNOS) and Connexin43 in Bladder Smooth Muscle Cells. J Biol Chem. 2011;286(48):41552–62.

30. Juan Y-S, Levin RM, Chuang SM, Hydery T, Li S, Kogan B, Schuler C, Huang C-H, Mannikarottu A. The Beneficial Effect of Coenzyme Q10 and Lipoic Acid on Obstructive Bladder Dysfunction in the Rabbit. J Urol. 2008;180(5):2234–40.

31. Maulik SK, Kumar S. Oxidative stress and cardiac hypertrophy: a review. Toxicol Mech Methods. 2012;22(5):359–66.

32. Pitre DA, Hassanain HH, Goldschmidt P, Bauer JA. A role for oxidative stress in urinary bladder dysfunction and remodeling: the use of transgenic model. FASEB J. 2002;16(4):A183.

33. Kanno Y, Mitsui T, Kitta T, Moriya K, Tsukiyama T, Hatakeyama S, Nonomura K. The inflammatory cytokine IL-1beta is involved in bladder remodeling after bladder outlet obstruction in mice. Neurourol Urodyn. 2016;35(3):377–81.

34. Xu L, Sun J, Lu R, Ji Q, Xu J-G. Effect of glutamate on inflammatory responses of intestine and brain after focal cerebral ischemia. World J Gastroenterol. 2005;11(5):733–6.

35. Roman-Ramos R, Almanza-Perez JC, Garcia-Macedo R, Blancas-Flores G, Fortis-Barrera A, Jasso EI, Garcia-Lorenzana M, Campos-Sepulveda AE, Cruz M, Alarcon-Aguilar FJ. Monosodium glutamate neonatal intoxication associated with obesity in adult stage is characterized by Chronic Inflammation and Increased mRNA expression of peroxisome proliferator-activated receptors in mice. Basic Clin Pharmacol. 2010;108: 406–13.

36. Hassan ZA, Arafa MH, Soliman WI, Atteia HH, Al-Saeed HF. The effects of monosodium glutamate on thymic and splenic immune functions and role of recovery (Biochemical and Histological study). J Cytol Histol. 2014;5:6.

37. Wang Z, Cheng Z, Cristofaro V, Li J, Xiao X, Gomez P, Ge R, Gong E, Strle K, Sullivan MP, et al. Inhibition of TNF-α improves the bladder dysfunction that is associated with type 2 diabetes. Diabetes. 2012;61(8):2134–45.

38. Heinrich M, Oberbach A, Schlichting N, Stolzenburg J-U, Neuhaus J. Cytokine effects on gap junction communication and connexin expression in human bladder smooth muscle cells and suburothelial myofibroblasts. PLoS One. 2011;6(6):e20792.

39. Zhai J, Bo Y, Lu Y, Liu C, Zhang L. Effects of coenzyme Q10 on markers of inflammation: a systematic review and meta-analysis. PLoS One. 2017;12(1): e0170172.

40. Singh K, Ahluwalia P. Studies on the effect of monosodium glutamate (MSG) administration on the activity of xanthine oxidase, superoxide dismutase and catalase in hepatic tissue of adult male mice. Indian J Clin Biochem. 2002;17(1):29–33.

41. Kushwaha V, Bharti G. Effect of Monosodium Glutamate (Msg) administration on some antioxidant enzymes in muscles of adult male mice. J Appl Biosci. 2015;41(1):54–6.

42. Kim JW, Jang HA, Bae JH, Lee JG. Effects of Coenzyme Q10 on bladder dysfunction induced by chronic bladder ischemia in a rat model. J Urol. 2012;189(6):2371–6.

43. Liu H-T, Wang Y-S, Kuo H-C. Nerve growth factor levels are increased in urine but not urothelium in patients with detrusor overactivity. Tzu Chi Med J. 2010;22(4):165–70.

44. Bullo M, Peerally MR, Trayhurn P, Folch J, Salas-Salvado J. Circulating nerve growth factor levels in relation to obesity and the metabolic syndrome in women. Eur J Endocrinol. 2007;157(3):303–10.

45. Abe Y, Akeda K, An HS, Aoki Y, Pichika R, Muehleman C, Kimura T, Masuda K. Proinflammatory cytokines stimulate the expression of nerve growth factor by human intervertebral disc cells. Spine (Phila Pa 1976). 2007;32(6):635–42.

46. Lamb K, Gebhart GF, Bielefeldt K. Increased nerve growth factor expression triggers bladder overactivity. J Pain. 2004;5(3):150–6.

47. Birder LA, Wolf-Johnston A, Griffiths D, Resnick NM. Role of urothelial nerve growth factor in human bladder function. Neurourol Urodyn. 2007;26(3):405–9.

48. Liu H-T, Chancellor MB, Kuo H-C. Urinary nerve growth factor levels are elevated in patients with detrusor overactivity and decreased in responders to detrusor botulinum Toxin-A injection. Eur Urol. 2009;56(4):700–7.

49. Cushing P, Bhalla R, Johnson AM, Rushlow WJ, Meakin SO, Belliveau DJ. Nerve growth factor increases connexin43 phosphorylation and gap junctional intercellular communication. J Neurosci Res. 2005;82(6):788–801.

50. Douard M, Robillard P, Deweirdt J, Baudrimont I, Dubois M, Marthan R, Savineau JP, Muller B, Guibert C, Freund-Michel V. Connexin-43 expression is increased by the nerve growth factor (NGF) and contributes to pulmonary arterial altered reactivity in pulmonary hypertension. Arch Cardiovasc Dis. 2018;10(2):248.

51. Sommersberg B, Bulling A, Salzer U, Frohlich U, Garfield RE, Amsterdam A, Mayerhofer A. Gap junction communication and connexin 43 gene expression in a rat granulosa cell line: regulation by Follicle-Stimulating Hormone1. Biol Reprod. 2000;63(6):1661–8.

52. Shu C, Huang W, Zeng Z, He Y, Luo B, Liu H, Li J, Xu J. Connexin 43 is involved in the sympathetic atrial fibrillation in canine and canine atrial myocytes. Anatol J Cardiol. 2017;18(1):3–9.

53. Negoro H, Kanematsu A, Doi M, Suadicani SO, Matsuo M, Imamura M, Okinami T, Nishikawa N, Oura T, Matsui S, et al. Involvement of urinary bladder Connexin43 and the circadian clock in coordination of diurnal micturition rhythm. Nat Commun. 2012;3:809.

9

A retrospective study of treatment persistence and adherence to mirabegron versus antimuscarinics, for the treatment of overactive bladder

Jameel Nazir[1*], Zalmai Hakimi[2], Florent Guelfucci[3], Amine Khemiri[4,7], Francis Fatoye[5], Ana María Mora Blázquez[6] and Marta Hernández González[6]

Abstract

Background: Persistence on-treatment with antimuscarinics in patients with overactive bladder (OAB) is reported to be sub-optimal. This retrospective, longitudinal, observational cohort study assessed treatment persistence with β_3-adrenoceptor agonists (i.e. mirabegron) and antimuscarinics, both classes of OAB pharmacotherapy, in patients with OAB in Spain.

Methods: Adults who received mirabegron or an antimuscarinic in routine clinical practice (1 June–31 October 2014), were identified from anonymised prescription data within the Spanish Cegedim Electronic Medical Records database. The primary endpoint, treatment persistence (time to treatment discontinuation [TTD] and the proportion of patients remaining on-treatment after 12 months), was unadjusted for potential confounders. Multivariate Cox regression models of persistence, adjusted for baseline characteristics, were used to compare differences in treatment groups. Adjusted subgroup analyses (target OAB drug, age, treatment status and sex) and sensitivity analyses (extending the time used to define treatment discontinuation from 30 days [base-case] to 45, 60 or 90 days without prescription renewal) were also performed.

Results: Overall, 1798 patients received mirabegron ($N = 1169$) or an antimuscarinic ($N = 629$); the mean age was 66. 42 years. Median TTD was longer for mirabegron versus antimuscarinics (90 vs 56 days) and a higher proportion of patients who received mirabegron were persistent after 12 months (20.2% vs 10.2%); multivariate analyses indicated significantly greater persistence with mirabegron versus antimuscarinics (hazard ratio [HR]: 1.52; 95% confidence interval [CI]: 1.37–1.70; $p < 0.001$). Significant differences were also observed in subgroup analyses of mirabegron versus individual antimuscarinics (median TTD: 90 vs [range] 28–60 days; HR range: 1.21–2.17; $p \leq 0.013$) and in all other subgroups assessed ($p < 0.001$). Sensitivity analysis showed that the median TTD for mirabegron increased by up to 31 days, and was significantly longer versus antimuscarinics across all adjusted periods (HR range: 1.43–1.53; all $p < 0.001$).

Conclusions: Patients with OAB in Spain who received mirabegron experienced longer persistence on-treatment than those who received antimuscarinics and the proportion of patients persistent on-treatment at 12 months with mirabegron was two-times higher versus antimuscarinics. These data may provide strategic insights for clinicians and policy makers involved in the management of OAB.

Keywords: Overactive bladder, Mirabegron, Antimuscarinics, Treatment persistence

* Correspondence: Jameel.Nazir@astellas.com
[1]Astellas Pharma Europe Ltd, 2000 Hillswood Drive, Chertsey KT16 0PS, UK
Full list of author information is available at the end of the article

Background

Overactive bladder (OAB) is characterised by urinary urgency, usually accompanied by frequency and nocturia, with or without urgency urinary incontinence, in the absence of urinary tract infection or other obvious pathology [1, 2]. The prevalence of OAB in Spain is approximately 20% in patients ≥40 years of age; OAB is most common in the elderly population, observed in more than one-quarter of Spanish adults >70 years of age [3].

Health-related quality of life (HRQoL) is profoundly affected in patients who experience OAB symptoms, as demonstrated by clinically meaningful impairments in HRQoL scores [4]. Aspects of life affected by OAB symptoms include sexual health, personal relationships, performing daily activities [5, 6], employment and productivity in the workplace [6, 7]. The major impact of symptoms is exemplified by a study of OAB in Spain, which reported that 96% of patients adopted non-medical coping strategies to help manage their daily and occupational activities, and up to 10% of work time was lost by patients experiencing urgency and urinary incontinence (UI) [8]. OAB is also associated with a substantial economic burden; the total annual direct economic impact (incremental costs) of OAB on the Spanish National Healthcare System is estimated to be around €366 million [7].

Following the use of conservative management strategies (recommended as initial treatment for OAB), oral pharmacotherapy with β_3-adrenoceptor agonists or antimuscarinic agents can improve OAB symptoms [9]. However, evidence from a large, retrospective analysis of medical and pharmaceutical claims database ($N = 167,907$) suggests that persistence (i.e. the duration of time from initiation to discontinuation of therapy [10]) and adherence (i.e. the extent to which a patient acts in accordance with the prescribed interval, and dose of a dosing regimen [10]) to antimuscarinics are low compared with pharmacological therapies used to treat other chronic diseases, including statins and oral diabetics [11]. A systematic literature review (SLR) and meta-analysis that assessed persistence and adherence to antimuscarinic therapy for OAB (14 retrospective database or self-report studies; $N = 190,279$) reported 12-month median persistence rates of 12.0–39.4%; persistence was evaluated up to 36 months and decreased over time [12]. Data from a review of 14 retrospective medical claims studies suggest that a high proportion (43–83%) of patients with OAB discontinued antimuscarinic treatment within the first 30 days [13]. In addition to poor tolerability, unmet treatment expectations, patient education and costs are cited as common reasons for discontinuing antimuscarinic treatment [14].

Mirabegron is a first-in-class licensed, selective, oral β_3-adrenoceptor agonist, which was approved for the treatment of OAB in Europe in December 2012 [15] and was first marketed in Spain in April 2014 [16]. Improved efficacy and similar tolerability for mirabegron compared with placebo has been demonstrated in several phase III studies [17–19]. Similar overall efficacy and improved tolerability regarding bothersome anticholinergic adverse events (AEs) was reported for mirabegron versus antimuscarinics in a network meta-analysis of 44 randomised controlled trials of OAB ($N = 27,309$) [20].

Significant improvements in persistence and adherence have been reported for mirabegron compared with antimuscarinics, in two large retrospective observational studies conducted in Canada and the United Kingdom (UK) [21, 22]. Persistence was also significantly greater for mirabegron versus tolterodine in a large, retrospective analysis of claims records of patients in the United States [23]. These findings may be due, in part, to a lower incidence of bothersome anticholinergic AEs, such as dry mouth, reported for mirabegron compared with antimuscarinics [20], which are frequent reasons for treatment discontinuation [24–26]. Other factors such as the information provided for the patient about their condition (i.e. patient education), patients' willingness to take long-term treatment, and treatment costs may also affect persistence and adherence in patients with OAB [14, 27–29].

Persistence and adherence in patients with OAB are associated with several clinical and economic benefits. Significant improvements in OAB symptoms and HRQoL have been reported in patients adherent to and those persistent on-treatment, respectively, compared with non-adherent or non-persistent patients [30, 31]. Moreover, economic models of OAB suggest that improvements in persistence with mirabegron versus antimuscarinics translate into reduced healthcare resource use, fewer lost work hours, and lower total costs [32, 33].

Data are available from two retrospective, observational studies which evaluated treatment persistence and adherence in patients receiving pharmacotherapy for OAB in Spain [34, 35]. However, limitations in the design of these studies include possible under-reporting of the incidence of OAB and a lack of evaluation of other variables besides pharmacological treatment. Multivariate analyses to adjust for the impact of baseline characteristics were included in the current study, which assessed treatment persistence and adherence observed with mirabegron versus several common antimuscarinics in patients with OAB in Spain.

Methods

Study design and objectives

This was a retrospective, longitudinal, observational cohort study of patients with OAB who received mirabegron or an antimuscarinic drug in routine clinical practice. Anonymised prescription records were collected from the Spanish Cegedim Electronic Medical

Records database, which holds information for approximately one million patients, submitted by primary and secondary care physicians in Spain.

The primary objective was to compare treatment persistence with mirabegron versus antimuscarinics in all eligible patients with OAB. Secondary objectives included: comparing treatment adherence with mirabegron versus antimuscarinics in all eligible patients; evaluating treatment persistence and adherence in different subgroups; and investigating the impact of different patient characteristics on treatment persistence and adherence.

Ethics committee approval for the study was obtained from the Hospital Clinic of Barcelona.

Study population

Eligible patients were ≥ 18 years of age and received a prescription for a target OAB drug between 1 June and 31 October 2014 (i.e. the selection period); the date of the first prescription of that drug was the index date (Additional file 1: Figure S1). Eligible patients were also required to have continuous enrolment during the pre- and post-index periods (12 months prior to and 12 months after the index date, respectively). Exclusion criteria were: prior prescription of the target OAB drug or a 5α-reductase inhibitor during the pre-index period, and prescription of another OAB drug (i.e. receipt of concomitant therapy) at the index date or up to 30 days afterwards; concomitant therapy was permitted > 30 days after the index date. Eligible drugs were identified using European Pharmaceutical Market Research Association (EphMRA) Anatomical Therapeutic Chemical (ATC) codes [36] (Additional file 2: Table S1).

Endpoints

Treatment persistence, the primary endpoint, was defined as the time from the index date until first discontinuation of the index drug (i.e. time to discontinuation [TTD]). An index drug was considered discontinued after a period of 30 days without prescription renewal.

Adherence, determined using the medical possession ratio (MPR), was assessed as a secondary endpoint. This was calculated by two methods: the sum of days' supply of the index drug, divided by 365 days (i.e. fixed-MPR), or divided by the TTD (i.e. variable-MPR). Patients were considered adherent with a MPR of ≥80%.

Statistical analyses

Treatment persistence and adherence (primary and secondary endpoints), assessed in all eligible patients, were not adjusted for potential confounding factors and data were reported descriptively. The unadjusted analyses of persistence were presented using Kaplan-Meier curves and reported as median TTD and the proportion of

patients persistent at the end of the 12-month post-index period. The unadjusted analyses of adherence were reported as mean MPR and the proportion of adherent patients at the end of the 12-month post-index period.

Multivariate analyses using Cox and linear regression models were used to analyse TTD and MPR, respectively. The target OAB drug (i.e. mirabegron or antimuscarinics) was the independent variable; adjustments were made for potential confounding baseline factors of treatment status (naïve or experienced) and age (45–64, 65–74 or ≥ 75 years for analyses of TTD; < 65 or ≥ 65 years for evaluation of MPR). Treatment-naïve patients received no prescriptions for an OAB drug during the 12 months prior to the index date, while treatment-experienced patients received prior prescription(s) for a different OAB drug to the index drug. The models were fitted by including all covariates that showed a significant relationship ($p < 0.10$) with TTD or fixed- and variable-MPR in univariate Cox or linear regression models. Additionally, a forward selection process was used in the multivariate analyses and any variables which did not maximise the quality of the models were excluded [37, 38].

Analyses of treatment persistence and adherence for mirabegron versus antimuscarinics (also using Cox and linear regression models, respectively) were performed, considering each individual antimuscarinic, and in the following patient subgroups: treatment-naïve or -experienced; < 65 or ≥ 65 years of age; and male or female. In addition, sensitivity analyses were performed to assess the impact of increasing the period without prescription renewal used to define TTD from 30 days (base case) to 45, 60 and 90 days. The sensitivity analyses were also adjusted for baseline characteristics.

Adjusted analyses were reported as hazard ratios (HRs) with 95% confidence intervals (CI) and p-values for TTD, or p-values only for MPR. For all adjusted comparisons, mirabegron was the reference comparator and a p-value of < 0.05 was considered statistically significant.

All analyses were performed using Statistical Analysis Software, version 9.3.

Results
Baseline demographics and characteristics

Overall, 1975 patients received a prescription for a target OAB drug during the selection period and 1798 were eligible for inclusion (Fig. 1). The most common reasons for exclusion were receipt of two or more different OAB drugs (i.e. concomitant therapy) at index date or up to 30 days afterwards ($N = 98$), receipt of the index drug during the pre-index period ($N = 50$), and < 18 years of age at the index date ($N = 36$). A total of 1169 (65.0%) eligible patients received mirabegron and 629 (35.0%)

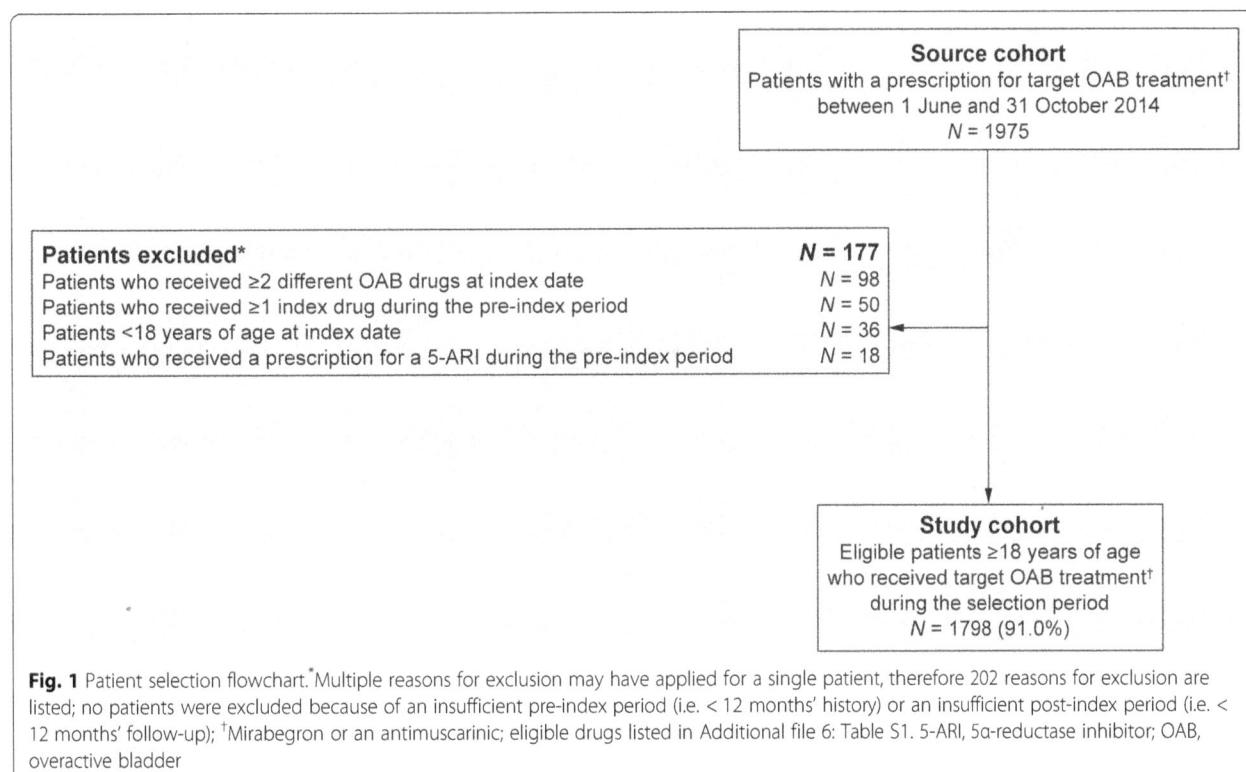

Fig. 1 Patient selection flowchart. *Multiple reasons for exclusion may have applied for a single patient, therefore 202 reasons for exclusion are listed; no patients were excluded because of an insufficient pre-index period (i.e. < 12 months' history) or an insufficient post-index period (i.e. < 12 months' follow-up); †Mirabegron or an antimuscarinic; eligible drugs listed in Additional file 6: Table S1. 5-ARI, 5α-reductase inhibitor; OAB, overactive bladder

received an antimuscarinic. Solifenacin was the most common prescribed antimuscarinic ($N = 266$; 14.8% of patients).

The mean age at index date was 66.42 years (Table 1); a higher proportion of patients were 65–80 years old in the mirabegron arm compared with the antimuscarinic arm (52.8% vs 44.0%), but a lower proportion were > 80 years old (11.8% vs 18.6%). Overall, 1021 (56.8%) patients were female; 637 (54.3%) and 384 (61.0%) in the mirabegron and antimuscarinic arms, respectively. Body mass index (BMI) data were available for 1185 patients, of whom, 545 (46.0%) were obese and 430 (36.3%) were overweight. Of 1289 (71.7%) treatment-naïve patients, a higher proportion was observed in the antimuscarinic arm compared with the mirabegron arm (85.7% vs 64.2%). Approximately two-thirds of patients in the mirabegron arm received their prescription in secondary care from a gynaecologist/urologist; around three-quarters of patients treated with an antimuscarinic received their prescription in primary care, from a general practitioner (GP).

Persistence
All eligible patients
Median TTD was longer with mirabegron versus antimuscarinic therapy (90 vs 56 days, respectively (Fig. 2). A higher proportion of patients prescribed mirabegron were persistent at 12 months ($N = 236$; 20.2%) compared with antimuscarinics ($N = 64$; 10.2%).

Multivariate analyses
Patients who received mirabegron were significantly less likely to discontinue treatment compared with those prescribed an antimuscarinic (HR: 1.52 [95% CI: 1.37–1.70]; $p < 0.001$) (Table 2). Patients < 75 years of age and treatment-naïve patients were significantly more likely to discontinue treatment compared with those ≥75 years of age and treatment-experienced patients, respectively (Table 2).

Subgroup analyses
Median TTD for mirabegron (90 days) was significantly longer versus each individual antimuscarinic (range: 28–60 days; HR range: 1.21–2.17; $p \leq 0.013$), and a higher proportion of patients were persistent at 12 months with mirabegron (20.2%) versus individual antimuscarinics (range: 3.2–13.9%) (Fig. 3). Among the antimuscarinics, solifenacin had the longest median TTD and the highest proportion of persistent patients. Treatment persistence was significantly longer with mirabegron versus all antimuscarinics in all the other subgroups: treatment naïve (HR: 1.47 [95% CI: 1.30–1.66]); treatment experienced (HR: 1.80 [95% CI: 1.41–2.31]); < 65 years (HR: 1.39 [95% CI: 1.17–1.69]); ≥65 years (HR: 1.60 [95% CI: 1.39–1.83]); male (HR: 1.75 [95% CI: 1.48–2.07]); and female (HR: 1.37 [95% CI: 1.18–1.58]) ($p < 0.001$ for all comparisons) (Additional file 3: Figure S2).

Table 1 Baseline characteristics in patients who received prescriptions for mirabegron or antimuscarinics[a]

	Mirabegron (N = 1169)	Antimuscarinics (N = 629)	Total (N = 1798)
Sex, N (%)			
Male	532 (45.5)	245 (39.0)	777 (43.2)
Female	637 (54.5)	384 (61.0)	1021 (56.8)
Age, mean (SD)	66.31 (13.41)	66.61 (14.71)	66.42 (13.88)
Age category, N (%)			
< 65 years	414 (35.4)	235 (37.4)	649 (36.1)
65–80 years	617 (52.8)	277 (44.0)	894 (49.7)
> 80 years	138 (11.8)	117 (18.6)	255 (14.2)
BMI, mean (SD)	30.15 (5.47)	29.88 (5.62)	30.06 (5.52)
BMI category, N (%)[b]			
Underweight (< 18.5)	4 (0.5)	5 (1.3)	9 (0.8)
Normal or healthy weight (18.5–24.9)	137 (17.3)	64 (16.2)	201 (17.0)
Overweight (25.0–29.9)	277 (35.1)	153 (38.7)	430 (36.3)
Obese (≥30.0)	372 (47.1)	173 (43.8)	545 (46.0)
Treatment status, N (%)			
Treatment-naïve	750 (64.2)	539 (85.7)	1289 (71.7)
Treatment-experienced	419 (35.8)	90 (14.3)	509 (28.3)
Prior treatment with α-blockers, N (%)[c]			
Yes	157 (13.4)	58 (9.2)	215 (12.0)
No	1012 (86.6)	571 (90.8)	1583 (88.0)
Prescriber at index date, N (%)			
Gynaecologist/urologist	749 (64.1)	131 (20.8)	880 (48.9)
GP	397 (34.0)	476 (75.7)	873 (48.6)
Other	23 (2.0)	22 (3.5)	45 (2.5)
Type of care for prescribed index drug, N (%)			
Primary	397 (34.0)	476 (75.7)	873 (48.6)
Secondary	23 (66.1)	22 (24.3)	45 (51.4)

BMI body mass index, GP general practitioner, SD standard deviation
[a]At index date
[b]Data based on 1185 patients (mirabegron: N = 790; antimuscarinics: N = 395)
[c]Data based on follow-up post-index date

Sensitivity analyses

Median TTD in patients prescribed mirabegron was increased from 90 days in the base-case analysis to 121 days, when the period without prescription renewal used to define treatment discontinuation was extended from 30 to 90 days (Additional file 4: Figure S3). This analysis had little impact on median TTD in patients who received an antimuscarinic (range: 56–60 days across all adjusted periods); median TTD was significantly longer for mirabegron versus antimuscarinics

across all of the adjusted time periods used to define treatment discontinuation (HR range: 1.43–1.53; $p < 0.001$ for all assessments).

Adherence
All eligible patients
Mean adherence using fixed-MPR was higher with mirabegron (38.69 [SD: 33.75] versus antimuscarinics (25.88 [SD: 28.14]) and the proportion of adherent patients was two-times higher with mirabegron versus antimuscarinics (22.0% versus 11.0%, respectively). Adherence measured using variable-MPR was similar between the two groups (Table 3). The results of the multivariate and subgroup analyses of MPR are described in Additional file 5, with results displayed in Additional file 6: Tables S2, Additional file 7: Tables S3, Additional files 8: Table S4.

Discussion
This retrospective study assessed treatment persistence and adherence in approximately 1800 patients with OAB in Spain, who received mirabegron or an antimuscarinic in routine clinical practice. Greater persistence was observed for mirabegron versus antimuscarinics in both the unadjusted (all eligible patients) and adjusted (multivariate) analyses, including a two-times larger proportion of persistent and adherent patients at 12 months in the mirabegron arm (primary and secondary endpoints). These findings were supported by the results of the sensitivity analyses and the data reported in various patient subgroups.

Overall, the results of our study add to the growing body of real-world evidence from several other countries, which indicates mirabegron provides greater treatment persistence compared with antimuscarinics in patients with OAB [21–23, 32]; 12-month persistence with mirabegron ranged from 33% to 39% in three of these studies [21, 22, 32]. Recent evidence from BE-LIEVE, a large, prospective, non-interventional study of 682 patients from eight European countries (NCT02 320773), reported that 53.8% of patients were persistent after 12 months on-treatment with mirabegron [39]; this was the highest 12-month persistence rate observed for mirabegron in real-world studies to date.

Median TTD and 12-month persistence rates for all OAB treatment reported in the current study were lower compared with recent retrospective, observational studies of treatment persistence with mirabegron and antimuscarinics conducted in different countries [21, 22, 40]. However, rates of 12-month persistence observed in the current study are comparable with some of the data reported in one other retrospective analysis (18%) [11, 23], and two systematic literature reviews of persistence in patients with OAB (12–39% and 10–25%) [12, 13]. National issues relating to clinical practice in Spain may have

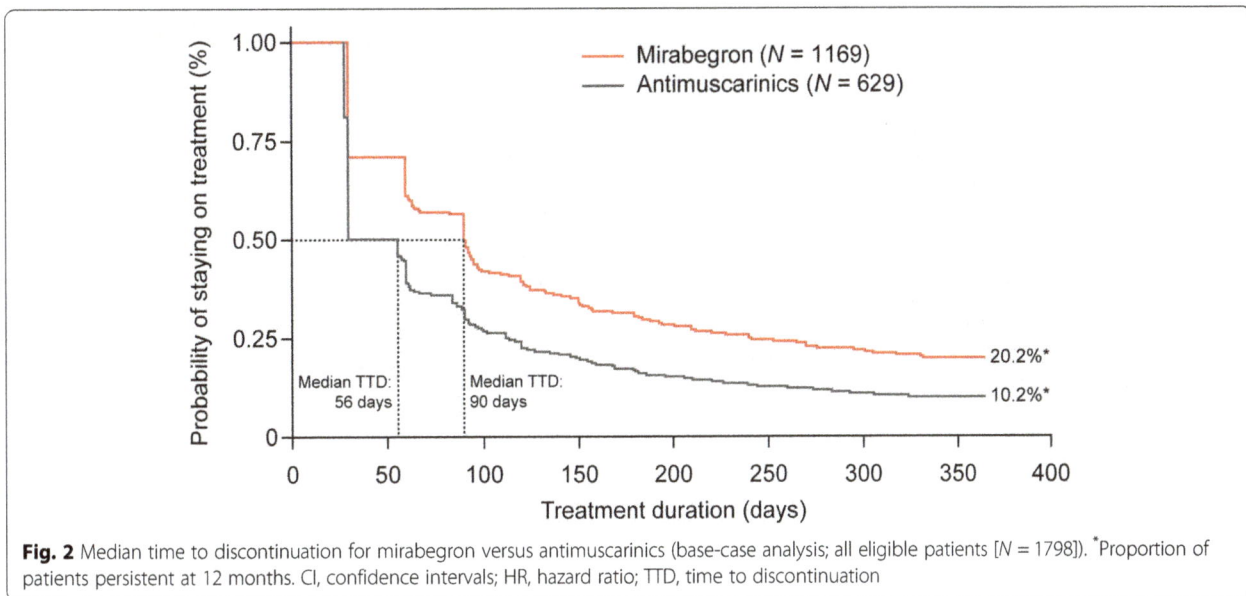

Fig. 2 Median time to discontinuation for mirabegron versus antimuscarinics (base-case analysis; all eligible patients [N = 1798]). *Proportion of patients persistent at 12 months. CI, confidence intervals; HR, hazard ratio; TTD, time to discontinuation

contributed to lower treatment persistence compared with some studies. For example, patients in Spain are expected to co-pay up-to 60% of drug costs [41]; cost is specified as one of several factors that might contribute to treatment discontinuation in the current European Association of Urology (EAU) guidelines for UI [9].

Two similar studies to evaluate persistence on-treatment in adults with OAB have been conducted in Spain, which reported higher rates of 12-month persistence on-treatment with solifenacin, fesoterodine or tolterodine monotherapy (range: 30.9–40.2%) compared with our study [34, 35]. These differences may be attributed to several factors: first, in both other studies, retrospective data were extracted from existing medical records from primary healthcare centres in parts of Catalonia and the Balearic Islands, compared with data representative of the overall Spanish population in our study. Second, our sensitivity analyses suggest that extending the period used to define treatment discontinuation results in greater persistence, and one of these other studies (Sicras-Mainar et al., 2014) used a considerably longer period to

define treatment discontinuation (52 weeks without prescription renewal) versus our study (30 days in the base case analysis) [34]. In the other prior Spanish study (Sicras-Mainar et al., 2015), OAB patients between 20 and 64 years of age who were active workers were included; therefore, it's possible these patients may have been healthier or had a better treatment response, compared with the patient population in our study which were selected using less-stringent criteria [35]. However, no stratification was performed to evaluate the potential impact of these patient characteristics.

A high proportion of patients included in our study (82.3%) were also overweight or obese according to BMI; these patients may be less likely to experience symptom improvement (and perhaps more likely to discontinue treatment) than those with lower BMI. Weight loss has been shown to reduce the number of UI episodes in overweight or obese women [42, 43], and is recommended by the EAU to reduce the risk of developing UI, or improve symptoms [9]. Similar to the current study, the mean BMI values in European patients with OAB

Table 2 Impact of covariates on time to discontinuation: multivariate Cox regression analysis adjusting for baseline characteristics in all eligible patients (N = 1798)[a]

	Target OAB drug received		Treatment status		Age, years		
	Mirabegron (N = 1169)[b]	Antimuscarinics (N = 629)	Naïve (N = 1289)	Experienced (N = 509)[b]	45–64 (N = 649)	65–74 (N = 595)	≥75 (N = 554)[b]
TTD							
Median, days	90	56	60	99	60	90	91
(95% CI)	90–92	30–56	60–61	92–121	56–60	68–91	90–99
HR (95% CI)	–	1.52 (1.37–1.70)[c]	1.35 (1.20–1.53)[c]	–	1.53 (1.35–1.74)[c]	1.15 (1.01–1.31)[d]	–

ATC Anatomical Therapeutic Chemical, CI confidence intervals, GP general practitioner, HR hazard ratio, OAB overactive bladder, TTD time to discontinuation
[a]At index date; HR, 95% CI and p-values generated using a stepwise Cox regression model including target OAB drug received, treatment status and age
[b]Reference comparator
[c]p < 0.001
[d]p = 0.039 (all other comparisons non-significant)

Target OAB drug (N = 1798)	12-month persistence, N (%)	Median TTD, days (95% CI)	HR (95% CI); p-value[‡]
Mirabegron (N = 1169)[*]	236 (20.2)	90 (90–92)	–
Tolterodine (N = 111)	10 (9.0)	28 (28–56)	2.17 (1.76–2.66); p < 0.0001
Fesoterodine (N = 141)	14 (9.9)	56 (28–62)	1.62 (1.35–1.96); p < 0.0001
Oxybutynin (N = 93)	3 (3.2)	30 (NR–NR)	1.78 (1.43–2.22); p < 0.0001
Solifenacin (N = 266)	37 (13.9)	60 (30–60)	1.21 (1.04–1.40); p = 0.013
Trospium (N = 18)	–[†]	30 (30–60)	NR

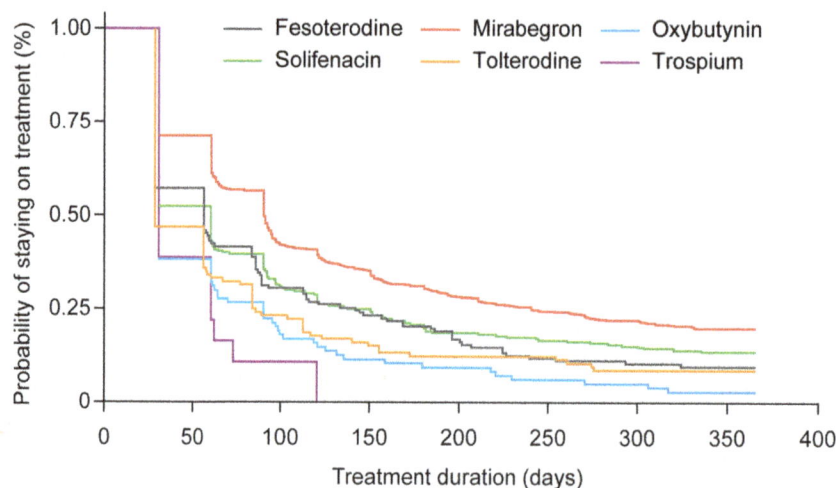

Fig. 3 Persistence with mirabegron compared with individual antimuscarinics: subgroup analysis. [*]Reference comparator; [†]Not evaluated due to small sample size; [‡]HRs, 95% CI and p-values generated using a Cox regression model with adjustment for age and treatment status. CI, confidence intervals; HR, hazard ratio; NR, not reached; OAB, overactive bladder; TTD, time to discontinuation

enrolled in phase II/III studies were also indicative of overweight [19, 44, 45]; the impact of patients' BMI on persistence and adherence was not evaluated in our study and this could perhaps be investigated in subsequent analyses.

In our study, the majority of patients (71.7%) were defined as treatment-naïve (i.e. they had not received any prescriptions for an OAB drug during the 12 months prior to the index date), which may have led to different expectations regarding efficacy and/or tolerability compared with treatment-experienced patients, and perhaps

Table 3 Summary of adherence to mirabegron compared with antimuscarinics (all eligible patients; N = 1798)

	Mirabegron (N = 1169)	Antimuscarinics (N = 629)
MPR-fixed		
Mean (SD)	38.69 (33.75)	25.88 (28.14)
Adherent[a], N (%)	257 (22.0)	69 (11.0)
MPR-variable		
Mean (SD)	97.65 (4.03)	98.03 (4.57)
Adherent[a], N (%)	1163 (99.5)	619 (98.4)

MPR medical possession ratio, SD standard deviation
[a]MPR of ≥80%

contributed to the observed low overall persistence. A proportionally smaller number of treatment-naïve patients were prescribed mirabegron vs antimuscarinics, and as reported in our study and other studies [21, 22, 46, 47], this may have had a positive impact on the persistence data – although treatment persistence was significantly longer with mirabegron versus all antimuscarinics in both the treatment naïve and treatment experienced subgroups. Most patients were prescribed antimuscarinics through primary care by a GP, while the majority of patients prescribed mirabegron received their prescription from a gynaecologist or urologist in secondary care. In the multivariate analysis of our study, the type of prescriber was not identified (during the stepwise selection process) as a covariate which produced a significant impact on TTD. However, we acknowledge there are two reports that indicate patients prescribed OAB treatment within a specialist setting experienced greater persistence compared with internal medicine/GP departments [48, 49].

Patients' medication-taking behaviour can be attributed to many different factors and one of these is the nature of the communication with their physician [50]; others include the patient's beliefs and values [50], expectations of treatment [14], perception of the severity of their condition [51], and other behavioural or societal factors [51]. To mitigate some of these factors having a negative impact on-treatment persistence and adherence, it is important that the patients' treating physician provides them with the appropriate information/education during initial consultations, involves the patient in decision making throughout the course of treatment, and helps to manage their expectations around efficacy and tolerability. Also, a wide variety of comorbidities (including other urological conditions, neurological diseases, endocrine disorders, respiratory dysfunctions, faecal motility disorders, and pelvic cancer) may cause or worsen OAB symptoms [27]. Therefore, individualised treatment for patients with OAB, taking all aspects of a patients' condition into account (i.e. treating OAB in the context of all comorbidities, rather than as a single condition) may be crucial for improving rates of persistence and adherence.

A higher proportion of patients in the current study (65.0%) received mirabegron compared with antimuscarinics (35.0%). Of the 629 patients prescribed an antimuscarinic, only trospium was prescribed to fewer than 90 patients and this antimuscarinic was not evaluated for 12-month persistence due to the small sample size ($N = 18$). The difference in the number of patients who received mirabegron and antimuscarinics may be attributed to mirabegron first being marketed in Spain in April 2014, fewer than two months prior to the start of the selection period [16]. It is possible that the proportional difference in prescriptions observed for mirabegron versus antimuscarinics may have contributed to the findings of our study, but this was not formally assessed.

Strengths of the study were the large sample size of approximately 1800 patients with OAB, and the collection of real-world data from a representative sample of patients treated in routine clinical practice in Spain. The main study limitation was the lack of significance estimates for the primary and secondary endpoints, which were not available as the protocol did not allow for adjustment of potential confounding factors in these specific analyses. However, significantly greater persistence was observed for mirabegron compared with antimuscarinics when Cox regression analyses were performed. Although the study tested for the confounding factors expected to be most important based on previous studies (and only those which had a significant association with TTD were included in our Cox regression models), the nature of retrospective database studies meant that all important confounding factors were unlikely to be captured, due to the analyses of limited secondary data (for example, information on the type of OAB symptoms or their severity were unavailable). Other limitations related to the database included persistence and adherence measured based on prescription data, rather than information being directly recorded by the treating physician; plus, several factors that could potentially impact treatment persistence were not recorded (e.g. physician compliance to management guidelines; severity of OAB symptoms; overall health/fragility of patients; physician bias for initial treatment/switching).

Also, the trends observed for fixed- and variable-MPR were not consistent and might have resulted from a proxy of the methodology used (i.e. denominators of 365 days and median TTD, respectively). Finally, persistence and adherence estimates may not have been completely accurate, as the study evaluated prescriptions issued, but information regarding collection or correct use of the prescribed medication according to the recommended regimen was not available; however, this would have likely impacted all patients, independent of the OAB treatment prescribed.

It is possible that the observed differences in persistence and adherence for mirabegron versus antimuscarinics in the current study, consistent with previous studies conducted in Canada and the UK [21, 22], could be attributed to an improved tolerability profile with mirabegron; in particular, a lower incidence of bothersome anticholinergic AEs such as dry mouth and constipation [20, 52]. However, as discussed above, many different factors are involved in patients' medication-taking behaviour. Recently published data from the BELIEVE study reported insufficient relief of symptoms, poor tolerability due to side effects, and the cost/amount of co-pay among the most common reasons for switching from or discontinuing treatment with mirabegron [39]. Future studies, including PERSPECTIVE (Clinicaltrials.gov: NCT02386072 [53] should offer additional insights into the underlying differences in treatment persistence and adherence across therapies used for OAB, possible reasons for treatment discontinuation and the potential impact on clinical practice (e.g. for clinical outcomes, economic impact and resource use).

Conclusions

Mirabegron is associated with greater treatment persistence and adherence in patients with OAB, compared with antimuscarinics. The differences in mechanism of action and efficacy/tolerability profile may contribute to this reported treatment benefit and supports data showing that mirabegron is an appropriate treatment option for patients with OAB. The real-world evidence from this longitudinal, observational cohort study of OAB in Spain may provide strategic insights for clinicians and policy makers involved in the management of patients with this chronic condition. However, further study is needed to understand the different factors that may contribute to low persistence and adherence on-treatment with OAB pharmacotherapy. Some of these factors may be mitigated by the patient's treating physician providing them with appropriate information during initial consultations, involving them in decision making throughout the course of treatment, helping to manage their expectations around efficacy and tolerability, and implementing an individualised treatment strategy.

Additional files

> **Additional file 1: Figure S1.** Study design. (TIF 1446 kb)
>
> **Additional file 2: Table S1.** Drugs available for selection using European Pharmaceutical Market Research Association (EphMRA) Anotomical Therapeutic Chemical (ATC) drug codes (1). (DOCX 14 kb)
>
> **Additional file 3: Figure S2.** Median TTD for mirabegron versus antimuscarinics (base-case analysis) in the following subgroups of patients: treatment-naïve (A); treatment-experienced (B); < 65 years of age (C); ≥65 years of age (D); male (E); and female (F). (TIF 2887 kb)
>
> **Additional file 4: Figure S3.** Median TTD when the 30-day period without prescription renewal used to define TTD was extended to 45 days (A); 60 days (B); and 90 days (C) (all eligible patients; N = 1798). (TIF 2722 kb)
>
> **Additional file 5** Summary of multivariate and subgroup analyses of MPR. (DOCX 16 kb)
>
> **Additional file 6: Table S2.** Impact of covariates on the medical possession ratio: multivariate linear regression analysis in all eligible patients (N = 1798). (DOCX 17 kb)
>
> **Additional file 7: Table S3.** Summary of adherence with mirabegron compared with antimuscarinics in subgroups defined by the target OAB drug received. (DOCX 17 kb)
>
> **Additional file 8: Table S4.** Summary of adherence with mirabegron compared with antimuscarinics in subgroups defined by treatment experience, age and gender. (DOCX 17 kb)

Abbreviations
AE: Adverse events; ATC: Anatomical Therapeutic Chemical; BMI: Body mass index; CI: Confidence intervals; EAU: European Association of Urology; EphMRA: European Pharmaceutical Market Research Association; GP: General practitioner; HR: Hazard ratio; HRQoL: Health-related quality of life; MPR: Medical possession ratio; NR: Not reached; OAB: Overactive bladder; SD: Standard deviation; SLR: Systematic literature review; TTD: Time to discontinuation; UI: Urinary incontinence; UK: United Kingdom

Acknowledgements
Medical writing support provided by David Griffiths, PhD, of Bioscript Medical. Sally Bowditch of Astellas Pharma Europe Ltd. provided input to the design of the study, as well as analysis and interpretation of data. Àgata Carreño of IMS Health and Quintiles (now IQVIA) provided statistical analysis support.

Authors' contributions
Conception and design: JN, ZH, FG, AK, FF, AMB and MHG. Acquisition of data: JN, ZH, AMB and MHG. Analysis and interpretation of the data: all authors (JN, ZH, FG, AK, FF, AMB and MHG). Drafting of the manuscript: all authors (JN, ZH, FG, AK, FF, AMB and MHG). Critical revision of the manuscript for important intellectual content: all authors (JN, ZH, FG, AK, FF, AMB and MHG). Statistical analysis: FG and AK. Obtaining funding: JN, ZH, AMB and MHG. Agreement to be accountable for all aspects of the work in ensuring that questions related to the accuracy or integrity of any part of the work are appropriately investigated and resolved: all authors (JN, ZH, FG, AK, FF, AMB and MHG). Read and approved the final manuscript: all authors (JN, ZH, FG, AK, FF, AMB and MHG).

Author details
[1]Astellas Pharma Europe Ltd, 2000 Hillswood Drive, Chertsey KT16 0PS, UK. [2]Astellas Pharma Europe B.V, Leiden, the Netherlands. [3]Creativ-Ceutical Ltd., London, UK. [4]Creativ-Ceutical Ltd., Tunis, Tunisia. [5]Manchester Metropolitan University, Manchester, UK. [6]Astellas Pharma S.A., Madrid, Spain. [7]Present Address: Keyrus Biopharma, Tunis, Tunisia.

References
1. Abrams P, Cardozo L, Fall M, Griffiths D, Rosier P, Ulmsten U, et al. The standardisation of terminology in lower urinary tract function: report from the standardisation sub-committee of the international continence society. Urology. 2002;61:37–49.

2. Haylen BT, de Ridder D, Freeman RM, Swift SE, Berghmans B, Lee J, et al. An international Urogynecological association (IUGA)/international continence society (ICS) joint report on the terminology for female pelvic floor dysfunction. Neurourol Urodyn. 2010;29:4–20.

3. Castro D, Espuna M, Prieto M, Badia X. Prevalence of overactive bladder in Spain: a population-based study. Arch Esp Urol. 2005;58:131–8.

4. Stewart WF, Van Rooyen JB, Cundiff GW, Abrams P, Herzog AR, Corey R, et al. Prevalence and burden of overactive bladder in the United States. World J Urol. 2003;20:327–36.

5. Nicolson P, Kopp Z, Chapple CR, Kelleher C. It's just the worry about not being able to control it! A qualitative study of living with overactive bladder. Br J Health Psychol. 2008;13:343–59.

6. Coyne KS, Sexton CC, Irwin DE, Kopp ZS, Kelleher CJ, Milsom I. The impact of overactive bladder, incontinence and other lower urinary tract symptoms on quality of life, work productivity, sexuality and emotional well-being in men and women: results from the EPIC study. BJU Int. 2008;101:1388–95.

7. Irwin DE, Mungapen L, Milsom I, Kopp Z, Reeves P, Kelleher C. The economic impact of overactive bladder syndrome in six western countries. BJU Int. 2009;103:202–9.

8. Rapariz M, Mora AM, Roset M. Impact of overactive bladder symptoms on work activity: The ACTIVHA study. Actas Urol Esp. 2017; https://doi.org/10.1016/jacuro201709005. [Epub ahead of print] 2017

9. Burkhard FC, Bosch JLHR, Cruz F, Lemack GE, Nambiar AK, Thiruchelvam N, Tubaro A. Guidelines on Urinary Incontinence. Available at: http://uroweb.org/guideline/urinary-incontinence/ (Access date: 27 Mar 2017).

10. Cramer JA, Roy A, Burrell A, Fairchild CJ, Fuldeore MJ, Ollendorf DA, et al. Medication compliance and persistence: terminology and definitions. Value Health. 2008;11:44–7.

11. Yeaw J, Benner JS, Walt JG, Sian S, Smith DB. Comparing adherence and persistence across 6 chronic medication classes. J Manag Care Pharm. 2009; 15:728–40.

12. Veenboer PW, Bosch JL. Long-term adherence to antimuscarinic therapy in everyday practice: a systematic review. J Urol. 2014;191:1003–8.

13. Sexton CC, Notte SM, Maroulis C, Dmochowski RR, Cardozo L, Subramanian D, et al. Persistence and adherence in the treatment of overactive bladder syndrome with anticholinergic therapy: a systematic review of the literature. Int J Clin Pract. 2011;65:567–85.

14. Benner JS, Nichol MB, Rovner ES, Jumadilova Z, Alvir J, Hussein M, et al. Patient-reported reasons for discontinuing overactive bladder medication. BJU Int. 2010;105:1276–82.

15. European Medicines Agency. Betmiga EPAR Product Information. Available at: http://www.ema.europa.eu/ema/index.jsp?curl=pages/medicines/human/medicines/002388/human_med_001605.jsp&mid=WC0b01ac058001d124/ (Access date: 16 May 2017).

16. BOTPLUS. National Spanish database from pharmacology colleges. Available at: https://botplusweb.portalfarma.com/botplus.aspx/ (Access date: 13 December 2017).

17. Herschorn S, Barkin J, Castro-Diaz D, Frankel JM, Espuna-Pons M, Gousse AE, et al. A phase III, randomized, double-blind, parallel-group, placebo-controlled, multicentre study to assess the efficacy and safety of the beta(3) adrenoceptor agonist, mirabegron, in patients with symptoms of overactive bladder. Urology. 2013;82:313–20.

18. Nitti VW, Auerbach S, Martin N, Calhoun A, Lee M, Herschorn S. Results of a randomized phase III trial of mirabegron in patients with overactive bladder. J Urol. 2013;189:1388–95.

19. Khullar V, Amarenco G, Angulo JC, Cambronero J, Hoye K, Milsom I, et al. Efficacy and tolerability of mirabegron, a beta(3)-adrenoceptor agonist, in patients with overactive bladder: results from a randomised European-Australian phase 3 trial. Eur Urol. 2013;63:283–95.

20. Maman K, Aballea S, Nazir J, Desroziers K, Neine ME, Siddiqui E, et al. Comparative efficacy and safety of medical treatments for the management of overactive bladder: a systematic literature review and mixed treatment comparison. Eur Urol. 2014;65:755–65.

21. Wagg A, Franks B, Ramos B, Berner T. Persistence and adherence with the new beta-3 receptor agonist, mirabegron, versus antimuscarinics in overactive bladder: early experience in Canada. Can Urol Assoc J. 2015;9: 343–50.

22. Chapple CR, Nazir J, Hakimi Z, Bowditch S, Fatoye F, Guelfucci F, et al. Persistence and adherence with mirabegron versus antimuscarinic agents in patients with overactive bladder: a retrospective observational study in UK clinical practice. Eur Urol. 2017;72:389–99.

A retrospective study of treatment persistence and adherence to mirabegron versus...

71

23. Nitti VW, Rovner ES, Franks B, Muma NM, Berner T, Fan A, et al. Persistence with mirabegron versus tolterodine in patients with overactive bladder. Am J Pharm Benefits. 2016;8:e25–33.

24. Athanasopoulos A, Giannitsas K. An overview of the clinical use of antimuscarinics in the treatment of overactive bladder. Adv Urol. 2011;2011: 820816.

25. Chapple CR, Fianu-Jonsson A, Indig M, Khullar V, Rosa J, Scarpa RM, et al. Treatment outcomes in the STAR study: a subanalysis of solifenacin 5 mg and tolterodine ER 4 mg. Eur Urol. 2007;52:1195–203.

26. Chapple CR, Khullar V, Gabriel Z, Muston D, Bitoun CE, Weinstein D. The effects of antimuscarinic treatments in overactive bladder: an update of a systematic review and meta-analysis. Eur Urol. 2008;54:543–62.

27. Corcos J, Przydacz M, Campeau L, Gray G, Hickling D, Honeine C, et al. CUA guideline on adult overactive bladder. Can Urol Assoc J. 2017;11:E142–e73.

28. Campbell UB, Stang P, Barron R. Survey assessment of continuation of and satisfaction with pharmacological treatment for urinary incontinence. Value Health. 2008;11:726–32.

29. Dmochowski RR, Newman DK. Impact of overactive bladder on women in the United States: results of a national survey. Curr Med Res Opin. 2007;23: 65–76.

30. Andy UU, Arya LA, Smith AL, Propert KJ, Bogner HR, Colavita K, et al. Is self-reported adherence associated with clinical outcomes in women treated with anticholinergic medication for overactive bladder? Neurourol Urodyn. 2015;35:738–42.

31. Kim TH, Choo MS, Kim YJ, Koh H, Lee KS. Drug persistence and compliance affect patient-reported outcomes in overactive bladder syndrome. Qual Life Res. 2016;25:2021–9.

32. Hakimi Z, Nazir J, McCrea C, Berling M, Fatoye F, Ramos B, et al. Clinical and economic impact of mirabegron compared with antimuscarinics for the treatment of overactive bladder in Canada. J Med Econ. 2017;20:614–22.

33. Nazir J, Berling M, McCrea C, Fatoye F, Bowditch S, Hakimi Z, et al. Economic impact of mirabegron versus antimuscarinics for the treatment of overactive bladder in the UK. PharmacoEconomics - Open. 2017;1:25–36.

34. Sicras-Mainar A, Rejas J, Navarro-Artieda R, Aguado-Jodar A, Ruiz-Torrejon A, Ibanez-Nolla J, et al. Antimuscarinic persistence patterns in newly treated patients with overactive bladder: a retrospective comparative analysis. Int Urogynecol J. 2014;25:485–92.

35. Sicras-Mainar A, Navarro-Artieda R, Ruiz-Torrejon A, Saez-Zafra M, Coll-de Tuero G. Impact of loss of work productivity in patients with overactive bladder treated with antimuscarinics in Spain: study in routine clinical practice conditions. Clin Drug Investig. 2015;35:795–805.

36. World Health Organization. ATC/DDD Index 2017. Drugs for urinary frequency and incontinence. Available at: https://www.whocc.no/atc_ddd_index/?code=G04BD (Access date: 11 May 2017).

37. Krall JM, Uthoff VA, Harley JB. A step-up procedure for selecting variables associated with survival. Biometrics. 1975;31:49–57.

38. Helmreich JE. Regression modeling strategies with applications to linear models, logistic and ordinal regression and survival analysis (2nd Edition). J Stat Softw. 2016;70(Book Review 2).

39. Freeman R, Foley S, Rosa J, Vicente E, Grill R, Kachlirova Z, et al. Mirabegron improves quality of life, treatment satisfaction and persistence in patients with overactive bladder - a multicentre, non-interventional, real-world, 12-month study. Curr Med Res Opin. 2017:1–9. https://doi.org/10.1080/03007995. [Epub ahead of print]

40. Wagg A, Compion G, Fahey A, Siddiqui E. Persistence with prescribed antimuscarinic therapy for overactive bladder: a UK experience. BJU Int. 2012;110:1767–74.

41. Errando-Smet C, Muller-Arteaga C, Hernandez M, Lenero E, Roset M. Healthcare resource utilization and cost among males with lower urinary tract symptoms with a predominant storage component in Spain: the epidemiological, cross-sectional MERCURY study. Neurourol Urodyn. 2017; https://doi.org/10.1002/nau.23293. [epub ahead of print]

42. Subak LL, Johnson C, Whitcomb E, Boban D, Saxton J, Brown JS. Does weight loss improve incontinence in moderately obese women? Int Urogynecol J Pelvic Floor Dysfunct. 2002;13:40–3.

43. Gozukara YM, Akalan G, Tok EC, Aytan H, Ertunc D. The improvement in pelvic floor symptoms with weight loss in obese women does not correlate with the changes in pelvic anatomy. Int Urogynecol J. 2014;25:1219–25.

44. Malone-Lee JG, Walsh JB, Maugourd MF. Tolterodine: a safe and effective treatment for older patients with overactive bladder. J Am Geriatr Soc. 2001;49:700–5.

45. Abrams P, Kelleher C, Staskin D, Rechberger T, Kay R, Martina R, et al. Combination treatment with mirabegron and solifenacin in patients with overactive bladder: efficacy and safety results from a randomised, double-blind, dose-ranging, phase 2 study (symphony). Eur Urol. 2015;67:577–88.

46. Kim TH, Lee KS. Persistence and compliance with medication management in the treatment of overactive bladder. Investig Clin Urol. 2016;57:84–93.

47. Wagg AS, Foley S, Peters J, Nazir J, Kool-Houweling L, Scrine L. Persistence and adherence with mirabegron vs antimuscarinics in overactive bladder: retrospective analysis of a UK general practice prescription database. Int J Clin Pract. 2017;71

48. Kalder M, Pantazis K, Dinas K, Albert US, Heilmaier C, Kostev K. Discontinuation of treatment using anticholinergic medications in patients with urinary incontinence. Obstet Gynecol. 2014;124:794–800.

49. Tran AM, Sand PK, Seitz MJ, Gafni-Kane A, Zhou Y, Botros SM. Does physician specialty affect persistence to pharmacotherapy among patients with overactive bladder syndrome? Int Urogynecol J. 2017;28:409–15.

50. Shingler SL, Bennett BM, Cramer JA, Towse A, Twelves C, Lloyd AJ. Treatment preference, adherence and outcomes in patients with cancer: literature review and development of a theoretical model. Curr Med Res Opin. 2014;30:2329–41.

51. Touchette D, Shapiro N. Medication compliance, adherence, and persistence: current status of behavioral and educational interventions to improve outcomes. J Manag Care Pharm. 2008;14:S2–S10.

52. Nitti VW, Khullar V, van Kerrebroeck P, Herschorn S, Cambronero J, Angulo JC, et al. Mirabegron for the treatment of overactive bladder: a prespecified pooled efficacy analysis and pooled safety analysis of three randomised, double-blind, placebo-controlled, phase III studies. Int J Clin Pract. 2013;67:619–32.

53. Clinicaltrials.gov. A Prospective, Observational, Multicenter Study of Patients Following Initiation of a New Course of Treatment for Overactive Bladder (OAB) (PERSPECTIVE). Available at: https://clinicaltrials.gov/ct2/show/NCT02386072?term=persistence+AND+overactive+bladder&rank=7/ (Access date: 19 May 2017).

10

Anticholinergic burden and comorbidities in patients attending treatment with trospium chloride for overactive bladder in a real-life setting: results of a prospective non-interventional study

A. Ivchenko[1], R.-H. Bödeker[2], C. Neumeister[3]* (iD) and A. Wiedemann[1]

Abstract

Background: Elderly people are representative for the patients most likely to be treated with anticholinergics for overactive bladder (OAB). They often receive further drugs with anticholinergic properties for concomitant conditions. This increases the risk for side effects, including central nervous system disorders. Data on comorbidities and baseline anticholinergic burden of OAB patients seen in urological practice is scarce. Therefore, we included an epidemiological survey on these issues in our study which assessed the effectiveness and tolerability of trospium chloride (TC) in established dosages under routine conditions.

Methods: Outpatients (≥ 65 years of age), for whom treatment with TC was indicated, were eligible to participate in this non-interventional, prospective study performed in 162 urological practices in Germany. Epidemiological questions were evaluated by the Anticholinergic Burden (ACB) scale and the Cumulative Illness Rating Scale for Geriatrics (CIRS-G) at baseline. Efficacy was assessed by changes in symptom-related variables of OAB after treatment. Dosage regimen, duration of treatment, adverse events, withdrawals, and ease of subdivision of the prescribed SNAP-TAB tablet were documented. Patients and physicians rated efficacy and tolerability of treatment. Statistics were descriptive.

Results: Four hundred fourty-five out of 986 (47.54%) patients in the epidemiological population had a baseline ACB scale score > 0, 100 (24.72%) of whom a score ≥ 3. The median CIRS-G comorbidity index score for all patients was 5. 78.55% (608/774) of patients in the efficacy population received a daily dose of 45 mg TC. 60.03% (365/608) of them took this dose by dividing the SNAP-TAB tablet in three equal parts. Before-after-comparisons of the core symptoms of OAB showed clear improvements. An influence of the dosage scheme (1 × 45 mg TC/d vs 3 × 15 mg TC/d) on clinical outcome could not be observed. Most urologists and patients rated TC treatment as effective and well tolerated. 44 (4.37%) out of 1007 patients in the safety collective ended their treatment prematurely, while 75 patients (7.45%) experienced adverse events.

Conclusions: Anticholinergic burden and comorbidities in elderly OAB patients are frequent. The acceptance of the SNAP-TAB tablet, which facilitates flexible dosing with TC, was high, which is supportive in ensuring adherence in therapy.

(Continued on next page)

* Correspondence: claudia.neumeister@dr-pfleger.de
[3]Department of Medical Science/Clinical Research, Dr. R. Pfleger GmbH,
Dr.-Robert-Pfleger-Strasse 12, 96052 Bamberg, Germany
Full list of author information is available at the end of the article

(Continued from previous page)

Keywords: Anticholinergic burden, Comorbidity index, CIRS-G, Overactive bladder, Elderly patients, Trospium chloride, Non-interventional study

Background

Trospium chloride, a synthetic quaternary antimuscarinic, is intended for symptomatic treatment of the overactive bladder syndrome, providing patients with a fast, reliable and considerable improvement or cure of the stressful symptoms: urinary incontinence, urgency and frequency [1–6]. The recommended daily dose is 45 mg TC (3 × 15 mg).[1] It is adequate for most patients with OAB. Flexible dosing up to daily doses of 90 mg TC is safe and well tolerated, permitting treatment to be tailored to the patient's optimal individual balance between efficacy and side effects [1, 7–9].

Increasing attention is paid to safety and compliance concerns, as older people show an increased prevalence of gradually declining human organ and body functions, resulting in physical, physiological and/or cognitive impairments, multi- and co-morbidities, and/or frailty [10]. They are exposed to an increasing number of medications (polypharmacy), often with known or unknown anticholinergic activity, including prescriptions and over-the-counter products [10, 11]. Estimates suggest that one third to half of commonly prescribed drugs for the elderly have anticholinergic properties [12]. Due to the pattern of receptor distribution and their mechanisms of action, anticholinergic drugs as well as many other drugs not usually denoted as anticholinergics, show their anticholinergic activity throughout the human body. This is often associated with a variety of adverse effects (AEs). The most common are peripheral AEs, such as dry mouth, blurred vision, constipation, and tachycardia, as well as central nervous system (CNS) AEs, including dizziness, sedation, falls, confusion, delirium and cognitive impairment [12–20]. These can, in turn, further worsen patient's mental and physical health status, often leading to dependence [21]. On the other hand, OAB is a common yet disabling condition with a considerably negative impact on the patient's quality of life, sleep, sexual function, work productivity and general mental health [11, 22–24]. Therefore, it is often associated with a significant increase in troublesome symptoms and comorbidities in those patients, such as falls, urinary tract infections, hypertension, diabetes [25–27], as well as higher odds for loneliness and depression [26, 28–30]. The causal relationship between many of these comorbid conditions as well as the question whether treatment of one condition improves or

exacerbates the other have thus far largely remained unclear [26]. Nevertheless, muscarinic receptor antagonists are universally accepted to be the first-line pharmacotherapy of OAB [31, 32].

Physicians prescribe drugs with primary or secondary anticholinergic properties based on their anticipated therapeutic benefits. Herein, they sometimes overlook that the concurrent use of several drugs with anticholinergic properties likely results in cumulating effects in the vulnerable elderly patients [12, 15, 21, 33]. This so-called anticholinergic burden (or anticholinergic load) can adversely impact both cognitive and functional status of patients further. Moreover, elderly individuals are thought to be particularly vulnerable to central nervous system AEs of anticholinergics due to age-associated morphological, biochemical, physiological and pathological changes in the brain [12, 34, 35]. A comprehensive systematic review examining associations between drugs with anticholinergic properties and adverse outcomes in older adults concluded that exposure to certain individual drugs with anticholinergic effects or increased overall anticholinergic exposure may increase the risk of falls, cognitive impairment and all-cause-mortality in these patients [36]. Therefore, physicians should carefully consider medical history and concomitant medications when initiating antimuscarinic treatment of OAB in elderly patients.

Generally, however, on the comorbidities and the baseline anticholinergic burden of OAB patients seen in daily urological practice very little information exists. To address this gap of knowledge, we included an epidemiological survey on these two issues in a non-interventional study (NIS) assessing treatment responses and tolerability to TC administered according to current routine treatment schemes in a diverse population of OAB outpatients. Evaluating the ease of subdivision of the SNAP-TAB tablet preparation, containing 45 mg of TC, by the elderly participants was a further objective of this study.

Methods

Study design

This open, prospective, observational study was conducted in 162 urology practices in Germany between November 2014 and October 2015. The number of patients that could be recruited by a single centre was limited to 10 to ensure that the data was not predominantly generated by few large practices, which could jeopardize the representativeness of the sample. The selection and number of study centres was set as is to reflect the most representative picture of "medical practice" in Germany possible. Regarding the data to be gathered in the epidemiological part of the study, 1250 patients were to be recruited into this study to obtain a final sample size of approximately 1000 patients for the analysis of epidemiological research questions. The TC therapy was prescribed by the participating urologists in the course of normal outpatient care, was commercially available and funded according to local practice in usual routine care. The study protocol, therefore, did not contain any specifications regarding dosing of TC or duration of treatment. Instead, the advising urologists were asked to follow the recommendations defined in the licensed approval by the national regulatory authorities. The contraindications, special warnings, precautions for use, interactions, information on use during pregnancy and lactation, effects on ability to drive and use machines, as well as undesirable effects specified in the Summary of Product Characteristics (SmPC) had to be observed.

Compliance with ethics

This post-registration trial conforms with § 67(6) of the German Drug Law. All procedures were carried out in accordance with the official recommendations regarding the conduct of non-interventional studies by the Federal Institute for Drugs and Medical Devices (BfArM) and the Paul-Ehrlich-Institute [37], and the recommendations for assuring Good Epidemiological Practice [38]. Accordingly, the study was notified to the federal authority and the relevant associations. Approval of an ethical committee was not required for such a non-interventional trial in Germany [§67(6) of the German Drug Law]. Nevertheless, the study protocol was submitted to the Ethics Committee of the Medical Chamber Westphalia-Lippe and the Westphalian Wilhelm University Münster, Germany, which gave a favourable recommendation prior to the start of the study (September 2014). All data and information collected in the scope of this study was gathered in accordance with the recommendations for baseline diagnosis specified in the AWMF Guideline No. 084/001 *Urinary Incontinence*, published by the German Geriatric Society [39]. The study was performed within the indication approved in the marketing authorization and under consideration of the contraindications and precautions defined therein [40]. Each physician had to decide on the OAB-therapy independently from the assignment of a patient's inclusion into the study. Patients were admitted only after they had given their written consent to the data protection policy at the first visit. Participants were free to withdraw at will at any time without giving

reasons and without incurring disadvantages. Documentation of study-related data of each patient was performed solely in accordance with routine urological assessments.

Patients and treatment

Elderly men and women (≥ 65 years of age) with symptoms of OAB for whom the attending urologist had decided to prescribe a TC preparation containing 45 mg active agent per tablet (Spasmex® 45 mg film-coated tablets) were included in this trial. Consistent with the non-interventional nature of the study, no further restrictions were applied in respect to the inclusion of patients or to the dose and duration of treatment. The preparation Spasmex® 45 mg is a modern SNAP-TAB tablet designed for easy and precise subdivision [41, 42].

Assessments

Participation in this trial included three visits per patient, defined as first, interim and last visit (= Visit 1, 2, 3), with a recommended minimum interval between visits of 10 days. The minimum duration of treatment was recommended to be no less than 6 weeks.

At Visit 1, patients were questioned regarding their comorbidities and their anticholinergic burden, using established scales and questionnaires. The Anticholinergic Cognitive Burden Scale, adapted to the German market, was selected to measure anticholinergic burden [19, 43, 44]. The level of burden caused by chronic illnesses was assessed using the German version of the Cumulative Illness Rating Scale for Geriatrics, which rates the severity of chronic diseases in 14 organ-specific categories on a five-point scale of 0 to 4 [45]. The illness ratings across all organ categories are subsequently summed up to create the comorbidity index (CMI).

The attending urologists entered the patient's data online via an encrypted website, using a validated German Internet-based input system (portal of MedSurv GmbH, Nidderau, Germany). They collected the following information at the specified time points and/or, if applicable, at the time of premature discontinuation of treatment: demography, medical history, pre-treatment of OAB, anticholinergic burden-related medications contributing to the ACB scale score, concomitant diseases contributing to the baseline CIRS-G score, further relevant comedication, OAB symptoms (number of voids/24 h, number of nocturnal voids/hour sleeping time, severity of urgency symptoms, occurrence and number of incontinence episodes, usual amount of urine leakage), prescribed dose and timing of administration of TC 45 mg, any adverse events as well as premature treatment termination. At Visits 2 and 3, physicians and patients were asked to assess effectiveness and tolerability of therapy using the following four categories: very good, good, poor, very poor. Additionally, at Visit 3 or time of premature discontinuation of treatment the investigator queried the patient to rate the ease of subdivision of the SNAP-TAB tablets on a four-point scale with the categories: very easy, easy, somewhat difficult, very difficult.

Data management and statistics

The validity of the anonymized submission data was checked for plausibility and completeness. Missing data on patient and physician assessments of treatment efficacy and tolerability and variables describing OAB symptoms at the last visit was replaced by the corresponding data collected at the interim visit in cases where the time difference between the first and the interim visit was at least 10 days. Adverse events were classified using the MedDRA coding system V19.1.

Transformation, preparation and exploratory analyses of data were carried out using the statistical software package SAS® V9.3 and 9.4, respectively. Since direct calculation of the exact confidence interval of the median was not possible with SAS, it was done using the DescTools package in R-version 3.3.1. The IML module was used to call R from SAS.

Data was analysed using descriptive statistical methods. The distributions of the qualitative and discrete quantitative variables were described in terms of absolute and relative frequencies based on sample size of the respective collective and were presented by three age classes and gender separately, and globally for all patients. The distributions of the continuous variables and quantitative discrete variables with a lot of values were described by sample size, number of missing values, minimum, 1. quartile (Q1), median, 3. quartile (Q3), maximum, and confidence interval (CI) of the median.

To answer the epidemiological research questions, we used logistic regression methods. Since the target variable, the ACB scale score, was extremely skewed to the right, we divided the variable "ACB score" into two classes (ACB = 0 and ACB > 0) before evaluating the data. Since a linear influence of age and CIRS-G score-derived comorbidity index on the probability of the presence of an anticholinergic burden could also not be assumed, the explanatory variable "age" was divided into three classes (65 years to < 75 years, 75 years to < 85 years, and ≥ 85 years), and the explanatory variable "comorbidity index" was divided into four quartile classes (0–2, 3–4, 5–7, and ≥ 8). Effects of the potential effect modifiers age, gender and CIRS-G derived comorbidity index as a measure of the number of health problems were then studied using logistic regression. Because the comorbidity index was also extremely right-skewed, we also transformed this index into a dichotomous variable (≤ 4 versus > 4) when handling the age–/gender-related question to the presence of comorbidity burden.

Efficacy outcomes were evaluated by change in the quantitative variables describing OAB symptoms which was defined as the score difference between the respective variable at Visit 1 and by using a new target variable constructed using the combined data from Visits 3 and 2 (last evaluable Visit minus Visit 1).

Post hoc subgroup analysis

After the statistical analysis was finished as laid down in the study protocol, a subgroup of the efficacy analysis set (n = 385 patients) consisting of two treatment groups according to the dosage regime "1 times a day 45 mg of TC" (n = 90 patients) or "3 times a day 15 mg of TC" (n = 295 patients) documented over the whole treatment period, was used to compare treatment outcomes in relation to the two administration schemes (Fig. 1). All analyses were descriptive and explorative in nature.

For between-group comparisons relating the main variables, we used effect size measures for evaluating the strength of the observed result. We calculated *Cohen's r* for the median *change of average number of voids/24 h between Visit 1 and the last evaluable visit*; and *Cramér's V* for the *combination in the occurrence of incontinence episodes at Visit 1 to the last evaluable visit*, as well as for the assessments of efficacy and tolerability by physicians and patients. For facilitating the interpretation of effect sizes, we used the defined reference values by Cohen [46] and Ellis [47].

Results

Participants

All 1007 recruited participants, including one patient who had been treated before the start of the study and whose data had been submitted retroactively, were included in the safety analysis. In accordance with the study protocol, data sets from 986 patients were available for the epidemiological analysis, and 774 were available for the efficacy analysis (Fig. 1).

Epidemiological population and research-related characteristics

Out of the 986 patients, 564 (57.2%) were women and 422 (42.8%) were men (Table 1). The median age in this population was 75.0 years (range: 65–97; Q1: 70.0, Q3: 79.0) with equal distributions by gender (Hodges-Lehmann estimator: 1 year, 95% CI: [0 years, 2 years]).

At Visit 1, data of 936 patients was analysed and scored on the ACB scale. Overall, 491 (52.46%) patients in the epidemiological population were not taking any drugs with potential anticholinergic effects, as reflected by an ACB scale score of 0; while 445 patients (47.54%; 95% CI [44.30%; 50.80%]) of all patients with evaluable ACB score data at Visit 1 had a baseline anticholinergic burden, as defined as an ACB scale score of > 0 (Fig. 2).

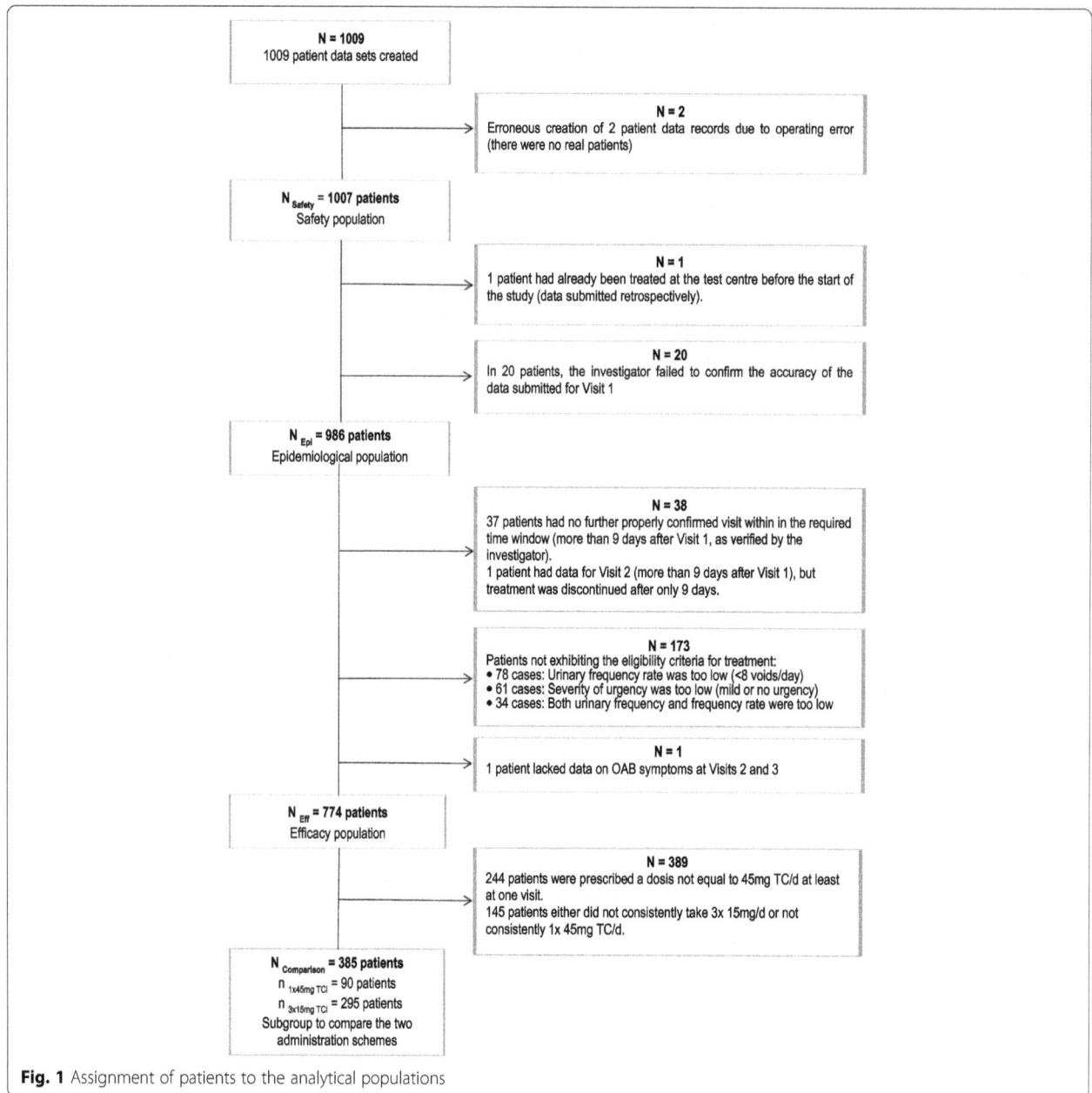

Fig. 1 Assignment of patients to the analytical populations

Table 1 Epidemiological population: Frequency distribution of age classes at the first visit, by sex, and globally

Sex	Patient age at Visit 1 (3 classes)						Total
	65 years to < 75 years		75 years to < 85 years		≥ 85 years		
	n	%	n	%	n	%	N
Female	281	49.82	239	42.38	44	7.80	564
Male	184	43.60	192	45.50	46	10.90	422
All patients	465	47.16	431	43.71	90	9.13	986

The total number of ACB-related drugs taken by the participants was 657. Of them, 479 (72.91%) had an ACB score of 1, 115 (17.50%) had a score of 2, and 63 (9.59%) were anticholinergics with an ACB score of 3. The most commonly used anticholinergic medication was metoprolol ($n = 159$), followed by TC ($n = 101$) and furosemide ($n = 66$).

The median comorbidity index, as calculated from the CIRS-G data for all patients of the epidemiological population, was 5 (exact 95% CI [4.0%; 5.0%]; sum of items 1–14, observed range 0–33), with 52.03% (513/986) of patients observed with a CMI of > 4. Most patients (837/986, 84.89%) did not have any relevant

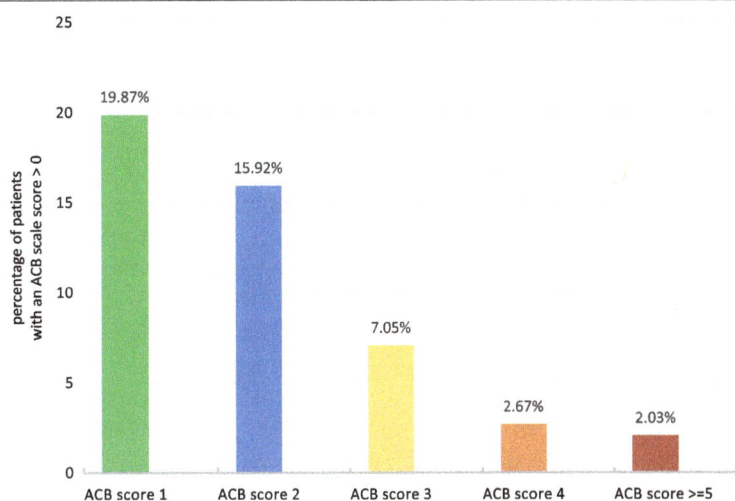

Fig. 2 Frequency distribution of patients with an ACB scale score > 0 at baseline (*n* = 445). The percent data refer to 936 patients of the epidemiological population. An ACB scale score of ≥3 was considered clinically relevant [19]

somatic morbidity (RSM, number of items with a rating of 3 or 4, except for psychiatric disorders = 0), 11.16% of patients (110/986) had a RSM of 1, 3.25% (32/986) a RSM of 2, and 0.71% (7/986) a RSM score between 3 and, at maximum, 5.

The data analysis of possible effect modifiers for the ACB score indicated that the chances of having an anticholinergic burden (ACB > 0) might be higher in patients aged ≥85 years and seemed to be higher in men than in women; additionally, the odds of having an anticholinergic burden seemed to increase with an increasing CMI (Table 2). Similarly, regarding the CIRS-G score-related comorbidity index in this population, the occurrence of having a CMI of > 4 seemed to increase with increasing age and women might have a lower likelihood than men.

Evaluation of efficacy

The population of the efficacy analysis set comprised 774 patients, 456 women and 318 men, with a median age of 75.0 years (range: 65–97; Q1: 70.0, Q3: 79.0) and equal distributions by sex (Hodges-Lehmann estimator for the difference between the location: 1 year, 95% CI: [0 years, 2 years]).

At study entry, 256 out of 764 patients (33.51%) suffered from OAB symptoms for years, 408 patients (53.40%) for months, and 100 patients (13.09%) reported symptoms occurring during the last weeks or days. 34.37% (266/774) of patients had received medical pre-treatment for their OAB syndrome; most frequently used drugs were anticholinergics (62.41%) and herbal drugs for urological disorders (11.28%). The reasons for switching of medication were "insufficient efficacy" in

Table 2 Epidemiological population: Effects of age and sex on ACB score and CMI

Effect	Category of interest versus reference category	Point estimate of the odds ratio	95% confidence interval (Wald's type)
A. Effects of age, gender and/or CIRS-G score-related comorbidity index on ACB score			
Sex	Female vs. male	0.72	[0.55; 0.94]
Age class	75 years to < 85 years vs. 65 years to < 75 years	1.13	[0.85; 1.50]
	≥ 85 years vs. 65 years to < 75 years	1.79	[1.08; 2.94]
CMI (4 classes)	Quartile 2 CMI 3–4 vs. Quartile 1 CMI 0–2	1.69	[1.13; 2.52]
	Quartile 3 CMI 5–7 vs. Quartile 1 CMI 0–2	2.03	[1.38; 2.99]
	Quartile 4 CMI ≥ 8 vs. Quartile 1 CMI 0–2	3.29	[2.23; 4.86]
B. Effects of age and/or gender on the comorbidity index			
Sex	Female vs. male	0.57	[0.44; 0.74]
Age class	75 years to < 85 years vs. 65 years to < 75 years	2.28	[1.74; 2.99]
	≥ 85 years vs. 65 years to < 75 years	2.79	[1.73; 4.51]

Odds ratio point estimates and confidence intervals calculated by comparing the respective category of interest with the reference category for the possible explanatory variables included in the model for the likelihood of having an anticholinergic burden (A) or a comorbidity index of > 4 (B)

221 out of 267 cases (82.77%) and "lack of tolerance" in 31 cases (11.61%).

At Visit 1, 78.55% (608/774) of patients were instructed to take a daily dose of 45 mg TC (Fig. 3). Of them, 60.03% (365/608) took the prescribed dose by dividing the SNAP-TAB tablet in three equal parts corresponding to 15 mg of TC each, to be taken in the morning, noon and night; 19.41% (118/608) took the whole 45 mg tablet as a single daily dose, and 20.56% (125/608) divided the tablet in two doses, one of 30 mg and one of 15 mg of TC.

At Visit 2, the physician decided on the patient's individual response to treatment whether a dose adjustment and/or a change in dosage regimen was necessary or not. In 81.61% (630/772) of patients, the prescribed daily dose remained unchanged (Fig. 4).

The median treatment period documented at the last evaluable visit ($n = 774$) was 64 days (min = 10 (predefined), max = 325; Q1: 46, Q3: 98). Treatment with TC improved symptoms of OAB as evaluated by before-and-after comparisons of different variables. The median change in the average *number of voids per 24 h*, as calculated by subtracting the outcome for Visit 1 from that for the last evaluable Visit, was – 4 (Q1: -6, Q3: -2; exact 95% CI [– 4 voids/24 h; – 4 voids/24 h]) for all patients included in the efficacy population (n = 774). The data analysis by logistic regression indicated that women were more likely to have a ≥ 4-void reduction in the average number of voids per 24 h than men (female vs. men: point estimate of the odds ratio (OR) 1.41, 95% $CI_{Wald's\ type}$ [1.05; 1.91]). Moreover, patients aged ≥75 years to < 85 years seemed to have a lower chance to experience this improvement than patients aged ≥65 years to < 75 years: OR 0.71 (95% $CI_{Wald's\ type}$ [0.52; 0.97]). The median change in the average *number of nocturnal voids/hour sleeping time in the last 7 days* was – 0.3 (Q1: -0.4, Q3: -0.1; $n = 769$). Under treatment, the *severity of urgency symptoms* decreased in 655 (84.63%, 95% CI [81.89%; 87.10%]) out of 774 patients.

38.50% (298/774) of the patients included in the efficacy analysis did not have any incontinence episodes by the time of the first and the last visit. Improvement in the *occurrence of incontinence episodes* was observed in 231 (29.84%, 95% CI [26.64%; 33.21%]) out of 774 individuals, 528 (68.22%) showed no change, and 15 (1.94%) reported worsening of accident occurrence. The *number of incontinence episodes* in this population ($n = 470$) decreased by a median of 5 incontinence episodes (Q1: -10, Q3: -2; 95% CI [– 5.0; – 4.0]). Six further patients confirmed the occurrence of incontinence episodes in the last 7 days before the respective visit but did not provide valid data describing the number of incontinence episodes or the amount of urine leakage. In 349 cases (74.26%) the *amount of urine leakage* decreased from Visit 1 to the last evaluable visit.

The post hoc subgroup analysis did not indicate a difference in treatment outcome between the two dosage regimens "1 x 45 mg TC/day" and "3 x 15 mg TC/day" for any of the efficacy variables. This was also obvious from the effect size measures relating to the variables, with *Cohen's r* = 0.103 for the median *change in the number of voids/24 h between Visit 1 and the last evaluable visit*, and *Cramér's V* = 0.050 for the *combination in the occurrence of incontinence episodes at Visit 1 to the last evaluable visit*. As the effect size of any variable was < 0.1 or only marginally greater than 0.1, this had to be considered a trivial effect in accordance with the conventions by Cohen [46] and Ellis [47].

Global assessment of effectiveness and tolerability

At the last evaluable visit, 91.21% of the physicians (706/774) assessed the effectiveness of the OAB treatment with TC 45 mg tablet as either "very good" or "good", as did 89.53% of patients (693/774). The question relating to therapy continuation with 45 mg of TC was answered affirmatively for 672 patients (89.36%); 57 patients (7.58%) required no further treatment and 23 (3.06%) were switched to another treatment modality.

Tolerability was assessed predominantly "very good" or "good" by 94.32% (730/774) of the physicians and by 90.96% (704/774) of the patients.

This trend was also observed in the post hoc analysis regarding the global assessment of effectiveness and tolerability across the two analysed dosage regimens; effectiveness: physicians – *Cramér's V* = 0.122, patients – *Cramér's V* = 0.161; tolerability: physicians – *Cramér's V* = 0.075, patients – *Cramér's V* = 0.107. Based on the reference values for effect size measures by Ellis [47], this

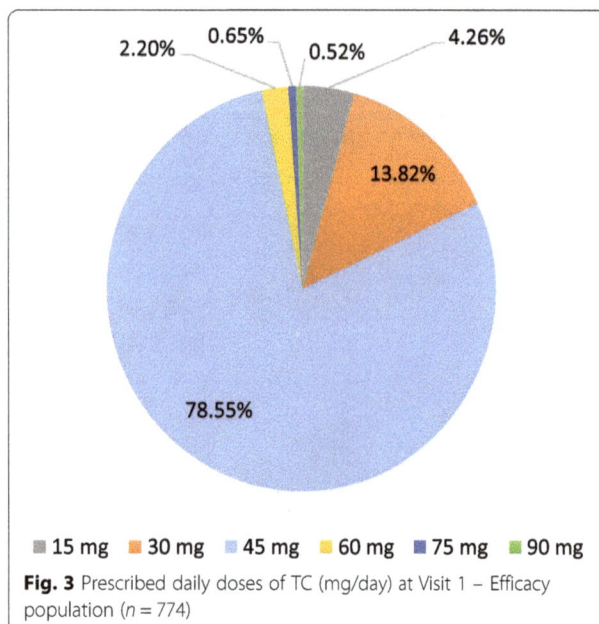

Fig. 3 Prescribed daily doses of TC (mg/day) at Visit 1 – Efficacy population (n = 774)

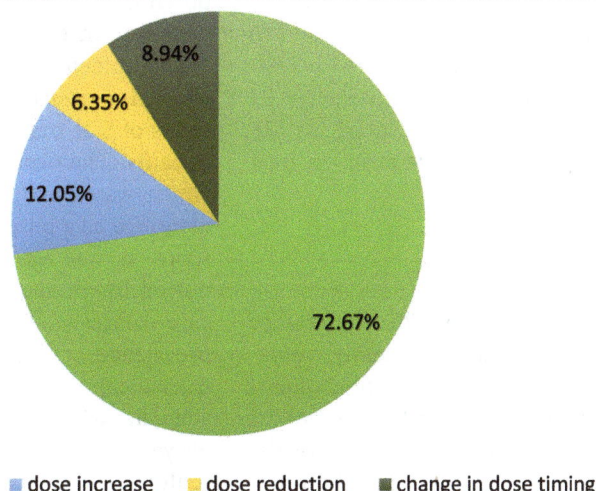

Fig. 4 Changes in dose or dosage regimen at Visit 2 (*n* = 772/774) – Efficacy population

indicated that the observed effect differences between the two treatment regimens were either irrelevant or very small at maximum.

Ease of subdivision analysis

The distribution of this variable is shown by age classes in Fig. 5. Since only 12.01% (91/758) of the patients rated the ease of subdivision as "difficult to divide" or "very difficult to divide", we constructed a new variable for the analysis by combining these two categories into one category and the other two categories ("very easy to divide" and "easy to divide") into a second. 87.99% (667/758; 95% CI [85.47%; 90.22%]) of the study participants (≥ 65 years of age) rated the ease of subdivision of the SNAP-TAB tablet into three equal parts as "very easy or easy to divide". An influence of age or gender of patients on the relative frequency at which the ease of

subdivision was rated like this could not be observed ($p_{Likelihood\ ratio}$ = 0.127).

Therapy withdrawals and adverse events

Treatment with TC was prematurely terminated in 44 (4.37%) out of 1007 patients recruited. The most common reason for withdrawal was "adverse event" (43.18%) followed by "lack of efficacy" (22.73%).

Overall, the attending physicians documented a total of 110 adverse events in 75 (7.45%) patients of the safety population; 82.72% of these were well-known side effects of TC listed in the SmPC. The most frequently reported AEs were dry mouth (4.87%) and constipation (1.49%). All other documented AEs occurred at a frequency of ≤0.5%. One serious AE was reported (postrenal failure), of which the causality to the study drug was assessed by the physician as unlikely. An at least possible causal

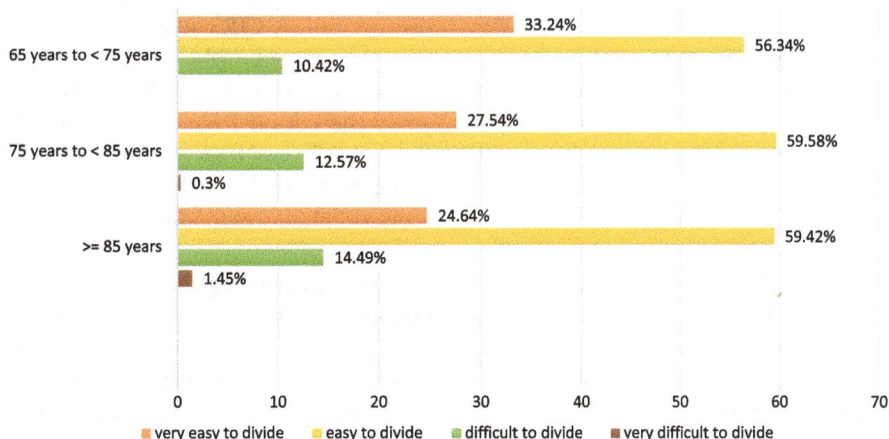

Fig. 5 Ease of subdivision analysis (*n* = 758) – Efficacy population. Frequency distribution of the "ease of subdivision rating at Visit 3 or, as applicable, at the time of premature discontinuation of treatment" by age classes

relationship between an AE and TC treatment was considered in 97 cases (88.18%) by the investigator, and in 91 cases (82.27%) by the marketing authorization holder. Treatment with the study drug was discontinued in 32 (29.09%) patients, the dosage was reduced in 16 (14.55%) patients, and no measures were taken to treat the AE in 49 (44.55%) cases.

Discussion

This non-interventional study examined the importance of real-life anticholinergic treatment of elderly outpatients with idiopathic OAB in view of their anticholinergic load and comorbidities, which to our knowledge was not done in any trial before it. The median age of the participants was 75 years; therefore, this population represents the group of adults most frequently affected by the OAB syndrome [13, 27, 48, 49]. 47.54% (445/936) of the elderly in our study were exposed to at least one anticholinergic medication at baseline, as indicated by an ACB scale score of > 0. Thereof 24.72% had an ACB score of ≥3, which is considered by Boustani et al. [19] as clinically relevant. Relating this to the total number of patients in the epidemiological group for which valuable information was available, the percentage of patients with an ACB scale score ≥ 3 was 11.75% (110/936). In a retrospective study of anticholinergic burden in a large cohort of hospitalized geriatric patients (89,579 analysed individuals with a median age of 82 years), 41,456 (46.3%) patients took at least one prescribed anticholinergic drug [50]. Of them, 24,569 (59.3%) had an ACB total score of 1, 5765 (13.9%) a score of 2, and 11,122 (26.8%) a score of 3 or more. Although we observed a population of outpatients in urological practice which is not directly comparable with the hospitalized population in the cohort study, and there is a difference in the median age of the patients in both studies, the magnitude of anticholinergic burden is broadly in line. The observed rate of prescriptions for drugs with anticholinergic properties in our study is also comparable with data from other previous studies, wherein rates vary between 25% in community-dwelling patients to up to 80% in nursing-home residents with cognitive impairments [14, 43, 51].

Several ranked lists have been compiled to assess anticholinergic burden of drugs. The ACB scale identifies the severity of anticholinergic AEs on cognition for many prescribed and over-the-counter medications in a single list [19]. Drugs are rated regarding their anticholinergic burden either through serum anticholinergicactivity or in vitro affinity to muscarinic receptors, and then scored according to their clinical relevance [36]. The study by Pasina et al. [21] found that the ACB scale might help to rapidly identify drugs potentially associated with cognitive impairment in a dose-response pattern.

The epidemiological survey in our study additionally showed a median CIRS-G score-based CMI for all patients of 5 at baseline, and a CMI of > 4 in 52.03% of all patients. The occurrence of a higher comorbidity index, which was found to increase with increasing age, was identified as a potential effect modifier for the ACB scale score, as was age of ≥85 years. These results are supported by an analysis of a large representative primary care dataset (1,751,841 patients) which showed that the prevalence of multimorbidity, defined in this study as the concomitant presence of ≥2 illnesses, increased substantially with age and was present in most people aged 65 years or older [52]. The percentage of subjects with multimorbidity was 64.9% (95% CI [64.7%, 65.1%]) in the group of 65–84 years olds compared to 81.5% (95% CI [81.1%, 81.9%]) in the group of ≥85 years olds. Laux et al. [53] observed a strong correlation between age, gender, multimorbidity (co-occurrence of ≥2 chronic diseases) and health care utilization in the context of the German CONTENT project, analysing the data from 39,699 patients. They discovered that the number of patients' chronic conditions have a significant impact on the number of different prescriptions ($\text{ß} = 0.226$, $P < 0.0001$) as well as on the number of referrals ($\text{ß} = 0.3$, $P < 0.0001$). In the 60–69 years age group, the average number ($\pm$ SE) of different prescriptions per patient was 4.45 ± 0.19 in men and 4.55 ± 0.16 in female, whereas the average number of prescriptions rose to 6.51 ± 0.69 and 6.57 ± 0.24, respectively, in the age group ≥80 years.

Currently, there are no CIRS-G based cut-offs for the illness severity and CMI established [54], making the classification of the observed results difficult. Miller et al. [55] identified a mean ($\pm$ SD) CMI of 4.5 ± 2.5 for a healthy elderly individual with a mean age of 71.1 ± 5.3 years ($n = 35$). In contrast, the total CIRS-G score ($\pm$ SD) was 12.7 ± 4.7 ($n = 76$) for people with Parkinson's disease [56]. A CIRS score of ≤6 is used to differentiate between patients who are eligible for intensive chemoimmunotherapy and those who are not [57]. If we apply the cut-off from Miller et al. [55] to our results, then slightly less than half (47.97%) of the study participants in the epidemiological group (473/986) had a CMI score of ≤4, corresponding with that of a healthy elderly subject.

Since anticholinergic activity affects both central and peripheral systems, these drugs are indicated in a wide spectrum of conditions. Multimorbidity and polypharmacy increase the cumulative anticholinergic burden and thus the risk for side effects, including the well-known risk for neurodegenerative disorders [12, 13, 19, 20, 35, 58, 59]. Apart from age-associated changes in pharmacokinetic and pharmacodynamic properties, elderly people may also be more sensitive to anticholinergic effects in the central nervous system because of age-related physiological and pathological changes at the brain [20, 34, 35]. An American population-based study in 12,423 men and women even showed that, comparable to the percentage of anticholinergic users in our study, 47% of the elders (≥ 65 years) used a medication with possible anticholinergic properties, which increased the cumulative risk of cognitive decline and mortality over 2 years in participants with normal or mildly impaired cognition at baseline [18]. Risacher et al. [60] observed that cognitively normal older adults (n = 402) taking medications with medium or high anticholinergic activity showed poorer memory and executive function, reduced cerebral glucose metabolism, whole-brain and temporal lobe atrophy, and increased clinical decline compared with non-users; these symptoms were most severe in those with the highest total anticholinergic burden scores. Using data from a well-established prospective cohort study, Chuang et al. [61] discovered that exposure to medications with mild anticholinergic activity in midlife is associated with greater risk of Alzheimer's disease and accelerated brain atrophy before cognitive impairment. In a population-based, longitudinal study of individuals 65 years or older, higher cumulative use of anticholinergics was associated with an increased risk for all-cause dementia and Alzheimer's disease [14]. In the cohort study by Pfistermeister et al. [50], anticholinergic drugs with an ACB score of 3 clearly contributed most to the patients' overall anticholinergic load for all patients having ACB total scores of ≥3. They further found a high anticholinergic burden to be associated with patients with severe cognitive impairment.

In contrast to all tertiary amines indicated in OAB, brain penetration of TC is highly restricted by the molecule's polar structure and its low lipophilicity, as well as by a P-glycoprotein mediated efflux in the endothelial cells of the blood-brain-barrier (BBB) [62, 63]; in a mouse model, TC permeation across the BBB was not increased with ageing [64]. A recent randomized placebo-controlled clinical study in 59 women aged 50 years and older being treated for OAB with 60 mg of TC per day for 4 weeks, measured no changes in cognitive function between the TC group and the placebo group [65]. Previous clinical studies investigating different indicators for cognitive function and neuropsychological effects, including electroencephalogram and sleep studies, have proven that TC is largely free of CNS effects [66–74]. The drug may therefore provide an effective approach to treating OAB without increasing the patient's central nervous anticholinergic burden.

This is also supported by the nature and the low frequency of AEs in our study. All documented AEs with an at least causal relationship are well-known side effects of oral TC. In general, TC was well tolerated which is reflected by the subjective assessments of physicians and patients. An observational study of TC 30 mg film-coated tablets in 4092 patients with OAB symptoms achieved comparable results: its tolerability was rated as "very good" or "good" by physicians in 90.2% of cases, and by patients in 87.1% [9].

The relevant changes in characteristic OAB symptoms, observed in the present trial after a median treatment period of 64 days and determined by before-after-comparisons of different variables, indicated that an oral dose of 45 mg TC per day is a potent treatment strategy, providing patients pronounced improvement or cure of the most bothersome symptoms of OAB. This has previously been proven in a previous 12-week, randomised, double-blind, phase IIIb study in 1658 patients with urinary urge incontinence evaluating the efficacy and tolerability of TC which demonstrated that urinary frequency and urge incontinence can be reduced significantly through a flexible dosing strategy [1, 7]. It has further been shown that these clinical effects are associated with improvements in several areas of health-related quality of life of those patients, suggesting a real clinically and personally relevant treatment success [1].

The majority of the patients in our trial (78.55%) - as in the preceding clinical study – were using the approved dose of 45 mg (3 × 15 mg) TC daily, which is defined in the current SmPC [75]. The flexible dosing strategy in our study allowed the physician together with the patient to decide at Visit 2 whether to increase, decrease or maintain the starting dose, or switch to another dosage regimen, until the end of the treatment period. 81.61% (630/772) of patients did not change their initial prescribed daily dose, and only 8.94% (69/772) of patients switched to another dosage regimen. This confirmed that a daily dose of 45 mg of TC is adequate for most patients with idiopathic OAB. This conclusion is supported further by the favourable assessment of efficacy by both the urologists and the patients, as well as the fact that the physicians answered the question relating to therapy continuation affirmatively for 672 out of 752 patients (89.36%) after the observational period. Pooled data from three non-interventional studies in a total of 9366 patients showed that flexible dosing of TC is commonly used in urological practice in Germany [76].

The post hoc analysis in our study, regarding the two dosage schemes "1 x 45 mg TC/day" and "3 x 15 mg TC/day", did not indicate a difference in clinical outcome for any of the variables. As was further shown in the present study, the SNAP-TAB tablet can be easily divided in three equal units, thereby providing a patient-friendly option in flexible drug dosing. This way of administration simplifies the optimal treatment with TC which should be individualised considering the patient's comorbidities and comedications, especially in the elderly, and based on the patient's individual responses to treatment, to ensure an optimal balance between efficacy and tolerability [1, 7–10]. Thus, in turn, it supports close patient adherence and persistence to treatment [76].

Due to its non-interventional and observational character the current trial has distinct advantages and disadvantages associated with it. Limitations are the heterogeneity of participants, the variable dosage regimen and the lack of a comparator group, such as tertiary amines. It must be noted that the epidemiological population in our NIS consisted only of elderly patients (although they account for most patients). While the urologists that attended asked follow-up questions (queries), the possibility that the ACB score data reported by the physicians may have been partly incomplete cannot be ruled out. Missing data for the efficacy analysis was handled by replacing missing values with the corresponding values documented at the last evaluable visit (Last-Observation-Carried-Forward method). Only those patients with evaluable data for the first and last visit and minimum of ≥10 days between the two visits were included in the sensitivity analysis for the variable of interest. This decreased the sample size by approximately 3%. Furthermore, the analysis of the data collected in this NIS and the interpretation of the results could solely be carried out in a descriptive manner.

On the plus side, our study follows national and international recommendations dealing with quality aspects of NIS. With its safety population of 1007 elderly patients and 162 attended urologists nationwide, it comprises a cross-section of the typical population of patients treated for symptoms of idiopathic OAB in daily practice. The open observational scenario highly reflects common use of the study drug. Moreover, the validated instruments, the ACB score and the German version of the CIRS-G scale, used in this NIS cover relevant epidemiological aspects related to the representative patient population. The NIS can therefore be a scientific instrument that completes the results of randomized controlled studies by contributing important data on the use of the drug in real-life practice, for example on medical prescription, dosage recommendations, patients' compliance, and on safety aspects [77]. The evaluation and demonstration of the adequate patient acceptability of a medicinal product is also presented as a major issue in the EMA Reflection Paper on the Pharmaceutical Development of Medicines for Use in the Older Population [10].

Conclusions

This NIS focussed on less-known epidemiological issues relating to comorbid conditions and anticholinergic burden from concomitant medications when treating idiopathic OAB. It adds evidence from daily therapeutically practice supporting the favourable benefit-risk profile of TC as reported from the randomized controlled trials. The use of the SNAP-TAB tablet containing 45 mg of TC was shown to be an effective, safe and easy to manage new type of drug administration that facilitates flexible dosing of TC to achieve the optimal patient-related balance between efficacy and tolerability in real-life practice.

Endnotes

[1]Trademark: *Spasmex®* 45 mg film-coated immediate-release tablets (Dr. R. Pfleger GmbH, Bamberg, Germany)

Abbreviations

ACB: Anticholinergic burden; AE(s): Adverse event(s); AWMF: Arbeitsgemeinschaft der Wissenschaftlichen Medizinischen Fachgesellschaften (Association of the Scientific Medical); BBB: Blood-brain-barrier; BfArM: Federal Institute for Drugs and Medical Devices; CI: Confidence interval; CIRS-G: Cumulative Illness Rating Scale for Geriatrics; CMI: Comorbidity index; CNS: Central nervous system; DRKS: German Register of Clinical Studies; EMA: European Medicines Agency; MedDRA: Medical Dictionary for Regulatory Activities; NIS: Non-interventional study; OAB: Overactive bladder; OR: Odds ratio; Q1/Q3: 1. quartile / 3. quartile; RSM: Relevant somatic morbidity; SmPc: Summary of Product characteristics; TC: Trospium chloride

Acknowledgements

Medical writing support was provided by Petra Schwantes, BioMedical Services, Germany.

Authors' contributions

All authors were involved in the study conception and project coordination. RHB was responsible for the statistical analysis. RHB, AI and AW were involved in the interpretation of data. CN and RHB wrote the study protocol and the study report. All authors read and approved the final manuscript.

Ethics approval and consent to participate

All procedures performed in this study were in accordance with the German Drug Law, with the joint recommendations of the Federal Institute for Drugs and Medical Devices (BfArM) and the Paul-Ehrlich-Institute relating to the conduct of non-interventional trials [37], and with the recommendations for assuring Good Epidemiological Practice [38]. Written informed consent regarding data protection was obtained from all patients before being included in the study. The Ethics Committee of the Medical Chamber Westphalia-Lippe and the Westphalian Wilhelm University Münster, Germany, approved the study protocol. This decision was provided to each urologist within the regulatory jurisdiction of the Ethics Committee. No further Ethics Committee was involved as ethics approval in general was not mandatory and all participating urologists were satisfied with the vote of the Ethics Committee of the Medical Chamber Westphalia-Lippe and Westphalian Wilhelm University Münster.This NIS was registered with the number DRKS00007109 at the German Register of Clinical Studies (DRKS) on October 29, 2014.

Author details

[1]Department of Urology, Evangelisches KrankenhausWitten gGmbH, UniversityWitten/Herdecke, Pferdebachstrasse 27, 58455 Witten, Germany. [2]Department of Statistics, Institute of Medical Informatics, University Clinic Giessen, Rudolf-Buchheim-Strasse 6, 35392 Gießen, Germany. [3]Department of Medical Science/Clinical Research, Dr. R. Pfleger GmbH, Dr.-Robert-Pfleger-Strasse 12, 96052 Bamberg, Germany.

References

1. Zellner M, Madersbacher H, Palmtag H, et al, and the P195 Study Group. Trospium chloride and oxybutynin hydrochloride in a German study of adults with urinary urge incontinence: results of a 12-week, multicenter, randomized, double-blind, parallel-group, flexible-dose noninferiority trial. Clin Ther 2009; 31: 2519–2539.

2. Ulshöfer B, Bihr AM, Bödeker RH, et al. Randomised, double-blind, placebo-controlled study on the efficacy and tolerance of trospium chloride in patients with motor urge incontinence. Clin Drug Invest. 2001;21(8):563–9.

3. Cardozo L, Chapple CR, Toozs-Hobson P, et al. Efficacy of trospium chloride in patients with detrusor instability: a placebo-controlled, randomised, double-blind, multicentre clinical trial. BJU. 2000;85:659–64.

4. Alloussi S, Laval KU, Eckert R, et al. Trospium chloride (Spasmo-lyt®) in patients with motor urge syndrome (detrusor instability): a double-blind, randomised, multicentre, placebo-controlled study. J. Clin Res. 1998;1:439–51.

5. Jünemann KP, Füsgen I, Svetlana T. Trospium chloride 40 mg – a placebo-controlled, randomised, double-blind clinical trial on the efficacy and tolerability for 3 weeks in patients with urge-syndrome. Eur Urol. 2000;37:84.

6. Jünemann KP, Füsgen I. Placebo-controlled, randomised, double-blind, multicentre clinical trial on the efficacy and tolerability of 1x40 mg and 2x40 mg trospium chloride (Spasmo-lyt®) daily for 3 weeks in patients with urge-syndrome. Neurourol Urodynam. 1999;18:375–6.

7. Bödeker RH, Madersbacher H, Neumeister C, Zellner M. Dose escalation improves therapeutic outcome: post hoc analysis of data from a 12-week, multicentre, double-blind, parallel-group trial of trospium chloride in patients with urinary urge incontinence. BMC Urol. 2010;10:15.

8. Wiedemann A, Neumann G, Neumeister C, et al. Efficacy and tolerability of add-on trospium chloride in patients with benign prostate syndrome and overactive bladder: a non-interventional trial showing use of flexible dosing. UroToday Int J. 2009;2(2) https://doi.org/10.3834/uij.1944-5784.2009.04.02.

9. Wiedemann A, Kusche W, Neumeister C. Flexible dosing of trospium chloride for the treatment of OAB – results of a non-interventional study in 4,092 patients. The Open Clinical Trials Journal. 2011;3:1–5.

10. EMA/CHMP/QWP/292439/2017 Rev.: 4.0. Reflection paper on the pharmaceutical development of medicines for use in the older population. EMA 18 May 2017. www.ema.europa.eu/docs/en_GB/document_library/Scientific_guideline/2017/08/WC500232782.pdf. Accessed 09-12-2017.

11. Wiedemann A, Füsgen I. Harninkontinenz bei Älteren. © pharma-aktuell Verlagsgruppe GmbH/Geriatrie-Report, Varel. Bamberg, Germany; 2017. (German)

12. Wagg A. The cognitive burden of anticholinergics in the elderly – implications for the treatment of overactive bladder. Eur Urol Rev. 2012; 7(1):42–9.

13. Lenherr SM, Cox L. Cognitive effects of anticholinergics in the geriatric patient population: safety and treatment considerations. Cur Bladder Dysfunct Rep. 2017;12:104–11.

14. Gray SL, Anderson ML, Dublin S, et al. Cumulative use of strong anticholinergics and incident dementia. A prospective cohort study. JAMA Intern Med. 2015;175(3):401–7.

15. Salahudeen MS, Duffull SB, Nishtala PS. Anticholinergic burden quantified by anticholinergic risk scales and adverse outcomes in older people: a systematic review. BMC Geriatr. 2015;15:31.

16. Marcum ZA, Wirtz HS, Pettinger M, et al. Anticholinergic medication use and falls in postmenopausal women: findings from the women's health initiative cohort study. BMC Geriatr. 2016;16:76.

17. Zia A, Kamaruzzaman S, Myint PK, Tan MP. Anticholinergic burden is associated with recurrent and injurious falls in older individuals. Maturitas. 2015; https://doi.org/10.1016/j.maturitas.2015.10.009. Accessed 10-05-2017

18. Fox C, Richardson K, Maidment ID, et al. Anticholinergic medication use and cognitive impairment in the older population: the medical research council cognitive function and ageing study. J Am Geriatr Soc. 2011;59:1477–83.

19. Boustani M, Cambell N, Munger S, et al. Impact of anticholinergics on the aging brain: a review and practical application. Aging Health. 2008;4(3):311–20.

20. Campbell N, Boustani M, Limbil T, et al. The cognitive impact of anticholinergics: a clinical review. Clin Interv Aging. 2009;4:225–33.

21. Pasina L, Djade CD, Lucca U, et al. Association of anticholinergic burden with cognitive and functional status in a cohort of hospitalized elderly: comparison of the anticholinergic cognitive burden scale and anticholinergic risk scale. Drugs Aging. 2013;30:103–12.

22. Kelleher CJ. Economic and social impact of OAB. Eur Urol. 2002;1:11–6.

23. Luscombe FA. Socioeconomic burden of urinary incontinence with focus on overactive bladder and tolterodine treatment. Rev Contemp Pharmacother. 2000;11:43–62.

24. Tubaro A. Defining overactive bladder: epidemiology and burden of disease. Urology. 2004;64(Suppl 6A):2–6.

25. Lua LL, Pathak P, Dandolu V. Comparing anticholinergic persistence and adherence profiles in overactive bladder patients based on gender, obesity, and major anticholinergic agents. Neurourol Urodyn. 2017;36:2123–31.

26. Coyne KS, Wein A, Nicholson S, et al. Comorbidities and personal burden of urgency urinary incontinence: a systematic review. Int J Clin Pract. 2013; 67(10):1015–33.

27. Irwin DE, Milsom I, Hunskaar S, et al. Population-based survey of urinary incontinence, overactive bladder, and other lower urinary tract symptoms in five countries: results of the EPIC study. Eur Urol. 2006;50:1306–15.

28. Stickley A, Santini ZI, Koyanagi A. Urinary incontinence, mental health and loneliness among community-dwelling older adults in Ireland. BMC Urol. 2017;17:29.

29. Lai HH, Shen B, Rawal A, Vetter J. The relationship between depression and overactive bladder/urinary incontinence symptoms in the clinical OAB population. BMC Urol. 2016;16:60.

30. Felde G, Ebbesen MH, Hunskaar S. Anxiety and depression associated with urinary incontinence. A 10-year follow-up study from the Norwegian HUNT study (EPINCONT). Neurourol Urodynam. 2017;36:322–8.

31. Corcos J, Przydacz M, Campeau L, et al. CUA guideline on adult overactive bladder. Can Urol Assoc J. 2017;11(5):E142–73. https://doi.org/10.5489/cuaj.4586. Accessed 09-20-2017

32. Andersson KE, Chapple CR, Cardozo L, et al. Pharmacological treatment of urinary incontinence. In: Abrams P, Cardozo L, Khoury S, Wein A, editors. Incontinence. 4th international consultation on incontinence. UK, Plymouth: Plymouth, Plymbridge Contributors Ltd; 2009. p. 631–700.

33. Lechevallier-Michel N, Molimard M, Dartigues JF, et al. Drugs with anticholinergic properties and cognitive performance in the elderly: results from the PAQUID study. Br J Clin Pharmacol. 2004;59(2):143–51.

34. Erdo F, Denes L, de Lange E. Age-associated physiological and pathological changes at the blood-brain-barrier: a review. J Cereb Blood Flow Metab. 2017;37(I):4–24.

35. Gerretsen P, Pollock BG. Cognitive risks of anticholinergics in the elderly. Aging Health. 2013;9(2):159–66.

36. Ruxton K, Woodman RJ, Mangoni AA. Drugs with anticholinergic effects and cognitive impairment, falls and all-cause mortality in older adults: a systematic review and meta-analysis. Br J Clin Pharmacol. 2015;80(2):209–20.

37. BfArM. Empfehlungen des Bundesinstituts für Arzneimittel und Medizinprodukte und des Paul-Ehrlich-Instituts zur Planung, Durchführung und Auswertung von Anwendungsbeobachtungen. 2010. http://www.bfarm.de/SharedDocs/Bekanntmachungen/DE/Arzneimittel/klinPr/bm-KlinPr-20100707-NichtinterventePr-pdf.pdf?__blob=publicationFile&v=5. Accessed 09-01-2017.

38. Hoffmann W, Latza U, Terschüren C. Leitlinien und Empfehlungen zur Sicherung von Guter Epidemiologischer Praxis (GEP). German: Deutsche Gesellschaft für Epidemiologie (DGEpi); 2008.

39. AWMF. Guideline No. 084/001. Harninkontinenz. German: Leitlinien der Deutschen Gesellschaft für Geriatrie; 2010.

40. Summary of Product Characteristics (SmPC). Spasmex® 45 mg film-coated tablets. Dr. R. Pfleger GmbH. Version 09/2013. www.fachinfo.de.

41. Van Santen E, Barends DM, Frijlink HW. Breaking of scored tablets: a review. Eur J Pharma Biopharm. 2002;53:139–45.

42. Wening K, Breitkreutz J. Oral drug delivery in personalized medicine: unmet needs and novel approaches. Int J Pharm. 2011;404:1–9.

43. Kolanowski A, Fick DM, Campbell J, et al. A preliminary study of anticholinergic burden and relationship to quality of life indicator, engagement in activities, in nursing home residents with dementia. J Am Med Dir Assoc. 2009;10(4):252–7.

44. Lertxundi U, Domingo-Echaburu S, Hernandez R, et al. Expert-based drug list to measure anticholinergic burden: similar names, different results. Psychogeriatrics. 2013;13:17–24.

45. Hock G, Nosper M. Manual CIRS-G. Cumulative Illness Rating Scale. Skala zur kumulierten Bewertung von Erkrankungen. V 2.1, MDK Rheinland-Pfalz 2003. English original paper: a manual of guidelines for scoring the cumulative illness rating scale (CIRS-G), by Miller MD & Towers A. Department of Geriatric Psychiatry, University of Pittsburgh, USA, 1991.

46. Cohen J. Statistical power analysis for the behavioral sciences. 2nd ed. Hillsdale, NJ: L. Erlbaum Associates; 1988.

47. Ellis PD. The essential guide to effect sizes: statistical power, meta-analysis, and the interpretation of research results. Cambridge: Cambridge University Press; 2010.

48. Irwin DE, Kopp ZS, Agatep B, et al. Worldwide prevalence estimates of lower urinary tract symptoms, overactive bladder, urinary incontinence and bladder outlet obstruction. BJU Int. 2011;108:1132–9.

49. Milsom I, Abrams P, Cardozo L, et al. How widespread are the symptoms of an overactive bladder and how are they manages? A population-based prevalence study. BJU Int. 2001;87:760–6.

50. Pfistermeister B, Tümena T, Gaßmann K-G, et al. Anticholinergic burden and cognitive function in a large German cohort of hospitalized geriatric patients. PLoS One. 2017; https://doi.org/10.1371/hournal.pone.0171353.

51. Koyama A, Steinman M, Ensrud K, et al. Long-term cognitive and functional effects of potentially inappropriate medications in older women. J Gerontol A Biol Sci Med Sci. 2014;69(4):423–9.

52. Barnett K, Mercer SW, Norbury M, et al. Epidemiology of multimorbidity and implications for health care, research, and medical education: a cross-sectional study. Lancet. 2012;380:37–43.

53. Laux G, Kuehlein T, Rosemann T, Szecsenyi J. Co- and multimorbidity patterns in primary care based on episodes of care: results from the German CONTENT project. BMC Health Serv Res. 2008;8:14.

54. Salvi F, Miller MD, Grilli A, et al. A manual of guidelines to score the modified cumulative illness rating scale and its validation in acute hospitalized elderly patients. J Am Geriatr Soc. 2008;56:1926–31.

55. Miller MD, Paradis CF, Houck PR, et al. Rating chronic medical illness burden in geropsychiatric practice and research: application of the cumulative illness rating scale. Psychiatry Res. 1992;41:237–48.

56. King LA, Priest KC, Nutt J, et al. Comorbidity and functional mobility in persons with Parkinson's disease. Arch Phys Med Rehabil. 2014;95(11):2152–7.

57. Cramer P. The management of fit, unfit, and high-risk CLL patients. New Evid Oncol. 2014;25:52–7.

58. Ancelin ML, Artero S, Portet F, et al. Non-degenerative mild cognitive impairment in elderly people and use of anticholinergic drugs: longitudinal cohort study. BMJ. 2006;332:455–9.

59. Turnheim K. When drug therapy gets old: pharmacokinetics and pharmacodynamics in the elderly. Exp Gerontol. 2003;38:843–53.

60. Risacher SL, McDonald BC, Tallman EF, et al. Association between anticholinergic medication use and cognition, brain metabolism, and brain atrophy in cognitively normal older adults. JAMA Neurol. 2016; https://doi.org/10.1001/jamaneurol.2016.0580.

61. Chuang Y-F, Elango P, Gonzalez CE, Thambisetty M. Midlife anticholinergic drug use, risk of Alzheimer's disease, and brain atrophy in community-dwelling older adults. Alzheimers Dement Transl Res Clin Intervent. 2017;3:471–9.

62. Geyer J, Gavrilova O, Petzinger E. The role of P-glycoprotein in limiting brain penetration of the peripherally acting anticholinergic overactive bladder drug trospium chloride. Drug Metab Dispos. 2009;37:1371–4.

63. Geyer J, Gavrilova O, Schwantes U. Differences in the brain penetration of the anticholinergic drugs trospium chloride and oxybutynin. UroToday Int J. 2010;3(1) https://doi.org/10.3834/uij.1944-5784.2010.02.12.

64. Kranz J, Petzinger E, Geyer J. Brain penetration of the OAB drug trospium chloride is not increased in aged mice. World J Urol. 2011;31(1):219–24.

65. Geller EJ, Dumond JB, Bowling JM, et al. Effect of trospium chloride on cognitive function in women aged 50 or older: a randomized trial. Female Pelvic Med Reconstr Surg. 2017;23(2):118–23.

66. Pietzko A, Dimpfel W, Schwantes U, Topfmeier P. Influences of trospium chloride and oxybutynin on quantitative EEG in healthy volunteers. Eur J Clin Pharmacol. 1994;47:337–43.

67. Todorova A, Vonderheid-Guth B, Dimpfel W. Effects of tolterodine, trospium chloride, and oxybutynin on the central nervous system. J Clin Pharmacol. 2001;41:636–44.

68. Diefenbach K, Arold G, Wollny A, et al. Effects on sleep of anticholinergics used for overactive bladder treatment in healthy volunteers aged ≥ 50 years. BJU Int. 2005;95(3):346–9.

69. Diefenbach K, Donath F, Maurer A, et al. Randomised, double-blind study of the effects of oxybutynin, tolterodine, trospium chloride and placebo on sleep in healthy young volunteers. Clin Drug Invest. 2003;23(6):395–404.

70. Staskin D, Kay G, Goldman H, et al. Central nervous system penetration and effect on memory: comparison of trospium chloride and oxybutynin in patients with overactive bladder and age-associated memory impairment. Neurourol Urodynam. 2012; https://doi.org/10.1002/nau.

71. Staskin D, Kay G, Tannenbaum C, et al. Trospium chloride has no effect on memory testing and is assay undetectable in the central nervous system of older patients with overactive bladder. Int J Clin Pract. 2010;64(9):1294–300.

72. Staskin D, Kay G, Tannenbaum C, et al. Trospium chloride is undetectable in the older human central nervous system. J Am Geriatr Soc. 2010;58(8):1618–9.

73. Staskin DR, Harnett MD. Effect of trospium chloride on somnolence and sleepiness in patients with overactive bladder. Curr Urol Rep. 2004;5:423–6.

74. Isik AT, Celik T, Bozoglu E, Doruk H. Trospium and cognition in patients with late onset Alzheimer disease. J Nutr Health Aging. 2009; https://doi.org/10.1007/s12603-009-0144-4.

75. Summary of Product Characteristics (SmPC) Spasmex® 45 mg film-coated tablets. Dr. R. Pfleger GmbH. 2017. http://www.fachinfo.de; 014933.pdf. Accessed 11-16-2017.

76. Schwantes U, Grosse J, Wiedemann A. Refractory overactive bladder: a common problem? Int Urogynecol J. 2015;26:1407–14.

77. Von Jeinsen BKJG, Sudhop T. A 1-year cross-sectional analysis of non-interventional post-marketing study protocols submitted to the German Federal Institute for Drugs and Medical Devices (BfArM). Eur J Clin Pharmacol. 2013;69:1453–66.

11

RRM1 predicts clinical outcome of high-and intermediate-risk non-muscle-invasive bladder cancer patients treated with intravesical gemcitabine monotherapy

Zhenxing Yang[1], Bingqiang Fu[2], Luqiang Zhou[1], Jie Xu[1], Ping Hao[3] and Zhenqiang Fang[1*]

Abstract

Background: The expression level of ribonucleotide reductase subunit M1 (RRM1) is closely related to the effect of gemcitabine-based therapy in advanced bladder cancer. However, the value of RRM1 expression in predicting progression-free survival in non-muscle-invasive bladder cancer (NMIBC) patients treated with intravesical gemcitabine chemotherapy has not been elucidated.

Methods: This study randomly assigned 162 patients to either the RRM1-known group or the unknown group. We collected cancer tissues from 81 patients to evaluate the mRNA expression of RRM1 by using liquid chip technology. All patients were diagnosed and then treated with intravesical gemcitabine monotherapy immediately after transurethral resection of the bladder tumour (TURBT).

Results: RRM1 expression was high in 21% (17/81) of patients. The RRM1 mRNA level was not correlated with sex, age, weight, performance status, or CUA/EAU risk ($p > 0.05$). Progression-free survival (PFS) was significantly longer for patients with low RRM1 expression than for patients with high and unknown RRM1 expression ($p = 0.009$). Additionally, the 1- and 2-year relapse rates also differed according to RRM1 expression level. The 1-year relapse rates for RRM1-low, RRM1-high and RRM1-unknown patients were 0, 17.7 and 6.2% ($p = 0.009$), while the 2-year relapse rates for these groups were 3.1, 29.4, and 11.1% ($p = 0.005$), respectively.

Conclusions: This preliminary study showed that low RRM1 expression was associated with longer progression-free survival and lower 1-year/2-year relapse rates in NMIBC patients treated with intravesical gemcitabine monotherapy, despite the need for further verification with large sample sizes and considering more mixed factors and biases.

Keywords: RRM1, Non-muscle-invasive bladder cancer, Gemcitabine

Background

Bladder tumours represent the ninth most prevalent malignancy in China, and they were responsible for an estimated 32,900 deaths in 2015 [1]. Approximately 70% of all bladder carcinomas are first diagnosed as non-muscle-invasive bladder cancer (NMIBC), including tumours of any grade at stages pTa, pT1, or carcinoma in situ (CIS) [2]. Unlike its muscle-invasive counterpart, NMIBC typically has a good prognosis. The EAU guidelines define NMIBC patients as low, intermediate, or high risk for recurrence (based upon stage, grade, tumour size, and multifocality) [3]. Patients with higher progression scores are more likely to progress to muscle invasion within 5 years. Transurethral resection of the bladder tumour (TURBT) is the diagnostic and gold standard treatment option for NMIBC. Despite visually complete resection, 30–80% of NMIBC patients will have disease recurrence, possibly due to invisible residual lesions or implantation of tumour cells during TURBT [4]. Current evidence suggests that subsequent instillations of intravesical chemotherapy are necessary for higher-risk disease [5]. Gemcitabine is a cell-cycle specific antimetabolite that is widely used in intravesical chemotherapy [6].

* Correspondence: fangzhenqiang123@126.com
[1]Department of Urology, Second Affiliated Hospital, Third Military Medical University, Chongqing 400037, China
Full list of author information is available at the end of the article

Ribonucleotide reductase subunit M1 (RRM1) is the largest catalytic subunit of ribonucleotide reductase (RR), which is the key enzyme catalysing the transformation of ribonucleoside diphosphates to deoxyribonucleoside diphosphates [7]. Gemcitabine is an analogue of deoxycytidine. The active forms of gemcitabine inhibit DNA synthesis by incorporating into the DNA chain or inhibiting RRM1 activity [8]. Gemcitabine has been widely used for the treatment of several aggressive solid tumour types, including non-small-cell lung cancer (NSCLC), bladder tumours, pancreatic tumours and nasopharyngeal carcinoma [9–12]. There are preclinical and clinical data indicating that high RRM1 protein levels in various cancers are associated with gemcitabine resistance [13, 14]. Moreover, several clinical studies have demonstrated the association between elevated RRM1 levels and unfavourable clinical outcomes in advanced bladder tumour patients treated with gemcitabinebased therapy [9, 15]. However, the relationship between RRM1 mRNA level and gemcitabine activity in NMIBC has not been addressed. In the current paper, we demonstrated the predictive and prognostic value of RRM1 in patients with NMIBC receiving intravesical gemcitabine chemotherapy.

Methods

Patients

This retrospective study enrolled 162 patients with histological confirmed NMIBC and intermediate/high-risk disease at the Second Affiliated Hospital of Third Military Medical University from November 2010 to January 2016. Tissue samples from patients were obtained after surgery. An Eastern Cooperative Oncology Group (ECOG) performance status (PS) of 0 to 2 was assessed in all enrolled patients. Patient inclusion criteria included the following: 1) an NMIBC patient diagnosis following the EAU guidelines; 2) intermediate or high-risk bladder cancer patients without lymph node metastasis or distant metastases; 3) all patients underwent transurethral resection of the bladder tumour plus subsequent instillations of intravesical gemcitabine chemotherapy; 4) first diagnosis of a bladder tumour without accepting any surgery or drug treatment; and 5) patients voluntarily participated in the study and signed the informed consent form. This study was conducted with the approval of the medical ethics committee of Second Affiliated Hospital of the Third Military Medical University. Each patient provided written informed consent before participation in the current investigation. Patient information on pathologic characteristics, treatment details, and survival was obtained from follow-up and surgical records. The major clinical endpoint in the current study was disease-free survival (DFS), and the secondary clinical outcomes were 1-year and 2-year relapse rates.

Treatment and response evaluation

All patients received intravesical gemcitabine monotherapy immediately after TURBT. A total of 1000 mg of gemcitabine was diluted in 40 ml of saline solution, and patients received weekly instillations for 8 consecutive weeks. The drug was held in the bladder for 60 min. The treatment cycle was then changed to once a month for one year. Follow-up was performed to assess the efficacy of the treatment for all involved patients. In general, in the first year, cystoscopy and urinary cytology were examined at 3-month intervals and then at 6-month intervals in the next year. Relapse was defined as a positive examination on cystoscopy. The first recurrence (disease-free survival) time was defined as the period between TURBT and positive finding during cystoscopy.

RRM1 mRNA expression analysis

In the current investigation, multiplex branched-DNA (bDNA) liquid chip technology was employed to perform RRM1 expression analyses at SurExam Medical Test Centre, Guangzhou, China, and these analyses are detailed in the paper published by Zhang [16]. Briefly, digested tissue was incubated with target gene-specific probe sets, and then fluorescence capture beads were added. Then, the mixture was hybridized with bDNA signal amplification probes for the purpose of signal amplification. In the end, the Luminex 200 system (Luminex Corp., Austin, Texas) was used to cluster the fluorescence value of each sample. Three standard genes were demonstrated as reference genes, including beta-2-microglobulin (B2M), transfer in receptor (TFRC), and TATA box-binding protein (TBP). All original data were subjected to standardize processing, which included raw data alignment (fastq file), duplication removal, quality control, etc., until we obtained clean data for subsequent analyses. All gene expression levels among patients were distributed across the whole samples, and then each patient received an RRM1 expression value. The median RRM1expression level was selected for the cutoff value. The expression level of RRM1 was considered high if its level was equal to or exceeded the cutoff value. All other mRNA values were considered low expression.

Statistical analysis

SPSS statistical software, version 19.0 (IBM Corporation, Armonk, New York, USA) was employed for data analysis. The χ^2 and Fisher exact tests were performed to identify associations between clinicopathologic variables and RRM1 status as appropriate. Survival curves were demonstrated by using the Kaplan-Meier method. A log-rank test was used to compare survival differences among groups. All statistical tests were two-sided, and a statistically significant difference was defined as $p < 0.05$.

Results

Patient features

Table 1 shows the baseline clinicopathologic features of the study population. The median age of the 162 patients was 60 years (range, 25–89 years), and there were 132 (81.5%) men and 30 (18.5%) women in the cohort. All patients were classified as having high-risk NMIBC and an ECOG PS 0~2. All patients underwent 1 year of intravesical gemcitabine chemotherapy after TURBT. The median patient follow-up was 30.5 months (range, 14–76 months). The patients were randomly assigned evenly to either the RRM1-known group (high and low expression of RRM1) or to the unknown group. There were 81 tumour samples successfully processed for RRM1 analysis, and 21.0% (17/81) of the patient demonstrated high RRM1 expression.

Relationship between clinicopathologic features and RRM1 expression

The expression of RRM1 was divided into high and low expression according to the cutoff value of RRM1, which was 0.557 (range 0.006–0.997). Of the 162 patients, RRM1 expression was high in 17 (10.5%) patients and low in 64 (39.5%) patients. The RRM1 level was unknown in the remaining 50% of patients. As shown in Table 2, the level of RRM1 expression was moderately associated with clinicopathologic features. There were no significant differences observed in sex ($p = 0.921$), age

Table 1 Patients' characteristics according to RRM1 expression

Features	N	RRM1 expression			χ^2值	p
		Low (%)	High (%)	Unknown (%)		
Gender						
Female	30	11 (17.2)	3 (17.6)	16 (19.8)	0.166	0.921
Male	132	53 (82.8)	14 (82.4)	65 (80.2)		
Age (years)						
≤ 60	85	39 (60.2)	12 (70.6)	34 (42.0)	3.542	0.170
> 60	77	25 (39.8)	5 (29.4)	47 (58.0)		
Weight (Kg)						
≤ 65	78	26 (40.6)	8 (47.1)	44 (56.4)	2.695	0.260
> 65	84	38 (59.4)	9 (52.9)	37 (44.0)		
ECOG Score						
0–1	157	62 (96.9)	17 (100.0)	78 (96.3)	0.645	0.724
2	5	2 (3.1)	0	3 (3.7)		
CUA/EAU risk group						
2	54	22 (34.4)	6 (35.3)	26 (32.1)	0.116	0.944
3	108	42 (65.6)	11 (64.7)	55 (67.9)		
Relapse						
Yes	23	3 (4.9)	5 (29.4)	15 (18.5)	9.223	**0.010**
No	139	61 (95.1)	12 (70.6)	66 (81.5)		

$p < 0.05$ is set in boldface

Table 2 The 1-year/2-year relapse rates according to RRM1 expression and clinicopathological features

	No	1-y R^a rate (%)	p	2-y R^a rate (%)	p
RRM1 level					
Low	64	0	**0.009**	3.1%	**0.005**
High	17	17.7%		29.4%	
Unknown	81	6.2%		11.1%	
Gender					
Female	30	13.3%	**0.040**	13.3%	0.500
Male	132	3.0%		9.1%	
Age (years)					
≤ 60	85	4.7%	0.569	10.6%	0.75
> 60	77	5.3%		9.1%	
Weight (Kg)					
≤ 65	78	13.3%	0.204	7.7%	0.369
> 65	84	4.8%		11.9%	
ECOG Score					
0–1	157	5.1%	0.774	10.2%	0.452
2	5	0		0	
CUA/EAU risk group					
2	54	1.9%	0.271	11.1%	0.710
3	108	6.5%		9.3%	

R: means relapse
$p < 0.05$ is set in boldface

($p = 0.170$), weight ($p = 0.260$), ECOG performance status ($p = 0.610$), or CUA/EAU risk between the three groups ($p = 0.944$). Surprisingly, when compared to patients with low (4.9%, 3/64) and unknown (18.5%, 15/81) RRM1 levels, patients with high RRM1 levels were more likely to relapse (29.4%, 5/17), $p = 0.010$.

Association between RRM1 level and clinical outcomes

After a median follow-up of 30.5 months, 14.2% (23/162) of the patients experienced disease progression, and all patients were alive. As shown in Fig. 1, PFS was significantly longer for patients with low RRM1 expression than for patients with high and unknown RRM1 expression, $p = 0.009$. However, median PFS could not be calculated because a majority of patients were disease-free at the end of follow-up.

Additionally, the 1-year and 2-year relapse rates also differed according to RRM1 expression and other clinical characteristics. The 1-year relapse rates for RRM1-low, RRM1-high and RRM1-unknown patients were 0, 17.7 and 6.2% ($p = 0.009$), respectively, while the 2-year relapse rates in these groups were 3.1, 29.4, and 11.1% ($p = 0.005$), respectively. Other clinical characteristics, such as age, weight, and performance status, showed little association with 1-year/2-year relapse rates. The female patients had higher 1-year relapse rates than the male patients (13.3% vs. 3.0%, $p = 0.04$).

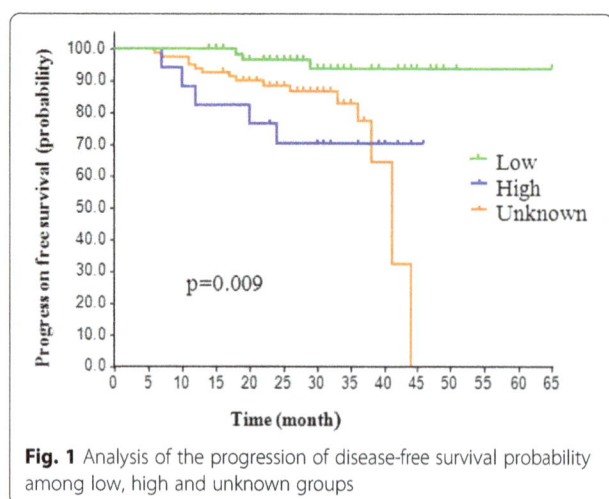

Fig. 1 Analysis of the progression of disease-free survival probability among low, high and unknown groups

Discussion

In clinical practice, the effects of chemotherapeutic agents or regimens vary among different individuals. Pharmacogenomics studies have shown that genetic factors play a vital role in curative effects. Therefore, identifying a biomarker is essential for establishing personalized treatments and improving treatment outcomes. Several recent studies have focused on evaluating predictive and/or prognostic markers for various tumours, including non-small-cell lung cancer (NSCLC), nasopharyngeal carcinoma and bladder carcinoma.

Our present study investigated the predictive and prognostic value of RRM1 in patients with NMIBC receiving intravesical gemcitabine chemotherapy. There were 162 NMIBC patients randomly assigned to either the RRM1-known group or the unknown group. The expression levels of RRM1 were significantly associated with age, sex, weight, ECOG performance status, or CUA/EAU risk, which is in accordance with prior results in advanced UC and NSCLC [9, 17]. Our data showed that high RRM1 expression was observed in less than 30% of tumours and was an unfavourable prognostic factor for PFS. Conversely, a low RRM1 level was found to be correlated with better PFS according to the Kaplan-Meier analysis. In addition, patients with low RRM1 expression showed the lowest 1-year/2-year relapse rate, while the RRM1-high patients had the highest relapse rates (17.1 and 29.4%, respectively). The association between RRM1 expression and prognosis in the present study was consistent with previous studies investigating other tumours treated with gemcitabine.

Previous studies associated with RRM1 expression in NSCLC patients largely demonstrated that low or negative RRM1 levels in patients with advanced NSCLC receiving gemcitabine-based regimens were correlated with higher response rates and a better prognosis [18]. In addition, there are also several studies that evaluated

the predictive and/or prognostic value of RRM1 expression level in patients with urothelial carcinoma (UC). In one study, high RRM1 expression in respectable MIBC patients aged < 70 years was associated with improved survival [19]. On the other hand, the RRM1 level in advanced BC patients receiving gemcitabine-based regimes was not correlated with response or OS, except time-to-progression (TTP) [20]. These discrepant results may be attributable to differences in the patients involved. Similar to our results, Kim et al. found that high RRM1 expression was associated with inferior prognosis and clinical outcome after platinum plus gemcitabine combination chemotherapy for advanced UC [9, 15]. In contrast with previous studies regarding RRM1 in UC with gemcitabine-based therapy, this is the first study of early BC (NMIBC) with intravesical gemcitabine monotherapy. Taken together, these studies suggest that low RRM1 expression may help identify patients who will significantly benefit from gemcitabine-based chemotherapy in early and advanced UC.

The role of RRM1 in gemcitabine resistance carries more significance in the MIBC population, in which gemcitabine chemotherapy in combination with cisplatin is the standard of care. The standard treatment of NMIBC, however, remains treatment with bacillus Calmette–Guerin (BCG). The role of gemcitabine as a standard intravesical treatment in non-BCG refractory patients is unclear, as recurrence rates have been shown to be significantly higher among high-risk patients treated with gemcitabine compared with those treated with BCG. BCG was the first choice in intravesical instillation treatment with intermediate- or high-risk NMIBC. The recurrence rate of BCG treatment is lower than that of gemcitabine intravesical chemotherapy. However, in China, the price of BCG is too high, approximately 6 times higher than the cost of gemcitabine treatment, and no medical insurance covers this cost. For economic reasons, most NMIBC patients generally give up using BCG treatment and use gemcitabine intravesical chemotherapy as a secondary choice. The purpose of current study was to maximize the efficacy of gemcitabine perfusion therapy in these patients.

Nevertheless, limitations must be considered in the current investigation. The current study is a single-centre study, and the number of RRM1-high patients investigated was relatively small ($N = 17$). In addition, the Kaplan-Meier analysis of RRM1-low and RRM1-unknown groups failed to reach median PFS despite having a median follow-up of 30.5 months (range, 14–76 months). One main reason for these limitations is that the prognosis of NMIBC patients is usually good. Therefore, further well-designed studies must enrol a larger sample size and have longer follow-up periods. In addition, the nature of the retrospective study means that there is a risk of selection bias, which is another limitation in our investigation, and a lack of secondary analysis (regression models) to confirm RRM1 as an independent variable associated with disease recurrence and progression should be avoided in future studies. Despite these limitations, the current study is clinically meaningful and suggests the important role of RRM1 mRNA expression in patients with NMIBC. To our knowledge, this is the first study evaluating RRM1 mRNA in NMIBC patients treated with intravesical gemcitabine monotherapy.

Conclusions

In conclusion, this preliminary study showed that low RRM1 expression was associated with longer progression-free survival and lower 1-year/2-year relapse rates in NMIBC patients treated with intravesical gemcitabine monotherapy, despite the need for further verification with large sample sizes and considering more mixed factors and biases.

Abbreviations
CUA: China Urological Association; EAU: European Association of Urology; NMIBC: Non-muscle-invasive bladder cancer; PFS: Progression-free survival; RRM1: Ribonucleotide reductase subunit M1; TURBT: Transurethral resection of the bladder tumour

Acknowledgements
Not applicable.

Authors' contributions
Z.F., J.X., and P.H. designed the investigation; Z.F. and J.X. provided the funding for the current research; Z.F. and L.Z. had access to all tissues samples; Z.F. and Z.Y.J.X. obtained statutory and ethics approvals; B.F. and Z.Y. contributed to data acquisition; Z.Y., B.F., and Z.F. performed the data preparation, quality control and analyses and checked the results. Y. and B.F. drafted the report. All authors contributed to writing the final report and approved the version to be published.

Author details
[1]Department of Urology, Second Affiliated Hospital, Third Military Medical University, Chongqing 400037, China. [2]SurExam Bio-Tech Co, Guangzhou 510663, Guangdong, China. [3]Department of Oncology, Second Affiliated Hospital, Third Military Medical University, Chongqing 400037, China.

References

1. Chen W, Zheng R, Baade PD, Zhang S, Zeng H, Bray F, Jemal A, Yu XQ, He J. Cancer statistics in China, 2015. CA Cancer J Clin. 2016;66(2):115–32.
2. Traboulsi SL, Kassouf W. Bladder cancer: a step closer to individualized treatment for bladder cancer. Nat Rev Urol. 2016;13(3):127–8.
3. Olivier Bosset P, Neuzillet Y, Paoletti X, Molinie V, Botto H, Lebret T. Long-term follow-up of TaG1 non-muscle-invasive bladder cancer. Urol Oncol. 2015;33(1):20 e21–7.
4. Porten SP, Leapman MS, Greene KL. Intravesical chemotherapy in non-muscle-invasive bladder cancer. Indian J Urol. 2015;31(4):297–303.
5. Sylvester RJ, Oosterlinck W, van der Meijden AP. A single immediate postoperative instillation of chemotherapy decreases the risk of recurrence in patients with stage ta T1 bladder cancer: a meta-analysis of published results of randomized clinical trials. J Urol. 2004;171(6 Pt 1):2186–90 quiz 2435.
6. Kim SI, Choo SH. Intravesical Chemotherapy. In: *Bladder Cancer*.edn: Elsevier; 2018. p. 263–76. https://doi.org/10.1016/B978-0-12-809939-1.00019-9.
7. Brissenden J, Caras I, Thelander L, Francke U. The structural gene for the M1 subunit of ribonucleotide reductase maps to chromosome 11, band p15, in human and to chromosome 7 in mouse. Exp Cell Res. 1988;174(1):302–8.
8. Mini E, Nobili S, Caciagli B, Landini I, Mazzei T. Cellular pharmacology of gemcitabine. Ann Oncol. 2006;17(Suppl5):v7–12.
9. Kim M, Ku JH, Kwak C, Kim HH, Lee E, Keam B, Kim TM, Heo DS, Lee SH, Moon KC. Predictive and prognostic value of ribonucleotide reductase regulatory subunit M1 and excision repair cross-complementation group 1 in advanced urothelial carcinoma (UC) treated with first-line gemcitabine plus platinum combination chemotherapy. PLoS One. 2015;10(7):e0133371.
10. Zhao LP, Xue C, Zhang JW, Hu ZH, Zhao YY, Zhang J, Huang Y, Zhao HY, Zhang L. Expression of RRM1 and its association with resistance to gemcitabine-based chemotherapy in advanced nasopharyngeal carcinoma. Chinese journal of cancer. 2012;31(10):476–83.
11. Lee JJ, Maeng CH, Baek SK, Kim GY, Yoo JH, Choi CW, Kim YH, Kwak YT, Kim DH, Lee YK et al: The immunohistochemical overexpression of ribonucleotide reductase regulatory subunit M1 (RRM1) protein is a predictor of shorter survival to gemcitabine-based chemotherapy in advanced non-small cell lung cancer (NSCLC). *Lung cancer (Amsterdam, Netherlands)* 2010, 70(2):205–210.
12. Aoyama T, Miyagi Y, Murakawa M, Yamaoku K, Atsumi Y, Shiozawa M, Ueno M, Morimoto M, Oshima T, Yukawa N, et al. Clinical implications of ribonucleotide reductase subunit M1 in patients with pancreatic cancer who undergo curative resection followed by adjuvant chemotherapy with gemcitabine. Oncol Lett. 2017;13(5):3423–30.
13. Davidson JD, Ma L, Flagella M, Geeganage S, Gelbert LM, Slapak CA. an increase in the expression of ribonucleotide reductase large subunit 1 is associated with gemcitabine resistance in non-small cell lung cancer cell lines. Cancer Res. 2004;64(11):3761–6.
14. Bergman AM, Eijk PP, Ruiz van Haperen VW, Smid K, Veerman G, Hubeek I, van den Ijssel P, Ylstra B, Peters GJ. in vivo induction of resistance to gemcitabine results in increased expression of ribonucleotide reductase subunit M1 as the major determinant. Cancer Res. 2005;65(20):9510–6.
15. Shilkrut M, Wu A, Thomas DG, Hamstra DA. Expression of ribonucleoside reductase subunit M1, but not excision repair cross-complementation group 1, is predictive in muscle-invasive bladder cancer treated with chemotherapy and radiation. Mol Clin Oncol. 2014;2(3):479–87.
16. Zhang Q, Sun T, Kang P, Qian K, Deng B, Zhou J, Wang R, Jiang B, Li K, Liu F, et al. Combined analysis of rearrangement of ALK, ROS1, somatic mutation of EGFR, KRAS, BRAF, PIK3CA, and mRNA expression of ERCC1, TYMS, RRM1, TUBB3, EGFR in patients with nonsmall cell lung cancer and their clinical significance. Cancer Chemother Pharmacol. 2016;77(3):583–93.
17. Simon G, Sharma A, Li X, Hazelton T, Walsh F, Williams C, Chiappori A, Haura E, Tanvetyanon T, Antonia S, et al. Feasibility and efficacy of molecular analysis-directed individualized therapy in advanced non-small-cell lung cancer. Journal of clinical oncology : official journal of the American Society of Clinical Oncology. 2007;25(19):2741–6.
18. Gong W, Zhang X, Wu J, Chen L, Li L, Sun J, Lv Y, Wei X, Du Y, Jin H et al: RRM1 expression and clinical outcome of gemcitabine-containing chemotherapy for advanced non-small-cell lung cancer: a meta-analysis. *Lung cancer (Amsterdam, Netherlands)* 2012, 75(3):374–380.
19. Harshman LC, Bepler G, Zheng Z, Higgins JP, Allen GI, Srinivas S. Ribonucleotide reductase subunit M1 expression in resectable, muscle-invasive urothelial cancer correlates with survival in younger patients. BJU Int. 2010;106(11):1805–11.
20. Bellmunt J, Paz-Ares L, Cuello M, Cecere FL, Albiol S, Guillem V, Gallardo E, Carles J, Mendez P, de la Cruz JJ, et al. Gene expression of ERCC1 as a novel prognostic marker in advanced bladder cancer patients receiving cisplatin-based chemotherapy. Ann Oncol. 2007;18(3):522–8.

12

Differential expression of histamine receptors in the bladder wall tissues of patients with bladder pain syndrome/interstitial cystitis – significance in the responsiveness to antihistamine treatment and disease symptoms

Hui Shan[1*], Er-Wei Zhang[2], Peng Zhang[3], Xiao-Dong Zhang[1], Ning Zhang[4], Peng Du[4] and Yong Yang[4]

Abstract

Background: Activation of mast cells plays an important role in the pathogenesis of bladder pain syndrome/interstitial cystitis (BPS/IC). Histamine, a mast cell-derived mediators, induced inflammation and hypersensitivity of the bladder. The present study investigated the expressions of histamine receptors in the bladder wall tissues of patients with BPS/IC, and its association with the effectiveness of antihistamine therapy and disease symptoms.

Methods: Bladder tissues were collected from 69 BPS/IC patients and 10 control female patients. The expression of H3R in BPS/IC was further examined in an independent cohort of 10 female patients with BPS/IC and another 10 age-matched female patients. Immunohistochemistry, Western blotting, and quantitative RT-PCR were performed to quantify the expressions of histamine receptors. Statistical analyses of the correlation of histamine receptor expression with antihistamine therapy outcome and severity of disease symptoms were also performed.

Results: The expression of four histamine receptors was significantly elevated in BPS/IC (H1R, $P < 0.001$; H2R, $P = 0.031$; H3R, $P = 0.008$; H4R, $P = 0.048$). Western blotting revealed that H3R were significantly reduced in the patients, whereas the mRNA levels of H3R were significantly increased. The patients were further divided into antihistamine responders ($n = 38$) and nonresponders ($n = 22$). No significant correlation was found in the expression of histamine receptors between responder and nonresponder groups. However, significant correlations between OLS and H1R ($P = 0.003$) and H3R ($P = 0.045$) were found.

Conclusion: The present study showed that expression of all the 4 histamine receptors were elevated in BPS/IC. There were no statistical significant correlations between the expression levels of the four different histamine receptors and the treatment outcome of antihistamine therapy (amtitriptyline or cimetidine).

Keywords: Bladder pain syndrome, Interstitial cystitis, Histamine receptors, Anti-histamine bladder

* Correspondence: shanhui902@163.com
[1]Department of Urology, Beijing Chaoyang Hospital, Capital Medical University, No.8 Gongti South Road, Beijing 100020, China
Full list of author information is available at the end of the article

Background

Bladder pain syndrome/Interstitial cystitis (BPS/IC), or bladder pain syndrome, is a complex bladder dysfunction characteristized by chronic (> 6 months) urinary bladder pain or discomfort, accompanied by other urinary symptom such as persistent urge to void [1]. BPS/IC can contribute to chronic pelvic pain and poor quality of life, which is now recognized as a serious medical condition. The disease occurs mostly in young and middle-aged women, with no known etiology. A survey conducted in US indicated that 575 in every 100,000 women had IC [2], and the prevalence rate of self-reported BPS/IC among community-dwelling adult women was around 4% [3].

Several etiologies have been proposed, including abnormalities in urine, infection, inflammation resulted from autoimmunity, activation of mast cells, neurogenic inflammation, and disturbance in permeability of the bladder wall [4]. Evidence from in vitro and clinical studies suggested that mast cells play a critical role in the pathogenesis and pathophysiology of BPS/IC [5, 6]. Upon the activation of mast cells, histamine is released; and the binding of histamine to the receptors on bladder wall could induce inflammation and hypersensitivity of the bladder [7, 8]. Treatments of BPS/IC include behavioral therapy, mucosal protection, histamine receptor antagonism, analgesia, and surgical treatment, whereas the most common interventions include bladder mucosal protective agents and anti-histamines [9].

There are four subtypes of histamine receptors: H1R, H2R, H3R, and H4R. It has been confirmed that the expression of all the four subtypes of histamine receptors were found in BPS/IC animal model, in which the receptors were expressed mainly in bladder epithelial cells. Significant differences were found in the expression of H1R, H2R, and H3R before and after BPS/IC [10]. However, it remains unclear on the pattern of expressions of the four histamine receptors in patients with IC. Also, it is not known whether there is an association between histamine receptor expression and efficacy of antihistamines.

In the current study, we analyze the correlation between expressions of histamine receptors and the severity of BPS/IC (as assessed by OLS score), as well as the effectiveness of antihistamine therapy.

Methods
Study population

The exploration study included the use of bladder tissues from 69 patients admitted to Beijing Chaoyang Hospital (Beijing, China) from 2005 to 2009 for treatment of interstitial cystitis. The diagnosis of BPS/IC was based on the guidelines published by the National Institute of Diabetes and Digestive and Kidney Diseases. Tissues were collected by biopsy forcep and were retrospectively analyzed. The study also collected bladder tissues as the control samples from 10 female patients with other urinary complications but no complaints of bladder pain. For the validation study, bladder tissues were collected from 10 patients with BPS/IC and 10 age-matched females with no BPS/IC but receiving surgical treatment for stress urinary incontinence. Tissues were collected by the use of cystoscopy from the trigone, and from the front, back, left and right walls of the bladder. The study design was approved by the ethnic committee of our hospital, with informed consents obtained from all the participants.

Antibodies and reagents

Antibodies against human histamine H1, H2, H3, and H4 receptors were purchased from Santa Cruz (Dallas, TX, USA). Rabbit polyclonal antibody antibody against human histamine H3 receptor was obtained from Life-Span Bioscience (Seattle, WA, USA). Chemiluminescent HRP substrate was from Chemicon (Temecula, CA, USA). Total RNA was isolated using RNA extraction kit from Ambion (Carlsbad, CA, USA), and was then transcribed and amplified using GoTaq® 2-Step RT-qPCR System (Promega, Madison, WI, USA).

Immunohistochemistry and quantitative image analysis

Formalin-fixed paraffin-embedded bladder tissues were sectioned, dewaxed, and stained with antibodies against human histamine receptors at 4 °C overnight. After the incubation with secondary antibody and washing, the reactivity signal was developed using DAB. Under microscopic observations (a magnification, 400x) three different fields were captured for signal quantitation. Image acquisition software Image Pro-Plus 6.0 was employed to measure the integral optical density (IOD) and area of each selected microscopic field. The mean density (MD) was then calculated as IOD/avea. Microscopic fields with MD values < 0.001 were determined as negative for human histamine receptors.

Western blotting and quantitative RT-PCR for H3R

The protein and gene expression of H3R in the validation cohort was examined using western blotting and quantitative RT-PCR, respectively. For western blotting, tissue homogenates were resolved by electrophoresis, transferred to PVDF membranes and probed with rabbit polyclonal antibody against H3R. Semi-quantitation of the band intensity of H3R was then performed using Quantity One software. For quantitative RT-PCR, H3R gene was amplified by STRATA3000 system with the level determined using $-2^{\Delta\Delta CT}$ approach.

Statistical analysis

Data analysis was done using statistical software SPSS version 19.0. Measurement data were presented as mean ± standard deviation, and were compared between groups using t-test. Statistically different comparison was indicated by P value <0.05.

Results

Differential expression of human histamine receptors in BPS/IC bladder tissues

The expression of four different histamine receptors in the bladder tissues of 69 patients with BPS/IC was examined using immunohistochemistry (Fig. 1). The receptors were mainly expressed in the mucosa of bladder, the interstitial blood vessels and the detrusor muscles. The IHC signals were quantified (Table 1). Compared to

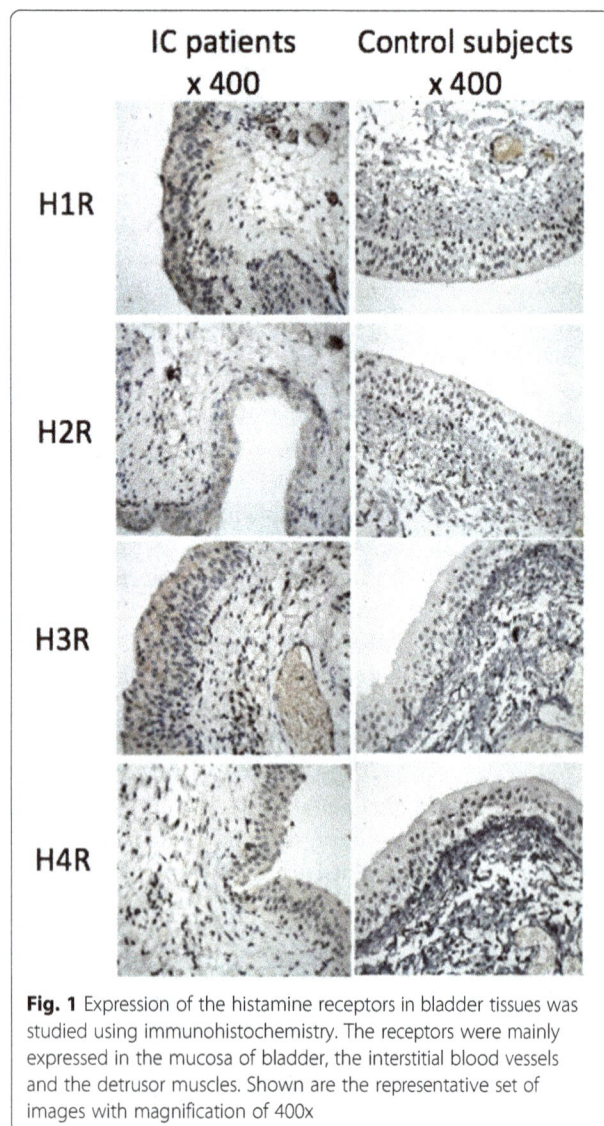

Fig. 1 Expression of the histamine receptors in bladder tissues was studied using immunohistochemistry. The receptors were mainly expressed in the mucosa of bladder, the interstitial blood vessels and the detrusor muscles. Shown are the representative set of images with magnification of 400x

the bladder tissues of subjects with no BPS/IC ($n = 10$), the expression of four histamine receptors was significantly elevated in BPS/IC (H1R, $P < 0.001$; H2R, $P = 0.031$; H3R, $P = 0.008$; H4R, $P = 0.048$).

H3R expression in an independent IC cohort

The expression of H3R in BPS/IC was further examined in an independent cohort of 10 female patients with BPS/IC and another 10 age-matched female patients receiving surgical treatment for stress urinary incontinence. The protein levels of H3R in the tissues were examined using western blotting. Western blotting revealed that H3R protein levels were significantly reduced in the bladder tissues of patients with BPS/IC comparing to those without BPS/IC ($P < 0.01$) (Fig. 2a). The gene expression of H3R in the tissues was studied using quantitative real-time PCR. Result demonstrated that the mRNA transcript levels of H3R were significantly increased in IC tissues when compared to those without IC (Fig. 2b).

Correlation of histamine receptor expression with antihistamine therapy outcome and OLS

After showing the elevation of four different histamine receptors in BPS/IC bladder tissues, we next investigated whether these expression would correlate the outcome of antihistamine treatment. Patients in this study received anti-histamine (amitriptyline or cimetidine) as first-line treatment, and those demonstrated an improvement of clinical symptoms (e.g. pain, urgency, and frequency) were classified as responders. We examined the histamine receptor expression in antihistamine responders ($n = 38$) and nonresponders ($n = 22$). In the responder group, there were 9 male and 29 female patients aged 25 to 80 years (average age, 50.59 ± 14.29 years), while in the nonresponder group, there were 2 male and 20 female patients aged 24 to 70 years (average age, 40.06 ± 12.63 years). Our analysis showed that the expression of histamine receptors between responder and nonresponder groups was statistically not significant (H1R, $P = 0.362$; H2R, $P = 0.082$; H3R, $P = 0.869$; H4R, $P = 0.292$) (Table 2).

The correlation between histamine receptor expression and symptom severity was also evaluated. The symptoms of BPS/IC were assessed using the O'Leary-Sant (OLS) questionnaire [11]. The mean OLS of the cohort was 29.39 ± 5.273. The correlations between the expression of individual receptor and OLS score were listed in Table 3. Significant correlations with OLS were found in H1R ($P = 0.003$) and H3R ($P = 0.045$).

Discussion

The present study examined the differential expression of 4 histamine receptors (H1R, H2R, H3R, and H4R) in the bladder tissues of patients with BPS/IC, showing all the receptors were significantly elevated in BPS/IC. Our

Table 1 Expression of histamine receptors in IC patients and in control subjects

Groups	Number of cases	H1R	H2R	H3R	H4R
IC patients	69	0.1389 ± 0.05115	0.0861 ± 0.01646	0.1124 ± 0.04665	0.1007 ± 0.02212
Control Subjects	10	0.0395 ± 0.00361	0.0633 ± 0.00809	0.0842 ± 0.01632	0.0576 ± 0.00982
P- value		0.000	0.031	0.008	0.048

analysis also suggested that although histamine receptors are biologically relevant to BPS/IC pathogenesis, there were no significant correlations between the expression levels of the four different histamine receptors and the treatment outcome of antihistamine therapy.

Despite the accumulated studies over the decades, the etiology of BPS/IC have yet to be fully studied [12]. Different hypothesized etiologies have been proposed, including abnormalities in urine, infection, inflammation resulted from autoimmunity, activation of

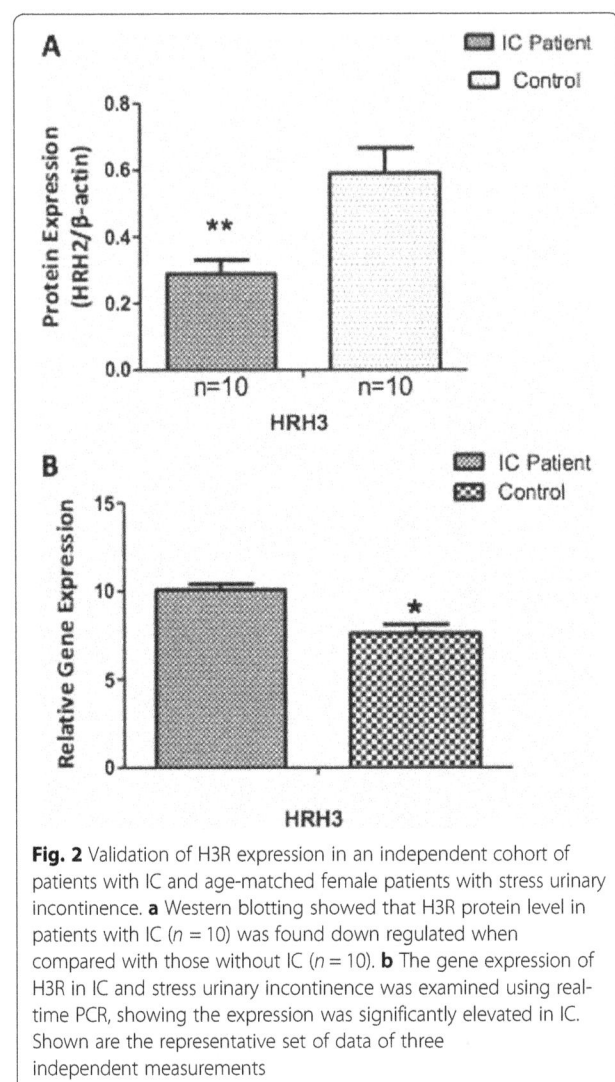

Fig. 2 Validation of H3R expression in an independent cohort of patients with IC and age-matched female patients with stress urinary incontinence. **a** Western blotting showed that H3R protein level in patients with IC ($n = 10$) was found down regulated when compared with those without IC ($n = 10$). **b** The gene expression of H3R in IC and stress urinary incontinence was examined using real-time PCR, showing the expression was significantly elevated in IC. Shown are the representative set of data of three independent measurements

mast cells, neurogenic inflammation, and disturbance in permeability of the bladder wall [4]. Epithelial antiproliferative factor plays a key role in inhibiting the growth of endothelial cell of the bladder. Baltimore et al. recently identified that the mutation of FZB8 gene would affect the normal functions of epithelial antiproliferative factor, disrupting the integrity of bladder mucosa, resulting in an increase in the permeability of the bladder [4, 7, 13]. Nevertheless, none of these hypotheses can fully explain the diverse clinical manifestations and differential drug responses among patients with BPS/IC.

The understanding on the pathophysiology is relatively clear comparing to the disease etiology. It has been widely accepted that BPS/IC is resulted from the chronic inflammation of the entire bladder wall, in which mast cells represent one of the key players. In patients with BPS/IC activated mast cells were found in the bladder of the patients [6]. By releasing histamine that binds to the receptors on bladder wall, the mast cells can induce inflammation and hypersensitivity of the bladder [7, 8]. In accordance with other previous studies, we herein demonstrated that all of the four histamine receptors were over expressed in the bladder wall of BPS/IC. Moreover, our examination clearly depicted the localisation of IHC signals mainly in the mucosa of bladder, with a lesser extent of reactivity could be detected in the interstitial blood vessels and the detrusor muscles. There results likely implicated that the mucosa of the bladder would be the major target of histamine released from the infiltrated mast cells, in turn, the major pathogenic sites of BPS/IC. Our study has therefore provided further evidences to support the hypothesis that BPS/IC would be resulted from the dysfunction of the bladder mucosa, and to strengthen the rationale of using antihistamine in the treatment of BPS/IC.

Histamine modulates diverse immunological responses through its activation on different histamine receptors. All the four histamine receptors are G-protein coupled receptors expressing in diverse tissues with distinct functions [14, 15]. H1R mediates inflammatory reaction [16], while H2R shows inhibitory effects on the apoptosis of mononuclear cells [17]. H3R mainly controls the inflammatory reactions by modulating the release of pro-inflammatory peptides [18],

Table 2 Expression of histamine receptors in responders and nonresponders

Groups	Number of cases	H1R	H2R	H3R	H4R
Responders	39	0.1364 ± 0.04775	0.0863 ± 0.01820	0.1127 ± 0.04903	0.1029 ± 0.02008
Non-responders	21	0.1407 ± 0.05580	0.0851 ± 0.01303	0.1201 ± 0.04578	0.0938 ± 0.02655
P-value		0.362	0.082	0.869	0.292

while H4R promotes the acute inflammatory responses through its enhancement on the migration of eosinophils and mast cells [19]. The pathogenic roles of H1 and H2 receptors in BPS/IC have been reported. H3R and H4R are relatively new histamine receptors, therefore, their roles in IC have remained largely unclear. In this study, we showed that the expressions of both H3R and H4R were increased in IC. The total protein of H3R, however, was reduced in an independent cohort of BPS/IC using Western blotting, suggesting a post-transcriptional modification of H3R.

We have not found significant differences in the expression of histamine receptors between responders and nonresponders. There were several possible explanations for the insignificant results: 1) the small sample size; 2) the expressions of all the four histamine receptors were relatively high in patients, however, only H1R and H2R antagonists were applied; 3) a drug treatment duration of 3 months is needed for antihistamine to achieve therapeutic effects. Some patients might fail to adhere to the medication schedule, thus the treatment outcome became sub-optimal. In future studies, H3R and H4R antagonists may be added to achieve sufficient inhibition of histamine receptors, and the correlation between the cystoscopic findings and expression of histamine receptors/ clinical outcome can be investigated. Further, H3R was significantly correlated with OLS, implicating the potential role of H3R in disease progression of BPS/IC.

Conclusion

In conclusion, the present study reported the increased expression of H1R, H2R, H3R, and H4R in BPS/IC. The expressions of the receptors were not statistically correlated with the outcome of antihistamine therapy (amtitriptyline or cimetidine); however, H1R and H3R were related to the disease severity as assessed by OLS, implicated the potential role of H3R in disease progression.

Table 3 Correlation of histamine receptor expression and OLS

		H1R	H2R	H3R	H4R
OLS	Correlation coefficient	0.360	0.026	0.244	−0.157
	P-value	0.003	0.837	0.045	0.202

Abbreviation
BPS/IC: Bladder pain syndrome/interstitial cystitis

Acknowledgements
None.

Authors' contributions
H S and EW Z contributed to the conception and design of the study; P Z contributed to the acquisition of data; XD Z and N Z performed the experiments; P D and Y Y contributed to the analysis of data; H S wrote the manuscript; All authors reviewed and approved the final version of the manuscript.

Author details
[1]Department of Urology, Beijing Chaoyang Hospital, Capital Medical University, No.8 Gongti South Road, Beijing 100020, China. [2]Department of Urology, The First Affiliated Hospital of Zhengzhou University, Zhengzhou, China. [3]Department of Urology, China Meitan General Hospital, Beijing, China. [4]Department of Urology, Beijing Cancer Hospital, Beijing, China.

References
1. van de Merwe JP, et al. Diagnostic criteria, classification, and nomenclature for painful bladder syndrome/interstitial cystitis: an ESSIC proposal. Eur Urol. 2008;53(1):60–7.
2. Rosenberg MT, Hazzard M. Prevalence of interstitial cystitis symptoms in women: a population based study in the primary care office. J Urol. 2005; 174(6):2231–4.
3. Ibrahim IA, et al. Prevalence of self-reported interstitial cystitis (IC) and interstitial-cystitis-like symptoms among adult women in the community. Int Urol Nephrol. 2007;39(2):489–95.
4. Teichman JM, Moldwin R. The role of the bladder surface in interstitial cystitis/painful bladder syndrome. Can J Urol. 2007;14(4):3599–607.
5. Sant GR, et al. The mast cell in interstitial cystitis: role in pathophysiology and pathogenesis. Urology. 2007;69(4 Suppl):34–40.
6. Theoharides TC, Kempuraj D, Sant GR. Mast cell involvement in interstitial cystitis: a review of human and experimental evidence. Urology. 2001;57(6 Suppl 1):47–55.
7. Jutel M, Blaser K, Akdis CA. Histamine receptors in immune regulation and allergen-specific immunotherapy. Immunol Allergy Clin N Am. 2006;26(2): 245–59 vii.
8. Thurmond RL, Gelfand EW, Dunford PJ. The role of histamine H1 and H4 receptors in allergic inflammation: the search for new antihistamines. Nature reviews. Drug Des Discov. 2008;7(1):41–53.
9. Theoharides TC, et al. Interstitial cystitis: bladder pain and beyond. Expert Opin Pharmacother. 2008;9(17):2979–94.
10. Neuhaus J, et al. Histamine receptors in human detrusor smooth muscle cells: physiological properties and immunohistochemical representation of subtypes. World J Urol. 2006;24(2):202–9.
11. O'Leary MP, et al. The interstitial cystitis symptom index and problem index. Urology. 1997;49(5A Suppl):58–63.
12. Toft BR, Nordling J. Recent developments of intravesical therapy of painful bladder syndrome/interstitial cystitis: a review. Curr Opin Urol. 2006;16(4):268–72.
13. Keay S, et al. Antiproliferative factor, heparin-binding epidermal growth factor-like growth factor, and epidermal growth factor in men with interstitial cystitis versus chronic pelvic pain syndrome. Urology. 2004; 63(1):22–6.
14. Breunig E, et al. Histamine excites neurones in the human submucous plexus through activation of H1, H2, H3 and H4 receptors. J Physiol. 2007; 583(Pt 2):731–42.

15. Strakhova MI, et al. Localization of histamine H4 receptors in the central nervous system of human and rat. Brain Res. 2009;1250:41–8.

16. Akdis CA, Blaser K. Histamine in the immune regulation of allergic inflammation. J Allergy Clin Immunol. 2003;112(1):15–22.

17. Jutel M, Akdis CA. Histamine as an immune modulator in chronic inflammatory responses. Clin Exp Allergy. 2007;37(3):308–10.

18. Cannon KE, Leurs R, Hough LB. Activation of peripheral and spinal histamine H3 receptors inhibits formalin-induced inflammation and nociception, respectively. Pharmacol Biochem Behav. 2007;88(1):122–9.

19. Coruzzi G, et al. Antiinflammatory and antinociceptive effects of the selective histamine H4-receptor antagonists JNJ7777120 and VUF6002 in a rat model of carrageenan-induced acute inflammation. Eur J Pharmacol. 2007;563(1–3):240–4.

Is hysterectomy beneficial in radical cystectomy for female patient with urothelial carcinoma of bladder? A retrospective analysis of consecutive 112 cases from a single institution

Haiwen Huang[1,2†], Bing Yan[3†], Meixia Shang[4], Libo Liu[1,2], Han Hao[1,2*] and Zhijun Xi[1,2*]

Abstract

Background: There is no criterion for determining whether female patients operated with cystectomy would benefit from hysterectomy. This study compares the oncological outcomes between female patients receiving uterus preserving cystectomy (UPC) and uterus excision cystectomy (UEC).

Methods: Retrospective review of 121 female patients with urothelial carcinoma of bladder undergoing UPC ($n = 63$) or UEC ($n = 49$) at a single institute between January 2006 and April 2017. Individual postoperative follow-up plans were performed for patients through outpatient visits. Overall survival (OS) and progression-free survival (PFS) estimates were analyzed using Kaplan-Meier method and multivariable Cox regression.

Results: The median follow-up time was 36 months (interquartile range 16–69). Among patients, 5 (4.1%) had uterus invasion. OS probability ($p = 0.939$) and PFS probability ($p = 0.565$) were similar in two groups. In multivariable Cox regression analysis, hysterectomy was not found to be a predictor of OS (hazard ratio 0.908, 95%CI 0.428–1.924, $p = 0.801$) and PFS (hazard ratio 1.109, 95%CI 0.439–2.805, $p = 0.826$) after adjusting for age, preoperative clinical stage, pathological stage, pathological nodal stage, neoadjuvant/adjuvant chemotherapy, location of the tumor, and surgical margin. No significant difference of overall survival probability was observed in the patients with organ-confined bladder cancer ($p = 0.675$) and in patients with no organ-confined bladder cancer ($p = 0.695$).

Conclusions: The results showed that the rate of uterus invasion was low in patients analyzed in this cohort. It was also found that hysterectomy was not an independent predictor of OS and PFS after radical cystectomy in patients with bladder cancer.

Keywords: Radical cystectomy, Urinary bladder neoplasms, Hysterectomy, Female

Introduction

Bladder cancer is the ninth most common cancer worldwide [1]. Despite the 4-fold higher incidence of bladder cancer among males than females, the latter have more advanced tumors at the time of diagnosis [2]. Radical cystectomy is the recommended treatment for recurrent high grade or muscle-invasive bladder cancer. Classical radical cystectomy in women involves en bloc removal of the bladder, entire urethra and adjacent vagina, uterus, distal ureters, and regional lymph nodes [3]. Recently, urological surgeons are considering whether hysterectomy is beneficial for women who undergo radical cystectomy.

The rationales of hysterectomy are the worse prognosis of female patients and in women there is no anatomical barrier in the vesicocervical areas (unlike in men, fascia of Denonvilliers prevent the spread of cancer from

* Correspondence: haohan1122@vip.sina.com; xizhijun@hsc.pku.edu.cn
†Haiwen Huang and Bing Yan contributed equally to this work.
[1]Department of Urology, Peking University First Hospital, 8 Xishiku Street, Xicheng District, Beijing 100034, China
Full list of author information is available at the end of the article

Is hysterectomy beneficial in radical cystectomy for female patient with urothelial carcinoma...

97

bladder and prostate to adjacent rectum) [4]. For patients with advanced urothelial carcinoma of bladder, hysterectomy sufficiently abrogates the tumor. However, previous studies reported that the involvement of the uterus in this condition was only 0.3–12.5% [5–10]. It has also been reported that the most commonly involved gynecologic organ is anterior vagina and not the uterus [5]. Furthermore, preserving the uterus is an important consideration for younger women who desire to retain their fertility, prevent the formation of pelvic prolapse and enterocele [7], as well as prevent the development of postoperative chronic urine retention [11].

Currently, there is no guideline for preserving the uterus during radical cystectomy. Previous studies have explored the risks of uterus involvement in bladder cancer [5, 8, 10]. In the present study, we compared the pathological outcomes and survival rate of women who underwent radical cystectomy with or without hysterectomy to determine whether hysterectomy is beneficial for such patients.

Patients and methods
Patient population
This study was approved by the institutional review board of our institute. A total of 1026 patients with urothelial carcinoma of bladder who underwent radical cystectomy (883 males and 143 females) at our institution from January 2006 to April 2017 were analyzed. Among 143 females, 12 patients who underwent hysterectomy before radical cystectomy and 19 patients who were lost to follow-up were excluded (Fig. 1). The indications for radical cystectomy were: $T_{2-4a}N_{0-x}M_0$ tumor, high risk and recurrent non-muscle-invasive tumors and BCG-resistant Tis, as well as extensive papillary disease that cannot be controlled with TUR-Bt and intravesical therapy alone. All patients were

diagnosed using computed tomography (CT), magnetic resonance imaging (MRI) or ultrasound (US) and also by pathological examinations including TUR or biopsy sampling. Cisplatin-based combination Neoadjuvant chemotherapy (NAC) was recommended for T_2-$T_{4a}N_0M_0$ bladder cancer patients and adjuvant chemotherapy (AC) was prescribed for patients with pT3/4 and/or pN+ disease if no neoadjuvant chemotherapy had been given, and the patients accepted NAC/AC steadily increased during the study period. The rate of NAC/AC increased from 10.6% in 2006–2011 to 16.9% in 2012–2017. Patients who were suspected with uterine and/or vaginal invasion received cystectomy with hysterectomy. For other patients, the decisions whether hysterectomy was required during radical cystectomy were based on stage of the tumors and patients' preferences, arrived after adequate discussions between patients and doctors. However, hysterectomy was performed if uterine and/or vaginal invasion was found. In total, 63 patients underwent uterus preserving cystectomy (UPC) whereas 49 patients underwent uterus excision cystectomy (UEC). All surgical complications that occurred within 30 days were classified according to the Clavien-Dindo classification system.

Outcomes measures
Pathological data
Postoperative specimens were analyzed by experienced pathologists of our hospital. Histologic type, tumor grade, tumor and nodal stage, the presence of lymphovascular invasion, perivesical organ and surgical margin status were included in the pathological reports.

Oncologic outcomes
Individual postoperative follow-up plans were performed for patients through outpatient visits. During the

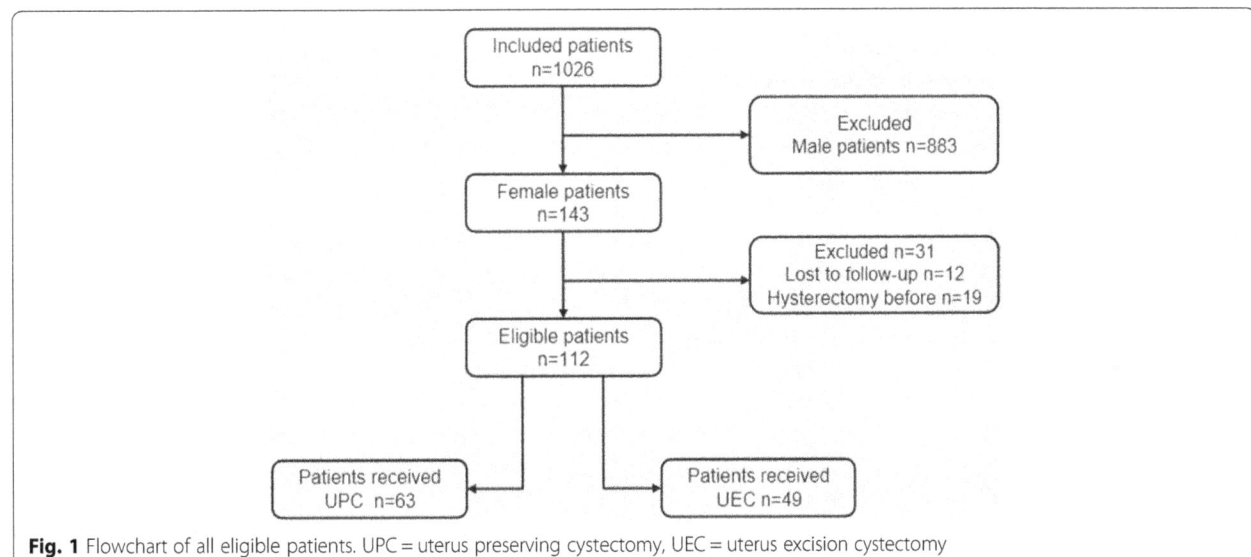

Fig. 1 Flowchart of all eligible patients. UPC = uterus preserving cystectomy, UEC = uterus excision cystectomy

follow-up period, history, physical examination, laboratory measurements of blood and urine were performed every 3 months in the first year, semi-annually in the second year and annually thereafter. At the same time, a CT scan was performed every 6 months until the third year and annually thereafter. Postoperative disease progression was characterized in terms of local recurrence (takes place in the soft tissues of original surgical site or in LNs), distant recurrence and urothelial recurrences.

Technique of uterus preserving cystectomy

Uterus preserving cystectomy can be performed though open or laparoscopic approaches. Initially, bilateral pelvic lymphadenectomy was performed. Thereafter, the peritoneum covering uterovesical pouch was incised to expose the posterior wall of bladder to access the trigone. Ligasure was used to transect the bilateral bladder pedicles. The uterine arteries and veins in front of distal ureters were preserved. There were autonomic nerves from the pelvic plexus existing on the posterolateral portion of the rectum and passing caudally on their way to the bladder neck and urethra to run dorsal to the distal ureter [11]. So it was necessary to be careful to dissect along bladder neck and proximal urethral, and avoid using electrocautery as soon as possible at this step. The anterior peritoneum of bladder was incised to access the retropubic space. Suture and ligature the dorsal vein of the clitoris together with the surrounding fascia. All sides of urethra were exposed, ensuring that proximal urethra was removed. This was followed by removal of the specimen and complete urinary diversion.

Data analysis

The clinicopathologic data of the two groups of patients was categorized based on whether hysterectomy performed. The normality of continuous variables was tested using Kolmogorov-Smirnov test. Independent-Samples t-test was used to compare continuous variables that followed a normal distribution (i.e., the age and time of operation as shown in Table 1). Mann-Whitney U test was used to compare continuous variables that did not follow normal distribution (i.e., BMI, bleeding volume during operation, intraoperative transfusion, postoperative stay and postoperative fasting time as shown in Table 1) between the two groups. For categorical variables, the x^2 test (or Fisher's exact test) was performed for disordered categorical variables (i.e., ORC/LRC, type of urinary diversion, preoperative clinical stage, pathologic stage, pathologic nodal stage, positive/negative surgery margin, and neoadjuvant/adjuvant chemotherapy [yes/no] as shown in Table 1). Mann-Whitney U test was performed to analyze ordered categorical variables (i.e., ASA score and Clavien-Dindo class as shown in Table 1). Kaplan-Meier curves were used to determine the

probability of overall survival and progress free survival among the patients. In addition, to decrease selection bias, the characteristics of survival/dead groups and progression/no-progression groups were compared to eliminate factors may affect the prognosis, after which multivariable Cox regression analysis of all patients was used to test for the effect of hysterectomy on risk of events of death and progress, adjusting for age, preoperative clinical stage (T0/Ta/Tis/T1, T2, T3,T4), pathologic stage (T0/Ta/Tis/T1, T2, T3/T4), pathologic nodal stage (N-, N+), neoadjuvant/adjuvant chemotherapy (yes,no), location of the tumor (posterior wall/trigone, other location) and surgery margin (negative, positive). All analyses were performed using IBM SPSS version23, and all p values are two-sided, $p < 0.05$ was considered statistically significant.

Result

Clinicopathologic data

This study enrolled 112 patients with urothelial carcinoma of bladder. Among them, 63 underwent uterus preserving cystectomy (UPC) and the rest were treated with uterus excision cystectomy (UEC). The two groups were well-matched with respect to baseline characteristics (Table 1). There was no significant difference between the two patient groups in terms of age, BMI, ASA, method of operation, type of urinary diversion, location of the tumor and neoadjuvant/adjuvant chemotherapy. But patients receiving uterus excision cystectomy had higher preoperative clinical stage ($p = 0.017$). Moreover, there was no difference between two groups in the time of operation, bleeding volume during operation, intraoperative transfusion, postoperative complications, postoperative stay and postoperative fasting time.

Regarding postoperative pathologic characteristics, uterus invasion was found in 5(4.1%) patients and were all from UEC group. There was no significant difference between the two groups with respect to pathologic stage ($p = 0.613$). But higher pathologic nodal stage can be found in UEC group ($p = 0.002$). There was no significant difference in the pathologic grade and surgical margin between the two groups. In the UPC group, two patients had positive margin of urethral, and one patient had positive margin of right ureter. And in the UEC group, one patient had positive margin of vagina, and one patient had positive margin of urethral.

Oncologic outcomes

The median follow-up period for patients was 36 months (interquartile range 16–69). At the last follow-up, the number of deaths in UPC group was 27 (42.9%) and that of UEC group was 20 (40.8%). A total of 15 (23.8%) patients of UPC group and 12 (24.5%) patients of UEC group experienced a progression. Kaplan-Meier curves were used to demonstrate OS probability and PFS

Table 1 The clinicopathologic characteristics of the patients performed uterus preserving cystectomy and uterus excision cystectomy

	UPC ($n = 63$)	UEC ($n = 49$)	p
Age (yr)	67.3 ± 12.2	67.7 ± 9.2	0.855[a]
BMI (kg/m^2)	22.9 (21.1–26.3)	23.9 (21.7–26.6)	0.205[b]
ASA score			0.961[b]
1	5 (7.9%)	1 (2.0%)	
2	46 (73.0%)	41 (83.7%)	
3	12 (19%)	7 (14.3%)	
ORC	46 (73.0%)	38 (77.6%)	0.582[c]
LRC	17 (27.0%)	11 (22.4%)	
Type of urinary diversion			0.100[c]
Cutaneous ureterostomy	29 (46.0%)	18 (36.7%)	
Ileal conduit	30 (47.6%)	31 (63.3%)	
Orthotopic neobladder	4 (6.3%)	0 (0%)	
Time of operation (mins)	294.8 ± 104.3	296.1 ± 120.0	0.950[a]
Bleeding volume during operation(L)	500 (200–800)	400 (200–650)	0.321[b]
Intraoperative transfusion(L)	200 (0–650)	200 (0–725)	0.762[b]
Clavien-Dindo class			0.061[b]
0	30 (47.6%)	32 (65.3%)	
1	2 (3.2%)	2 (4.1%)	
2	30 (47.6%)	14 (28.6%)	
3	0 (0%)	0 (0%)	
4	1 (1.6%)	0 (0%)	
5	0 (0%)	1 (2%)	
Postoperative stay (days)	11 (8–17)	9 (8–12)	0.076[b]
Postoperative fasting time (days)	5 (3–5)	5 (3–6)	0.537[b]
Location of the tumor			0.399[c]
Posterior wall or trigone	43 (68.3%)	37 (75.5%)	
Other location	20 (31.7%)	12 (24.5%)	
Preoperative clinical stage			0.017[c]
Ta and Tis and T1	18 (28.6%)	12 (24.5%)	
T2	26 (41.3%)	16 (32.7%)	
T3	19 (30.2%)	14 (28.6%)	
T4	0 (0%)	7 (14.3%)	
Pathologic stage			0.613[c]
Ta and Tis and T1	18 (28.6%)	10 (20.4%)	
T2	22 (34.9%)	19 (38.8%)	
T3 and T4	23 (36.5%)	20 (40.8%)	
Pathologic nodal stage			0.002[c]
N0	60 (95.2%)	37 (75.5%)	
N+	3 (4.8%)	12 (24.5%)	
Pathologic grade			1.000[c]
Low grade	7 (11.1%)	5 (10.2%)	
High grade	55 (87.3%)	44 (89.8%)	
Negative margin	60 (95.2%)	47 (95.9%)	1.000[c]

Table 1 The clinicopathologic characteristics of the patients performed uterus preserving cystectomy and uterus excision cystectomy *(Continued)*

	UPC (*n* = 63)	UEC (*n* = 49)	*p*
Positive margin	3 (4.8%)	2 (4.1%)	
No neoadjuvant/adjuvant chemotherapy	55 (88.7%)	39 (81.3%)	0.271[c]
Neoadjuvant/adjuvant chemotherapy	7 (11.3%)	9 (18.8%)	

UPC uterus preserving cystectomy, *UEC* uterus excision cystectomy, *BMI* Body Mass Index, *ASA* American Society of Anesthesiologists, *ORC* open radical cystectomy, *LRC* laparoscopic radical cystectomy, [a]Independent-Samples T test, [b]Mann-Whitney U test, [c]x^2 test (or Fisher's exact test)

probability after UPC and UEC for all patients (shown in Fig. 2a and b). The 5-years OS and PFS were 0.622 and 0.777 in UPC group vs 0.596 and 0.694 in UEC group, respectively. There were no significant differences in the OS probability (*p* = 0.939) and PFS probability (*p* = 0.565) between the two groups.

However, there were more T4 patients and pathological nodal stages in UEC group compared to UPC group. To decrease selection bias, the clinicopathologic characteristics of the survival/dead cases were compared. The analysis revealed that there were significant differences in age (*p* = 0.014), pathologic stage (*p* = 0.014), pathologic nodal stage (*p* = 0.043), and neoadjuvant/adjuvant chemotherapy (*p* = 0.004) between survival and dead cases (Table 2). Similarly, a comparison of the clinicopathologic characteristics of progression and no-progression cases revealed that there were significant differences in pathologic nodal stage (*p* = 0.006), and neoadjuvant/adjuvant chemotherapy (*p* = 0.002) between the two groups (Table 3). Subsequently, multivariable Cox regression analysis was performed to adjust factors that may influence long-term prognosis of

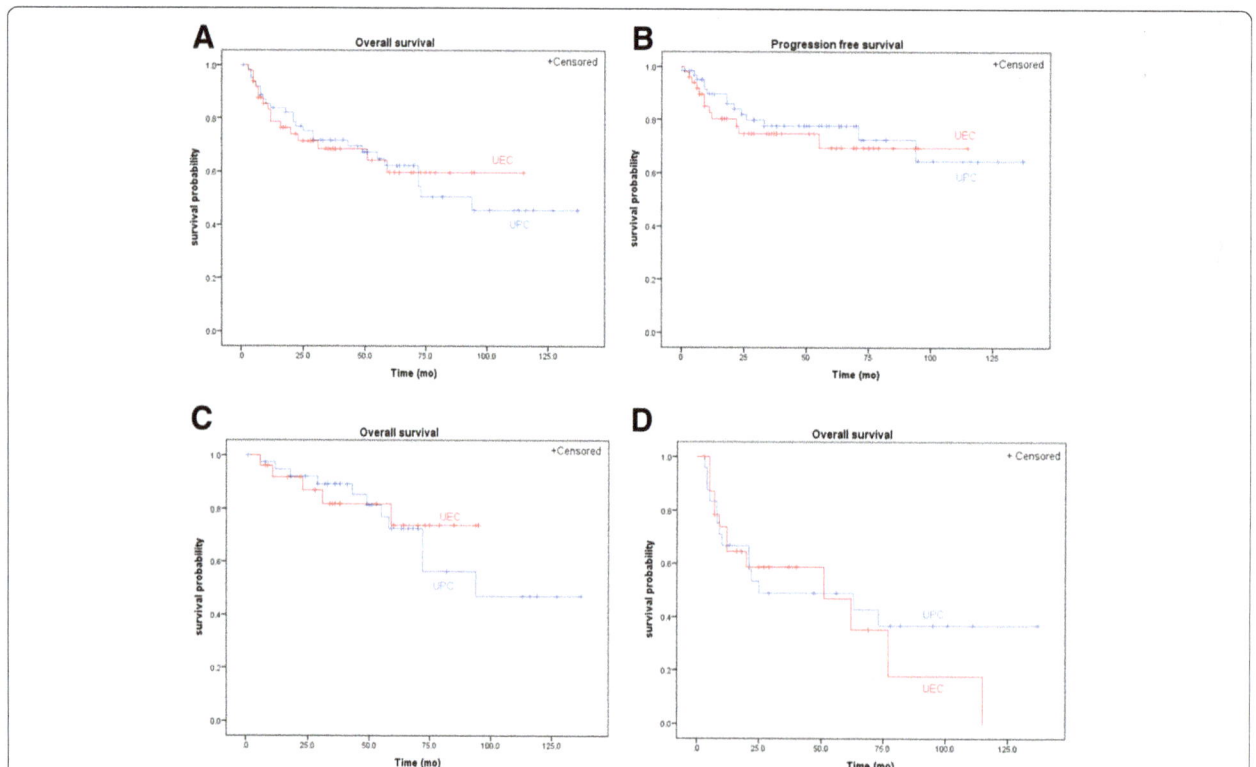

Fig. 2 a Kaplan-Meier curves of overall survival probability in all patients. The 5-years OS were 0.622 vs 0.596 between two groups, and there were no significant differences in the OS probability (*p* = 0.939). **b** Kaplan-Meier curves of progression-free survival probability in all patients. The 5-years PFS were 0.777 vs 0.694 between two groups, and there were no significant differences in the PFS probability (*p* = 0.565). **c** Kaplan-Meier curves of overall survival probability in organ-confined patients. The 5-years OS were 0.723 vs 0.735 between two groups, and there were no significant differences in the OS probability (*p* = 0.675). **d** Kaplan-Meier curves of overall survival probability in no-organ confined patients. The 5-years OS were 0.489 vs 0.469 between two groups, and there were no significant differences in the OS probability (*p* = 0.695). (UPC = uterus preserved cystectomy, UEC = uterus excision cystectomy)

Table 2 The clinicopathologic characteristics of the patients of survival group and dead group

	Survival ($n = 71$)	Dead ($n = 41$)	p
Age (yr)	65.5 ± 11.5	70.8 ± 9.2	0.014[a]
BMI (kg/m^2)	23.7 (21.4–26.6)	23.4 (20.8–26.2)	0.570[b]
ORC	50 (70.4%)	34 (82.9%)	0.141[c]
LRC	21 (29.6%)	7 (17.1%)	
Location of the tumor			0.107[c]
Posterior wall or trigone	47 (66.2%)	33 (80.5%)	
Other location	24 (33.8%)	8 (19.5%)	
Pathologic stage			0.014[c]
Ta and Tis and T1	21 (29.6%)	7 (17.1%)	
T2	30 (42.3%)	11 (26.8%)	
T3 and T4	20 (28.2%)	23 (56.1%)	
Pathologic nodal stage			0.043[c]
N0	65 (91.5%)	32 (78.0%)	
N+	6 (8.5%)	9 (22.0%)	
Negative margin	69 (97.2%)	38 (92.7%)	0.159[c]
Positive margin	2 (2.8%)	3 (7.3%)	
No neoadjuvant/adjuvant chemotherapy	66 (93.0%)	29 (72.5%)	0.004[c]
Neoadjuvant/adjuvant chemotherapy	5 (7.0%)	11 (26.8%)	

BMI Body Mass Index, *ASA* American Society of Anesthesiologists, *ORC* open radical cystectomy, *LRC* laparoscopic radical cystectomy, [a]Independent-Samples T test, [b]Mann-Whitney U test, [c]χ^2 test (or Fisher's exact test)

Table 3 The clinicopathologic characteristics of the patients of no progression group and progression group

	No-progression ($n = 86$)	Progression ($n = 26$)	p
Age (yr)	69.00 (61.00–76.00)	70.50 (63.75–78.00)	0.370[b]
BMI (kg/m^2)	23.0 (21.2–26.3)	24.6 (22.3–27.0)	0.100[b]
ORC	65 (75.6%)	19 (73.1%)	0.796[c]
LRC	21 (24.4%)	7 (26.9%)	
Location of the tumor			0.777[c]
Posterior wall or trigone	62 (72.1%)	18 (69.2%)	
Other location	24 (27.9%)	8 (30.8%)	
Pathologic stage			0.159[c]
Ta and Tis and T1	25 (29.1%)	3 (11.5%)	
T2	31 (36.0%)	10 (38.5%)	
T3 and T4	30 (34.9%)	13 (50.0%)	
Pathologic nodal stage			0.006[c]
N0	79 (91.9%)	18 (69.2%)	
N+	7 (8.1%)	8 (30.8%)	
Negative margin	83 (96.5%)	24 (92.3%)	0.329[c]
Positive margin	3 (3.5%)	2 (7.7%)	
No neoadjuvant/adjuvant chemotherapy	79 (91.9%)	17 (65.4%)	0.002[c]
Neoadjuvant/adjuvant chemotherapy	7 (8.1%)	9 (34.6%)	

BMI Body Mass Index, *ASA* American Society of Anesthesiologists, *ORC* open radical cystectomy, *LRC* laparoscopic radical cystectomy, [a]Independent-Samples T test, [b]Mann-Whitney U test, [c]χ^2 test (or Fisher's exact test)

patients, and the results are shown in Tables 4 and 5. It was found that hysterectomy was not an independent predictor of overall survival (hazard ratio 0.908, 95%CI 0.428–1.924, $p = 0.801$) and progression-free survival (hazard ratio 1.109, 95%CI 0.439–2.805, $p = 0.826$) after adjusting for age, preoperative clinical stage (T0/Ta/Tis/ T1, T2, T3,T4), pathologic stage (T0/Ta/Tis/T1, T2, T3/ T4), pathologic nodal stage (N-, N+), neoadjuvant/adjuvant chemotherapy (yes,no), location of tumor (posterior wall/trigone, other location) and surgery margin (negative, positive).

Furthermore, patients with organ-confined tumors (≤pT2bN0M0) were used in the survival analysis and those with on-organ confined tumors were used for sensitivity analysis to eliminate inclusion bias. and no significant difference of overall survival probability was observed in the patients with organ-confined bladder cancer ($p = 0.675$) and in patients with no organ-confined bladder cancer ($p = 0.695$). (Fig. 2c and d).

Discussion

Currently, radical cystectomy is the mainstream treatment for recurrent high grade or muscle-invasive bladder cancer. Unlike in male patients, radical cystectomy in female patients includes total anterior pelvic exenteration encompassing the bladder, urethra, anterior vagina and uterus. This type of resection is recommended for patients with vaginal or uterus invasion. However, uterus invasion is rare according to the prevailing literature on postoperative pathological data. Among 160 female patients who underwent radical cystectomy, Gregg et al. found that 20 (12.5%) had uterus invasion [5], which is the highest rate reported so far (0.3–7.5%) [6–10]. In our cohort, among 112 patients who underwent radical cystectomy, only 5 (4.5%) had uterus invasion. According to Kluth, the prognosis of female patients is poorer compared to that of men, further explaining why resection is necessary for female patients. Moreover, it was stated that female gender was an independent risk factor for death from this disease (hazard ratio = 1.17 [range 1.05 to 1.31], $p = 0.005$) [12]. From the anatomical perspective, in women, there is no natural anatomical barrier between the bladder and uterus to prevent tumor invasion [4]. Therefore, majority of urological surgeons hold the view that hysterectomy seems to be a reasonable part of cystectomy, especially for postmenopausal women and those who no longer have the desire to preserve their fertility.

Table 4 Univariable/Multivariable Cox regression analysis of variables associated with overall survival after cystectomy

Variable	univariable cox regression analysis			multivariable cox regression analysis		
	Hazard Ratio	95% CI	p	Hazard Ratio	95% CI	p
Age (continuous)	1.034	1.003–1.067	0.034	1.027	0.994–1.061	0.108
Preoperative stage			0.113			0.927
Ta and Tis and T1	–	referent	–	–	Referent	–
T2	1.317	0.552–3.141	0.535	0.814	0.281–2.359	0.705
T3	2.496	1.064–5.851	0.035	1.050	0.355–3.100	0.930
T4	2.608	0.683–9.951	0.161	0.862	0.174–4.264	0.856
Pathologic stage			0.005			0.129
Ta and Tis and T1	–	referent	–	–	referent	–
T2	1.375	0.530–3.568	0.513	1.315	0.456–3.792	0.613
T3 and T4	3.341	1.427–7.822	0.005	2.508	0.876–7.174	0.087
Pathologic nodal stage						
N0	–	referent	–	–	Referent	–
N+	2.725	1.285–5.778	0.009	1.896	0.791–4.544	0.152
No chemotherapy	–	referent	–	–	Referent	–
Chemotherapy	2.979	1.486–5.973	0.002	1.860	0.848–4.081	0.121
Location of the tumor						
other location	–	referent	–	–	Referent	–
posterior wall/trigone	2.028	0.934–4.402	0.074	1.902	0.834–4.339	0.126
Negative margin	–	referent	–	–	Referent	–
Positive margin	3.938	1.177–13.172	0.026	1.463	0.381–5.628	0.580
No hysterectomy	–	referent	–	–	Referent	–
Hysterectomy	0.976	0.520–1.832	0.976	0.908	0.428–1.924	0.801

Table 5 Univariable/Multivariable Cox regression analysis of variables associated with progression free survival after cystectomy

Variable	univariable cox regression analysis			multivariable cox regression analysis		
	Hazard Ratio	95% CI	p	Hazard Ratio	95% CI	p
Age (continuous)	1.024	0.986–1.064	0.216	1.013	0.971–1.056	0.556
Preoperative stage			0.168			0.437
Ta and Tis and T1	–	referent	–	–	referent	–
T2	2.011	0.630–6.419	0.238	0.983	0.236–4.102	0.981
T3	3.516	1.114–11.099	0.032	1.529	0.369–6.341	0.558
T4	1.509	0.167–13.609	0.714	0.286	0.025–3.296	0.316
Pathologic stage			0.055			0.541
Ta and Tis and T1	–	referent	–	–	referent	–
T2	2.904	0.792–10.654	0.108	2.003	0.460–8.721	0.355
T3 and T4	4.600	1.300–16.270	0.018	2.419	0.507–11.543	0.268
Pathologic nodal stage						
N0	–	referent	–	–	Referent	–
N+	4.372	1.883–10.150	0.001	4.067	1.424–11.610	0.009
No chemotherapy	–	referent	–	–	Referent	–
Chemotherapy	4.705	2.075–10.670	<0.001	2.950	1.131–7.694	0.027
Location of the tumor						
other location	–	referent	–	–	Referent	–
Posterior wall/trigone	1.004	0.436–2.313	0.992	0.737	0.292–1.859	0.518
Negative margin	–	referent	–	–	Referent	–
Positive margin	3.369	0.778–14.584	0.104	1.500	0.253–8.904	0.656
No hysterectomy	–	referent	–	–	Referent	–
Hysterectomy	1.254	0.578–2.718	0.567	1.109	0.439–2.805	0.826

Due to technological advancement of endoscopy technology and the duration of application, many urological surgeons prefer minimally invasive surgery in the management of bladder cancer [13]. In present study, 28 (25%) patients received laparoscopic radical cystectomy (LRC), and during the study period, more patients chose minimally invasive surgery technique. The number of patients who received LRC increased from 14.9% in 2006–2011 to 32.3% in 2012–2017. This is because urological surgeons prefer surgical approaches that improve patients' postoperative quality of life. For this reason, the use of pelvic organ-preserving techniques has increased tremendously. The need to understand the pelvic structure and improve surgical techniques has driven the emergence of new techniques, such as those aimed at preserving neurovascular bundle, vagina, uterus or variations of any the stated techniques [14]. In present study, 63(56.3%) patients received uterus preserved cystectomy.

Uterus sparing radical cystectomy decreases the rate of sexual dysfunction, preserves fertility and improves the voiding function of orthotopic neobladder [15].

However, in this study, 9 patients were below 50 years old, but we did not ascertain the number of those who wanted to retain their fertility. Nevertheless, not many patients wanted to retain their fertility, in fact many patients chose uterus preserving surgery to avoid losing another organ. Classic radical cystectomy may damage neurovascular bundles along the lateral vaginal wall, which may compromise sexual arousal and orgasm. Female Sexual Function Index can be preserved if autonomic nerves are left intact, but it can be severely diminished when such nerves are removed [16]. For patients receiving orthotopic neobladder, leaving the uterus and vaginal intact will provide proper support to the neobladder and prevent herniation of posterior wall of the pouch through the vaginal. This decreases the rate of postoperative chronic urinary retention and hence improve the voiding function [17, 18]. In this study, a high percent of patients received cutaneous ureterostomy diversion and only 4 patients chose orthotopic neobladder for urinary diversion. Yet, we were alert to the fact that ileal conduits and neobladder reconstruction are better options, especially for patients with a lower stage of disease. As more laparoscopic operations were performed in our institution, more orthotopic neo-bladder were applied.

Some previous study investigated the risks of uterus invasion to determine which group of patients is likely to benefit from uterus preserving cystectomy. A study by Varkarakis performed in Austria, retrospectively reviewed 54 women who had clinical organ confined transitional cell bladder cancer. In their study, preoperative risk factors could not be identified, although 3 cases of tumor invasion to internal genitalia (1 uterus and 2 vaginal) were observed in the dome and base of bladder [7]. Choi et al. reported that tumor location of the trigone or bladder neck at TUR-Bt, maximum tumor size ≥4.8 cm at CT, and hydronephrosis at CT were independent predictors of female organ involvement [8]. A study by Ali-El-Dein indicated that high grade of the bladder tumor and positive lymph node status were positive predictors of secondary gynecologic organ involvement [10]. Gregg et al. stated that lack of trigonal or bladder floor tumor, intraoperative palpable posterior mass, and clinical lymphadenopathy were associated with absence of female pelvic organ involvement. Hence, unifocal, organ-confined tumors (≤cT2b) away from the bladder neck, trigone, and bladder base seem to be suited for reproductive organ-sparing radical cystectomy [15]. In this study, there was no definite indication for uterus-sparing radical cystectomy. Hysterectomy was performed in radical cystectomy based on the consensus between doctors and patients. Hysterectomy was also performed in cases where preoperative examinations revealed a suspected uterine invasion or when uterine invasion was found during intraoperation. In present study, one patient, who had no uterine invasion from preoperative examination, was changed to uterus excision cystectomy because uterine invasion was found during operation. It should be noted that patients in the two groups were matched in terms of age, BMI and ASA, and the decisions had no relationship with the surgeons' preference (data not show).

As a treatment for malignant tumors, the main goal of radical cystectomy is to achieve oncological control. This study involved a long-term follow-up duration to assess the oncological outcomes after UPC. Among 112 female patients with bladder cancer, 63 (56.3%) were operated with UPC and 49 (43.7%) received UEC. No significant differences were observed between two groups in overall survival and progression-free survival rates. However, the group of UEC, comprising more cases of T4 and more cases with higher pathological nodal stage, whose prognosis was supposed to be worse than that of the group of UPC. Therefore, to reduce selection bias, we used multivariable Cox regression analysis to adjust for the factors that may affect the patients' prognosis— age, preoperative clinical stage (T0/Ta/Tis/T1, T2, T3,T4),

pathologic stage (T0/Ta/Tis/T1, T2, T3/T4), pathologic nodal stage (N-, N+), neoadjuvant/adjuvant chemotherapy (yes,no), location of the tumor (posterior wall/trigone, other location), and surgery margin (negative, positive). The results showed that hysterectomy was not an independent predictor of overall survival (hazard ratio 0.908, 95%CI 0.428–1.924, p = 0.801) and progression-free survival (hazard ratio 1.109, 95%CI 0.439–2.805, p = 0.826). Further analysis revealed that, in patients with organ-confined tumors (≤cT2bN0M0), there were no significant differences in overall survival (p = 0.675) and progression-free survival (p = 0.985) between UPC and UEC groups. Hence, we infer that hysterectomy is not suitable for female patients with organ-confined bladder cancer. Similarly, for patients with advanced tumor, there were no significant differences in the overall survival and progression-free survival between two groups. We postulate that hysterectomy may not be effective in patients with advanced tumor because of poor prognosis. However, this concept need to be clarified in further studies. In this study, the 5-year OS was 0.622 and 0.596 in UPC and UEC groups, respectively, and was slightly lower compared to 65–83% reported in previous studies [14]. This was attributed to the lower percent of patients receiving neoadjuvant/adjuvant chemotherapy in this study. In our case, many patients refused chemotherapy because of its adverse events.

There are some limitations to consider in this study. A key limitation is that this is a retrospective design with some inherent selection bias. In addition, the decision whether to perform hysterectomy in radical cystectomy was based on discussions between doctors and patients. Application of uterine preserving surgery was not based on clear guidelines. Patients with advanced tumors were more likely to choose hysterectomy. Therefore, this study may have some selection biases and confounding biases. We adopted a multivariable Cox regression analysis to adjust for factors that may affect patients' prognosis instead of a Kaplan-Meier analysis with matched groups because the lower prevalence of the bladder cancer in women contributed to the relatively small sample size. Moreover, due to patients' privacy and the retrospective nature of this study, we did not include other outcomes such as changes in sexual and urinary function, rate of prolapse, and postoperative fertility.

Conclusion

The results showed that the rate of uterus invasion was low in patients analyzed in this cohort. It was also found that hysterectomy was not an independent predictor of OS and PFS after radical cystectomy in patients with bladder cancer.

Is hysterectomy beneficial in radical cystectomy for female patient with urothelial carcinoma...

105

Additional file

Additional file 1: Information of the patients. This data includes relevant information of all patients enrolled in this study, including Clinicopathologic data and oncologic outcomes. (XLSX 24 kb)

Abbreviations

AC: Adjuvant chemotherapy; ASA: American Society of Anesthesiologists; BMI: Body Mass Index; CT: Computed tomography; LRC: Laparoscopic radical cystectomy; MRI: Magnetic resonance imaging; NAC: Neoadjuvant chemotherapy; ORC: Open radical cystectomy; OS: Overall survival; PFS: Progression-free survival; UEC: Uterus excision cystectomy; UPC: Uterus preserving cystectomy; US: Ultrasound

Acknowledgements

Not applicable.

Authors' contributions

HH1 collected the patients data, analyzed the data, and drafted and revised the manuscript; BY collected the patients data and analyzed the data; MS was a major contributor in data analysis; LL collected the data and provided pathological support; HH2 collected the data; ZX was a major contributor in data analysis and revising the manuscript. All authors read and approved the final manuscript. (HH1 corresponding to Haiwen Huang and HH2 corresponding to Han Hao).

Author details

[1]Department of Urology, Peking University First Hospital, 8 Xishiku Street, Xicheng District, Beijing 100034, China. [2]Institute of Urology, Peking University, National Urological Cancer Center, 8 Xishiku Street, Xicheng District, Beijing 100034, China. [3]Department of Urology, Xingtai People's Hospital, 16 Hongxing Street, Qiaodong District, Xingtai 054001, China. [4]Department of Medical Statistics, Peking University First Hospital, 8 Xishiku Street, Xicheng District, Beijing 100034, China.

References

1. Antoni S, Ferlay J, Soerjomataram I, Znaor A, Jemal A, Bray F. Bladder Cancer incidence and mortality: a global overview and recent trends. Eur Urol. 2017;71(1):96–108.
2. Dobruch J, Daneshmand S, Fisch M, Lotan Y, Noon AP, Resnick MJ, Shariat SF, Zlotta AR, Boorjian SA. Gender and bladder Cancer: a collaborative review of etiology, biology, and outcomes. Eur Urol. 2016;69(2):300–10.
3. Stenzl A, Nagele U, Kuczyk M, Sievert K-D, Anastasiadis A, Seibold J, Corvin S. Cystectomy – technical considerations in male and female patients. EAU Updat Ser. 2005;3(3):138–46.
4. Weissbart SJ, Smith AL. Hysterectomy in the Urologist's practice. Curr Urol Rep. 2017;18(1).
5. Gregg JR, Emeruwa C, Wong J, Barocas DA, Chang SS, Clark PE, Cookson MS, Penson DF, Resnick MJ, Scarpato KR, et al. Oncologic outcomes after anterior Exenteration for muscle invasive bladder Cancer in women. J Urol. 2016;196(4):1030–5.
6. Chang SS, Cole E, Smith JA Jr, Cookson MS. Pathological findings of gynecologic organs obtained at female radical cystectomy. J Urol. 2002; 168(1):147–9.
7. Varkarakis IM, Pinggera G, Antoniou N, Constantinides K, Chrisofos M, Deliveliotis C. Pathological review of internal genitalia after anterior exenteration for bladder cancer in women. Evaluating risk factors for female organ involvement. Int Urol Nephrol. 2007;39(4):1015–21.
8. Choi SY, Yoo S, Han JH, Jeong IG, Hong B, Hong JH, Ahn H, Kim C-S, You D. Predictors of female genital organ involvement in radical cystectomy for urothelial carcinoma of the bladder: a single-center retrospective analysis of 112 female patients. Int J Surg. 2017;47:101–6.
9. Salem H, El-Mazny A. Primary and secondary malignant involvement of gynaecological organs at radical cystectomy for bladder cancer: review of literature and retrospective analysis of 360 cases. J Obstet Gynaecol. 2012; 32(6):590–3.
10. Ali-El-Dein B, Abdel-Latif M, Mosbah A, Eraky I, Shaaban AA, Taha NM, Ghoneim MA. Secondary malignant involvement of gynecologic organs in radical cystectomy specimens in women: is it mandatory to remove these organs routinely? J Urol. 2004;172(3):885–7.
11. Ali-El-Dein B, Mosbah A, Osman Y, El-Tabey N, Abdel-latif M, Eraky I, Shaaban AA. Preservation of the internal genital organs during radical cystectomy in selected women with bladder cancer: a report on 15 cases with long term follow-up. Eur J Surg Oncol (EJSO). 2013;39(4):358–64.
12. Kluth LA, Rieken M, Xylinas E, Kent M, Rink M, Roupret M, Sharifi N, Jamzadeh A, Kassouf W, Kaushik D, et al. Gender-specific differences in clinicopathologic outcomes following radical cystectomy: an international multi-institutional study of more than 8000 patients. Eur Urol. 2014;66(5): 913–9.
13. Tang K, Li H, Xia D, Hu Z, Zhuang Q, Liu J, Xu H, Ye Z. Laparoscopic versus open radical cystectomy in bladder cancer: a systematic review and meta-analysis of comparative studies. PLoS One. 2014;9(5):e95667.
14. Veskimäe E, Neuzillet Y, Rouanne M, MacLennan S, Lam TBL, Yuan Y, Compérat E, Cowan NC, Gakis G, van der Heijden AG, et al. Systematic review of the oncological and functional outcomes of pelvic organ-preserving radical cystectomy (RC) compared with standard RC in women who undergo curative surgery and orthotopic neobladder substitution for bladder cancer. BJU Int. 2017;120(1):12–24.
15. Niver BE, Daneshmand S, Satkunasivam R. Female reproductive organ-sparing radical cystectomy: contemporary indications, techniques and outcomes. Curr Opin Urol. 2015;25(2):105–10.
16. Bhatt A, Nandipati K, Dhar N, Ulchaker J, Jones S, Rackley R, Zippe C. Neurovascular preservation in orthotopic cystectomy: impact on female sexual function. Urology. 2006;67(4):742–5.
17. Puppo P, Introini C, Calvi P, Naselli A. Prevention of chronic urinary retention in orthotopic bladder replacement in the female. Eur Urol. 2005; 47(5):674–8 discussion 678.
18. Finley DS, Lee U, McDonough D, Raz S, deKernion J. Urinary retention after orthotopic neobladder substitution in females. J Urol. 2011;186(4):1364–9.

14

The impact of perivesical lymph node metastasis on clinical outcomes of bladder cancer patients undergoing radical cystectomy

Meenal Sharma[1], Takuro Goto[1,2], Zhiming Yang[1] and Hiroshi Miyamoto[1,2,3*] (iD)

Abstract

Background: Perivesical lymph nodes (PVLNs) are occasionally isolated during grossing of cystectomy specimens. However, the prognostic implications of the involvement of PVLNs in bladder cancer patients, especially those with comparisons to pN0 disease, remain poorly understood.

Methods: A retrospective review identified 115 radical cystectomy cases where PVLNs had been histologically assessed. These cases were then divided into 4 groups – Group 1 ($n = 76$): PVLN-negative/other pelvic lymph node (non-PVLN)-negative; Group 2 ($n = 5$): PVLN-positive/non-PVLN-negative; Group 3 ($n = 17$): PVLN-negative/non-PVLN-positive; and Group 4 ($n = 17$): PVLN-positive/non-PVLN-positive.

Results: pT stage at cystectomy was significantly higher in Group 3 ($P = 0.013$), Group 4 ($P < 0.001$), Groups 2 and 4 ($P < 0.001$), or Groups 2–4 ($P < 0.001$) than in Group 1. However, the number of positive PVLNs (mean: 1.8 vs. 2.1; $P = 0.718$) or the rate of extracapsular extension in the PVLNs (40% vs. 65%, $P = 0.609$) was not significantly different between Group 2 and Group 4. Kaplan-Meier analysis and log-rank test revealed significantly ($P < 0.05$) higher risks of disease progression (Group 3/Group 4), cancer-specific mortality (Group 2/Group 3/Group 4), and overall mortality (Group 4), compared with Group 1. Multivariate analysis further showed metastasis to both PVLN and non-PVLN (Group 4), PVLN (Groups 2 and 4), or PVLN and/or non-PVLN (Groups 2–4) as an independent prognosticator for cancer-specific mortality and overall survival. There were also insignificant ($P = 0.096$) and significant ($P = 0.036$) differences in cancer-specific survival and overall survival, respectively, between Group 3 versus Group 4, and the trend of the latter was confirmed by subset multivariate analysis (hazard ratio = 3.769; $P = 0.099$).

Conclusions: Worse prognosis was observed in bladder cancer patients with isolated PVLN metastasis (vs. pN0 disease especially for cancer-specific survival), PVLN metastasis with or without non-PVLN metastasis (vs. pN0 disease), and concurrent PVLN and non-PVLN metastases (vs. PVLN-negative/non-PVLN-positive disease especially for overall survival). These findings indicate the importance of thorough histopathological assessment of PVLNs in radical cystectomy specimens.

Keywords: Cancer-specific survival, Mortality, Pelvic lymph node metastasis, Progression-free survival, Staging, Urothelial carcinoma

---

* Correspondence: hiroshi_miyamoto@urmc.rochester.edu
[1]Department of Pathology and Laboratory Medicine, University of Rochester Medical Center, Rochester, NY, USA
[2]James P. Wilmot Cancer Institute, University of Rochester Medical Center, Rochester, NY, USA
Full list of author information is available at the end of the article

Background

Urinary bladder cancer, which is mostly a urothelial carcinoma, is one of the most frequently diagnosed neoplasms worldwide [1]. Muscle-invasive disease with which approximately 30% of patients initially present accounts for the majority of mortalities associated with bladder cancer [2, 3]. Additionally, it has been well documented that metastasis to the regional lymph node(s) represents a critical prognostic factor in patients with bladder cancer. Meanwhile, radical cystectomy usually with pelvic lymph node dissection remains the mainstay of treatment for locally advanced bladder cancer.

Previous studies have addressed the clinical impact of the extent and boundaries of lymph node dissection during radical cystectomy on patient outcomes [4–7]. By contrast, the prognostic implications of perivesical lymph node (PVLN) involvement by bladder cancer metastasis remain far from being fully understood. It has been variably reported that PVLNs are isolated in 0–46% of patients via grossing and histological assessment of cystectomy specimens, presumably dependent on surgical technique and tissue processing [8–13]. Metastasis to the PVLNs has also been found in 3–21% of the cystectomy cases for bladder cancer in which PVLNs are identified [8, 11–13]. Importantly, in the latest edition of the American Joint Committee on Cancer (AJCC) TNM staging for bladder cancer (8th Edition implemented on January 1, 2018) [14], PVLN metastasis was definitively classified as N1 (single node involvement) or N2 (multiple node involvement). However, no recent studies have assessed the clinical significance of PVLN involvement in patients with bladder cancer, especially with comparisons to N0 disease. We here comparatively studied the outcome of groups of patients with or without positive PVLN and/or non-PVLN who underwent radical cystectomy and pelvic lymphadenectomy for bladder cancer.

Methods

We searched our Surgical Pathology database for radical cystectomy/cystoprostatectomy cases performed between July 2004 and March 2019. Of these, 115 primary bladder cancer cases (93 males and 22 females; age range: 25–88 years; mean age: 68.5 years; median age: 69 years) where PVLNs had been histologically assessed were identified. All these 115 patients underwent pelvic lymph node dissection. The cystectomy specimens were grossly reviewed for the presence of PVLNs and processed primarily by pathology assistants and/or pathology residents who were supervised by attending pathologists. Histologically, an aggregate of lymphoid tissue at least partially encapsulated was defined as a lymph node. Clearing techniques or solvents, as well as special stains, for isolating PVLNs were not used. We also retrieved clinical and histopathological findings as well as follow-up data (median: 24 months; 5 cases lost to follow-up and 4 recent cases) from all 115 patients. Neoadjuvant systemic chemotherapy prior to cystectomy or adjuvant systemic chemotherapy/immunotherapy following cystectomy was performed in 21 or 25 patients, respectively.

Data were analyzed, using the Student's t-test for continuous variables and the Fisher's exact test for non-continuous variables. The rates of progression-free survival, cancer-specific survival, and overall survival were calculated by the Kaplan-Meier method, and comparison was made by log-rank test. Tumor progression was defined as the development of recurrent or metastatic tumors after cystectomy. In addition, the Cox proportional hazards model was used to determine statistical significance of prognostic factors in a multivariate setting. P values less than 0.05 were considered to be statistically significant.

Results

We analyzed 115 radical cystectomy cases where PVLNs (range: 1–14; mean: 2.3; median: 2) were histologically assessed. Twenty-two (19%) and 34 (30%) patients had metastases to the PVLNs and other pelvic lymph nodes (non-PVLNs), respectively. Of the latter cases, 3 had pN3 disease, but none had isolated metastasis to the common iliac lymph nodes. Seventeen (15%) patients showed concurrent metastases to both PNLN and non-PVLN. For further analyses, these cases were divided into 4 groups based on the status of lymph node metastasis – Group 1 ($n = 76$): PVLN-negative/non-PVLN-negative; Group 2 ($n = 5$): PVLN-positive/non-PVLN-negative; Group 3 ($n = 17$): PVLN-negative/non-PVLN-positive; and Group 4 ($n = 17$): PVLN-positive/non-PVLN-positive.

Table 1 summarizes the clinicopathological features of the 4 cohorts of patients. Clinical stage prior to neoadjuvant chemotherapy and subsequent cystectomy was significantly higher (≥III) in Group 4 (35%, $P = 0.021$), Groups 2 and 4 (29%, $P = 0.039$), or Groups 2–4 (28%, $P = 0.034$) than in Group 1 (11%). Similarly, pT stage at cystectomy was significantly higher (≥pT3) in Group 3 (71%, $P = 0.013$), Group 4 (94%, $P < 0.001$), Groups 2 and 4 (86%, $P < 0.001$), or Groups 2–4 (79%, $P < 0.001$) than in Group 1 (36%). In addition, adjuvant therapy was more often administered in Group 4 (47%, $P = 0.006$), Groups 2 and 4 (41%, $P = 0.010$), or Groups 2–4 (36%, $P = 0.010$) than in Group 1 (14%). However, there were no significant differences in age, sex, neoadjuvant chemotherapy, histology [conventional urothelial carcinoma vs. variants including squamous differentiation ($n = 14$), glandular differentiation or adenocarcinoma ($n = 3$), small cell carcinoma ($n = 3$), and micropapillary ($n = 5$), nested ($n = 2$), or sarcomatoid ($n = 3$) feature], and surgical margin status between groups. Meanwhile, the

Table 1 Clinicopathological features of patients undergoing radical cystectomy and pelvic lymphadenectomy

	Group 1 PVLN(−)/non-PVLN(−)	Group 2 PVLN(+)/non-PVLN(−)	Group 3 PVLN(−)/non-PVLN(+)	Group 4 PVLN(+)/non-PVLN(+)	P value
No. of patients	76	5	17	17	
Age (mean ± SD, years)	67.6 ± 12.5	73.8 ± 11.0	70.8 ± 8.9	68.9 ± 9.7	> 0.1[a]
Sex					> 0.1[a]
Male	60 (79%)	4 (80%)	13 (76%)	16 (94%)	
Female	16 (21%)	1 (20%)	4 (24%)	1 (6%)	
Clinical stage (prior to cystectomy)					0.021[b] (G1 vs G4); 0.039[b] (G1 vs G2&G4); 0.034[b] (G1 vs G2-G4)
≤ II	61 (80%)	4 (80%)	13 (76%)	10 (59%)	
≥ III	8 (11%)	1 (20%)	4 (24%)	6 (35%)	
Unknown	7 (9%)	0 (0%)	0 (0%)	1 (6%)	
Neoadjuvant chemotherapy					> 0.1[a]
No	65 (86%)	4 (80%)	12 (71%)	13 (76%)	
Yes	11 (14%)	1 (20%)	5 (29%)	4 (24%)	
Histology					> 0.1[a]
Conventional	56 (74%)	5 (100%)	14 (82%)	10 (59%)	
Variants	20 (26%)	0 (0%)	3 (18%)	7 (41%)	
pT stage					0.013 (G1 vs G3); < 0.001 (G1 vs G4); < 0.001 (G1 vs G2&G4); < 0.001 (G1 vs G2-G4)
≤ 2	49 (64%)	2 (40%)	5 (29%)	1 (6%)	
≥ 3	27 (36%)	3 (60%)	12 (71%)	16 (94%)	
Surgical margin					> 0.1[a]
No	71 (93%)	4 (80%)	17 (100%)	14 (82%)	
Yes	5 (7%)	1 (20%)	0 (0%)	3 (18%)	
Adjuvant therapy					0.006 (G1 vs G4); 0.010 (G1 vs G2&G4); 0.010 (G1 vs G2-G4)
No	65 (86%)	4 (80%)	12 (71%)	9 (53%)	
Yes	11 (14%)	1 (20%)	5 (29%)	8 (47%)	

Abbreviation: *PVLN* perivesical lymph node
[a]all comparisons performed between two groups
[b]≤ II vs ≥ III

number of positive PVLNs and the size of largest tumor focus in the PVLN were not significantly different between Groups 2 and 4 (Table 2). The rate of extracapsular extension in positive PVLNs in Group 4 (65%) was higher than that in Group 2 (40%), although the difference was not statistically significant ($P = 0.609$).

We further investigated possible associations between the status of PVLN/non-PVLN metastasis and patient outcomes after radical surgery. The median follow-up periods for overall survival in alive patients were: 50 (Group 1); 72.5 (Group 2); 6 (Group 3); and 20 (Group 4) months. Kaplan-Meier analysis coupled with log-rank

Table 2 Characteristics of PVLNs

	Group 2 PVLN(+)/non-PVLN(−)	Group 4 PVLN(+)/non-PVLN(+)	P value
No. of patients	5	17	
No. of PVLN [mean / median (range)]	5.0 / 4 (1–14)	3.1 / 2 (1–12)	0.472
No. of positive PVLN [mean / median (range)]	1.8 / 1 (1–4)	2.1 / 1 (1–12)	0.718
Largest tumor focus [mean / median (range), cm]	0.8 / 0.8 (0.2–1.1)	0.7 / 0.8 (0.1–2.4)	0.989
Extracapsular extension	2 (40%)	11 (65%)	0.609

Abbreviation: *PVLN* perivesical lymph node

test revealed significantly worse prognosis in Group 2 (cancer-specific survival), Group 3 (disease-free/cancer-specific survival), and Group 4 (progression-free/cancer-specific/overall survival), compared with Group 1 (Fig. 1). Significantly higher risks of disease progression/mortality were also seen in patients with lymph node metastasis (Groups 2, 3, and 4), either PVLN or non-PLVN metastasis (Groups 2 and 3; except overall survival), or PVLN metastasis (Groups 2 and 4), compared to those with pN0 disease (Group 1). Interestingly, there were insignificant ($P = 0.096$) and significant ($P = 0.036$) differences in cancer-specific survival and overall survival, respectively, between Groups

3 versus 4. Similarly, insignificantly worse overall survival ($P = 0.072$) was seen in PVLN-positive cases (Groups 2 and 4), compared with Group 3. No statistically significant differences in patient outcomes between Groups 2 versus 3 and Groups 2 versus 4 were observed. Meanwhile, neoadjuvant and adjuvant therapies were associated with significantly lower rates of progression-free survival and progression-free/cancer-specific survival, respectively (see Table 3).

To determine whether the involvement of PVLNs and/or non-PVLNs was an independent prognosticator in bladder cancer patients undergoing radical cystectomy, multivariate analysis was performed with the Cox model

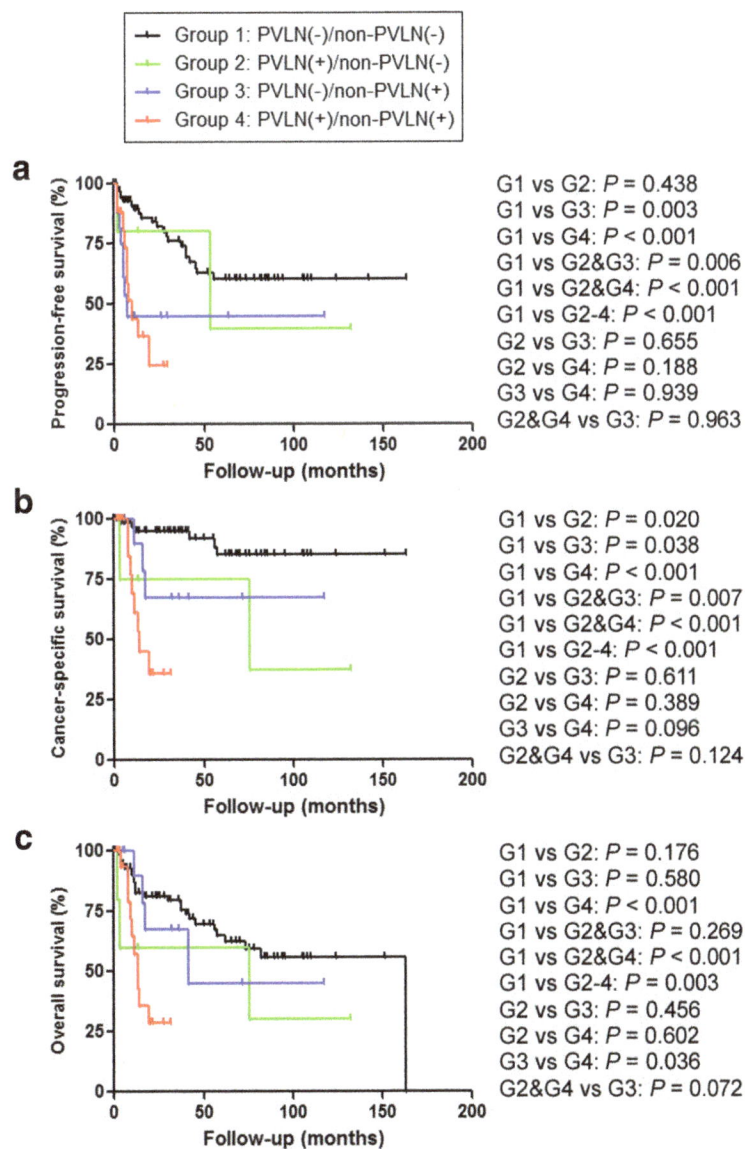

Fig. 1 Progression-free survival (**a**), cancer-specific survival (**b**), or overall survival (**c**) in bladder cancer patients undergoing radical cystectomy and pelvic lymphadenectomy according to the status of PVLN and non-PVLN metastases (i.e. Groups 1–4). Comparisons between two groups were made by log-rank test

Table 3 Univariate and multivariate analyses of survival in patients undergoing radical cystectomy and pelvic lymphadenopathy

	Progression-free survival				Cancer-specific survival				Overall survival			
	Univariate		Multivariate		Univariate		Multivariate		Univariate		Multivariate	
	HR (95% CI)	P value	HR (95% CI)	P value	HR (95% CI)	P value	HR (95% CI)	P value	HR (95% CI)	P value	HR (95% CI)	P value
Lymph node status												
Group 1; PVLN(−)/ non-PVLN(−)	1 (reference)		1 (reference)		1 (reference)		1 (reference)		1 (reference)		1 (reference)	
Group 2; PVLN(+)/ non-PVLN(−)	2.086 (0.325–13.38)	0.438	0.559 (0.117–2.665)	0.465	33.28 (1.719–644.3)	0.020	3.570 (0.525–24.27)	0.193	3.224 (0.593–17.54)	0.176	1.977 (0.496–7.874)	0.334
Group 3; PVLN(−)/ non-PVLN(+)	6.191 (1.869–20.51)	0.003	1.523 (0.570–4.068)	0.401	8.894 (1.128–70.34)	0.038	3.166 (0.630–15.93)	0.162	1.403 (0.423–4.657)	0.580	1.657 (0.509–5.398)	0.402
Group 4; PVLN(+)/ non-PVLN(+)	22.62 (6.259–81.76)	< 0.001	1.448 (0.571–3.671)	0.435	142.6 (25.61–794.0)	< 0.001	7.667 (1.894–31.05)	0.004	12.36 (3.751–40.72)	< 0.001	3.474 (1.376–8.771)	0.008
Age (years)												
≤ 69	1 (reference)		NA		1 (reference)		NA		1 (reference)		NA	
≥ 70	1.237 (0.662–2.313)	0.505			1.074 (0.431–2.675)	0.878			1.581 (0.847–2.951)	0.150		
Sex												
Male	1 (reference)		1 (reference)		1 (reference)		1 (reference)		1 (reference)		1 (reference)	
Female	0.601 (0.279–1.297)	0.195	1.066 (0.379–2.996)	0.904	0.289 (0.091–0.917)	0.035	< 0.001 (0-Infinity)	0.997	0.543 (0.248–1.191)	0.128	0.503 (0.170–1.486)	0.214
Neoadjuvant chemotherapy												
No	1 (reference)		1 (reference)		1 (reference)		1 (reference)		1 (reference)		1 (reference)	
Yes	2.994 (1.117–8.028)	0.029	2.484 (1.036–5.952)	0.041	0.865 (0.214–3.504)	0.840	0.615 (0.121–3.134)	0.559	0.636 (0.243–1.664)	0.356	0.507 (0.150–1.710)	0.274
Histology												
Conventional	1 (reference)		1 (reference)		1 (reference)		1 (reference)		1 (reference)		1 (reference)	
Variants	0.951 (0.441–2.050)	0.898	0.475 (0.183–1.234)	0.126	1.525 (0.490–4.746)	0.466	1.723 (0.488–6.083)	0.398	2.039 (0.947–4.386)	0.069	1.442 (0.614–3.391)	0.401
pT stage												
≤ 2	1 (reference)		1 (reference)		1 (reference)		1 (reference)		1 (reference)		1 (reference)	
≥ 3	5.547 (2.917–10.55)	< 0.001	5.829 (2.238–15.18)	< 0.001	6.293 (2.494–15.88)	< 0.001	2.716 (0.623–11.87)	0.184	3.392 (1.796–6.406)	< 0.001	2.057 (0.842–5.024)	0.113
Surgical margin												
Negative	1 (reference)		1 (reference)		1 (reference)		1 (reference)		1 (reference)		1 (reference)	
Positive	7.764 (2.086–28.89)	0.002	1.766 (0.681–4.578)	0.242	4.713 (0.752–29.53)	0.098	2.640 (0.588–11.86)	0.205	4.051 (1.148–14.30)	0.030	2.472 (0.949–6.443)	0.064
Adjuvant therapy												
No	1 (reference)		1 (reference)		1 (reference)		1 (reference)		1 (reference)		1 (reference)	
Yes	5.929 (2.700–13.02)	< 0.001	1.867 (0.891–3.914)	0.098	5.372 (1.835–15.73)	0.002	1.205 (0.429–3.387)	0.724	1.365 (0.644–2.896)	0.417	0.619 (0.289–1.324)	0.216

Abbreviations: HR hazard ratio, *CI* confidence interval, *PVLN* perivesical lymph node, *NA* not assessed

for all the variables assessed for univariate analysis except age showing no prognostic significance in any comparisons. Metastasis to both PVLN and non-PVLN (Group 4) was independently associated with poor cancer-specific survival and overall survival (Table 3). Patients undergoing neoadjuvant and adjuvant therapies were also significantly (*P* = 0.041) and insignificantly (*P* = 0.098), respectively, associated with disease progression. Multivariate analysis in subgroups of patients further showed that metastasis to PVLN [Groups 2 and 4; hazard ratio (HR) = 5.898, 95% confidence interval (CI) = 1.424–24.42; *P* = 0.014 for cancer-specific survival; HR =

2.690, 95% CI = 1.109–6.525, *P* = 0.029 for overall survival] or either PVLN or non-PVLN or both (Groups 2–4; HR = 5.053, 95% CI = 1.474–17.32, *P* = 0.010 for cancer-specific survival; HR = 2.493, 95% CI = 1.130–5.501, *P* = 0.024 for overall survival), compared with no metastatic disease (Group 1), was an independent predictor. In addition, those with PVLN-positive/non-PVLN-positive disease (Group 4) tended to have worse overall survival (HR = 3.769; 95% CI = 0.777–18.28; *P* = 0.099), but not cancer-specific survival (HR = 3.195; 95% CI = 0.637–16.15; *P* = 0.160), compared to those with PVLN-negative/non-PVLN-positive disease (Group 3).

Discussion

Several studies have addressed the role of assessing the PVLNs histopathologically in radical cystectomy specimens [8–13]. In only two of the studies [8, 13], the prognostic significance of PVLN metastasis from bladder cancer has been simultaneously investigated. To the best of our knowledge, however, no studies have definitively compared the outcomes of bladder cancer patients with N0 disease versus isolated PVLN metastasis. Thus, the primary aim of the present study was to determine the impact of PVLN involvement on oncologic outcomes of patients who underwent radical cystectomy for bladder cancer.

In a study by Bella et al. [8], PVLN was isolated in 32 (16%) of 198 cases undergoing radical cystectomy and pelvic lymphadenectomy for clinically organ-confined bladder urothelial carcinoma, and metastasis to the PVLN was seen in 14 of the patients. Outcome analysis further showed that overall survival ($P = 0.002$), disease-specific survival ($P = 0.013$), and disease-free survival ($P < 0.001$) were significantly worse in patients with PVLN-positive disease than in those with PVLN-negative disease and that PVLN metastasis was an independent predictor of overall mortality ($P = 0.016$) or disease-specific mortality ($P = 0.025$). However, each of the PVLN-positive or PVLN-negative cohort included both other pelvic lymph node positive and negative cases. Meanwhile, significant differences in overall survival ($P = 0.001$), disease-specific survival ($P = 0.010$), and disease-free survival ($P = 0.023$) between metastatic cases to other pelvic lymph node(s) with versus without PVLN involvement were observed. In a more recent study [13], Hu et al. identified the PVLN in 936 (46%) of 2017 tissue specimens from radical cystectomy/pelvic lymphadenectomy (performed in 1971–2009) in 197 (10%) of which metastatic carcinoma was present. On univariate analysis, concurrent metastases to the PVLN and other pelvic lymph node ($n = 96$) were associated with significantly worse recurrence-free survival or overall survival, compared with metastasis only to the PVLN ($n = 101$) or other pelvic lymph node ($n = 268$) in the entire cohort of patients, whereas the associations of survival of the concurrent metastases group ($n = 43$) with that of the other lymph node metastasis only group ($n = 110$), but not with that of the isolated PVLN metastasis group ($n = 12$), were statistically significant in the contemporary subset (2002–2009 cases). Similarly, multivariate analysis in the entire patients ($n = 465$) showed significantly worse prognosis of concurrent PVLN/other lymph node metastases, but not isolated PVLN metastasis, compared with other lymph node metastasis only/PVLN-negative cases. These two studies might have contributed to the definitive classification of PVLN involvement as N1/N2 in the current AJCC staging for bladder cancer [14]. In

accordance with these findings [8, 13], we found significantly or marginally worse prognosis in bladder cancer patients with PVLN metastasis, compared to those with PVLN-negative/non-PVLN-positive disease (i.e. Groups 4 vs. 3, Groups 2 & 4 vs. 3), although a slightly higher proportion of patients in Group 4 showed unfavorable histopathological findings, including variant histology, locally advanced stage (≥pT3), and positive surgical margin, compared with those in Group 3. Of note, isolated PVLN metastasis (Group 2) was associated with a significantly higher risk of cancer-specific mortality, compared with pN0 disease (Group 1), although it was found not to be an independent factor when analyzed in a multivariate setting. Additionally, as expected, PVLN metastasis (Groups 2 and 4), as well as PVLN and/or non-PVLN metastasis (Groups 2–4), was found to be an independent predictor of cancer-specific mortality or overall survival. Further validation studies with larger cohorts, including patients with isolated PVLN metastasis as well as no PVLN/non-PVLN metastasis, are thus warranted. It may also be interesting to assess the relationship between the location of positive PVLNs and patient outcomes.

The numbers of lymph nodes histopathologically assessed have been shown to have prognostic implications in bladder cancer patients undergoing radical cystectomy and pelvic lymphadenectomy and even in those with distant metastasis [15, 16]. Nonetheless, the count of pelvic lymph nodes is critically dependent on not only the extent of their dissection or surgical technique but also tissue processing at surgical pathology. Similarly, varied numbers of the PVLNs isolated from cystectomy specimens have been reported in different studies [8–13]. Then, maximum effort to isolate the PVLNs is particularly important when grossing radical cystectomy specimens. Meanwhile, in a study using tissues from lymphadenectomy during radical cystectomy [17], no metastasis was found in considerable numbers of additional lymph nodes that were not grossly identified but were isolated via submission of the entire fatty specimens for histological examination.

Classical understanding of lymphatic drainage of bladder cancer is that positive primary lymph nodes, including obturator, internal and external iliac, and sacral nodes, as well as PVLN in a subset of patients [18], drain into the common iliac region and subsequently lead to distant metastasis, as skip metastases are extremely rare [9, 19]. It has been further hypothesized that bladder cancer drainage within the regional lymph nodes is bidirectional and that some patients have lymphatic drainage from the PVLN to lymphatics other than the primary regional nodes described above [13]. These may explain why bladder cancer patients with PVLN-positive and other pelvic lymph node-positive disease show poorer outcomes than those with PVLN-negative and other pelvic lymph node-positive disease.

There are several limitations in our investigation. First, due to its retrospective design, the present study is subject to potential selection bias. In particular, our database search was solely dependent on the diagnosis of "PVLN" included in the pathology reports of radical cystectomy cases. Pathologists at our institution might not have always reported the presence of PVLNs even if they were found. Moreover, there was no standard protocol for identifying the PVLNs in radical cystectomy specimens. Therefore, we might have missed a considerable number of cases with PVLN. Second, the number of the isolated PVLN metastasis group (Group 2) is relatively small, which may especially affect statistical analyses. Significantly worse prognosis in patients with PVLN metastasis (Groups 2 and 4; $n = 22$) might also have been principally due to that in patients with concurrent PVLN and non-PVLN metastasis (Group 4; $n = 17$). Third, at least 4 surgeons performed radical cystectomy and pelvic lymphadenectomy for our patient cohort, and their surgical techniques, including the extent of node dissection, might thus have varied. Despite the limitations of this study, however, our data showing considerable or no significant differences in patient outcomes between the PVLN-negative/other node-positive and PVLN-positive/other node-positive groups (i.e. Groups 3 vs. 4) or between the PVLN-positive/other node-negative and PVLN-negative/other node-positive groups (i.e. Groups 2 vs. 3), respectively, are consistent with previous observations in a larger-scale study [13]. More strikingly, we are likely the first to demonstrate that patients with isolated PVLN metastasis (Group 2) had a significantly higher risk of cancer-specific mortality, compared to those with pN0 disease (Group 1), at least after definitive classification of PVLN metastasis as pN1 or pN2.

Conclusions

As previously reported, bladder cancer metastasis limited to the PVLNs can occur. In the present study involving 115 bladder cancer patients undergoing radical cystectomy and pelvic lymph node dissection, we mainly demonstrated that: 1) pT stage at cystectomy was significantly higher in PVLN-positive cases than in pN0 cases; 2) the number of positive PVLN and the rate of extracapsular extension in the PVLN were not significantly different between the isolated PVLN-positive and concurrent non-PVLN-positive groups; and 3) PVLN metastasis was associated with a higher risk of mortality especially in those with concurrent other node-positive disease. Importantly, worse prognosis was observed in bladder cancer patients with isolated PVLN metastasis (vs. pN0 disease) and those with concurrent PVLN/

non-PVLN metastases (vs. PVLN-negative/non-PVLN-positive disease). These outcome data may support the AJCC 8th edition bladder cancer staging system, while it possibly needs to be slightly amended for the classification of the PVLN as a regional node. Our findings also indicate the importance of diligent histopathological examination of radical cystectomy specimens to identify the PVLNs.

Abbreviations
AJCC: American Joint Committee on Cancer; CI: confidence interval; HR: hazard ratio; non-PVLN: other pelvic lymph node; PVLN: perivesical lymph node

Acknowledgements
Not applicable.

Authors' contributions
HM conceived the study and MS and HM were involved in its design. HM extracted data and MS, TG and ZY analyzed and interpreted them. MS, TG and ZY contributed to drafting the manuscript and HM edited it. All of the authors read and approved the final manuscript.

Author details
¹Department of Pathology and Laboratory Medicine, University of Rochester Medical Center, Rochester, NY, USA. ²James P. Wilmot Cancer Institute, University of Rochester Medical Center, Rochester, NY, USA. ³Department of Urology, University of Rochester Medical Center, Rochester, NY, USA.

References
1.	Bray F, Ferlay J, Soerjomataram I, Siegel RL, Torre LA, Jemal A. Global cancer statistics 2018: GLOBOCAN estimates of incidence and mortality worldwide for 36 cancers in 185 countries. CA Cancer J Clin. 2018;68(6):394–424.
2.	Antoni S, Ferley J, Soerjomataram I, Znaor A, Jemal A, Bray F. Bladder cancer incidence and mortality: a global overview and recent trends. Eur Urol. 2017;71(1):96–108.
3.	Zuiverloon TCM, van Kessel KEM, Bivalacqua TJ, Boormans JL, Ecke TH, Grivas PD, et al. Recommendations for follow-up of muscle-invasive bladder cancer patients: a consensus by the international bladder cancer network. Urol Oncol. 2018;36(9):423–31.
4.	Konety BR, Joslyn SA, O'Donnell MA. Extent of pelvic lymphadenectomy and its impact on outcome in patients diagnosed with bladder cancer: analysis of data from the surveillance, epidemiology and end results program data base. J Urol. 2003;169(3):946–50.
5.	Herr HW, Faulkner JR, Grossman HB, Crawford ED. Surgical factors influence bladder cancer outcomes: a cooperative group report. J Clin Oncol. 2004; 22(14):2781–9.
6.	May M, Herrmann E, Bolenz C, Brookman-May S, Tiemann A, Moritz R, et al. Association between the number of dissected lymph nodes during pelvic lymphadenectomy and cancer-specific survival in patients with lymph node-negative urothelial carcinoma of the bladder undergoing radical cystectomy. Ann Surg Oncol. 2011;18(7):2018–25.
7.	Bi L, Huang H, Fan X, Li K, Xu K, Jiang C, et al. Extended vs non-extended pelvic lymph node dissection and their influence on recurrence-free survival in patients undergoing radical cystectomy for bladder cancer: a systematic review and meta-analysis of comparative studies. BJU Int. 2014;113(5b):E39–48.
8.	Bella AJ, Stitt LW, Chin JL, Izawa JI. The prognostic significance of metastatic perivesical lymph nodes identified in radical cystectomy specimens for transitional cell carcinoma of the bladder. J Urol. 2003;170(6):2253–7.
9.	Abol-Enein H, El-Baz M, Abd El-Hameed MA, Abdel-Latif M, Ghoneim MA. Lymph node involvement in patients with bladder cancer treated with radical cystectomy: a patho-anatomical study – a single center experience. J Urol. 2004;172(5):1818–21.
10.	Bochner BH, Cho D, Herr HW, Donat M, Kattan MW, Dalbagni G. Prospectively packaged lymph node dissections with radical cystectomy: evaluation of node count variability and node mapping. J Urol. 2004;172(4):1286–90.
11.	Vazina A, Dugi D, Shariat SF, Evans J, Link R, Lerner SP. Stage specific lymph node metastasis mapping in radical cystectomy specimens. J Urol. 2004; 171(5):1830–4.

12. Jensen JB, Ulhøi BP, Jensen KME. Lymph node mapping in patients with bladder cancer undergoing radical cystectomy and lymph node dissection to the level of the inferior mesenteric artery. BJU Int. 2010;106(2):199–205.

13. Hu B, Satkunasivam R, Schuckman A, Sherrod A, Cai J, Miranda G, et al. Significance of perivesical lymph nodes in radical cystectomy for bladder cancer. Urol Oncol. 2014;32(8):1158–65.

14. Amin MB, Edge SB, Greene FL, et al. AJCC Cancer staging manual. 8th ed. New York: Springer; 2017. p. 765–74.

15. Li F, Hong X, Hou L, Lin F, Chen P, Pang S, et al. A greater number of dissected lymph nodes is associated with more favorable outcomes in bladder cancer treated by radical cystectomy: a meta-analysis. Oncotarget. 2016;7(38):61284–94.

16. Mazzone E, Preisser F, Nazzani S, Tian Z, Fossati N, Gandaglia G, et al. More extensive lymph node dissection improves survival benefit of radical cystectomy in metastatic urothelial carcinoma of the bladder. Clin Genitourin Cancer. 2019;17(2):105–13 e2.

17. Gordetsky J, Scosyrev E, Rashid H, Wu G, Silvers C, Golijanin D, et al. Identifying additional lymph nodes in radical cystectomy lymphadenectomy specimens. Mod Pathol. 2012;25(1):140–4.

18. Liedberg F, Chebil G, Davidsson T, Gudjonsson S, Månsson W. Intraoperative sentinel node dissection improves nodal staging in invasive bladder cancer. J Urol. 2006;175(1):84–9.

19. Dorin RP, Daneshmand S, Eisenberg MS, Chandrasome S, Cai J, Miranda G, et al. Lymph node dissection technique is more important than lymph node count in identifying nodal metastases in radical cystectomy patients: a comparative mapping study. Eur Urol. 2011;60(5):946–52.

15

Association between De Ritis ratio (aspartate aminotransferase/alanine aminotransferase) and oncological outcomes in bladder cancer patients after radical cystectomy

Yun-Sok Ha[1,2], Sang Won Kim[1,2], So Young Chun[1,2], Jae-Wook Chung[1,2], Seock Hwan Choi[1,2], Jun Nyung Lee[1,2], Bum Soo Kim[1,2], Hyun Tae Kim[1,2], Eun Sang Yoo[1,2], Tae Gyun Kwon[1,2], Won Tae Kim[3], Wun-Jae Kim[3] and Tae-Hwan Kim[1,2]*

Abstract

Background: New biological prognostic predictors have been studied; however, some factors have limited clinical application due to tissue-specific expression and high cost. There is the need for a promising predictive factor that is simple to detect and that is closely linked to oncological outcomes in patients with urothelial bladder cancer (BC) who have undergone radical cystectomy (RC). Therefore, we investigated the clinical prognostic value of the preoperative De Ritis ratio (aspartate aminotransferase/alanine aminotransferase) on oncological outcomes in patients with urothelial BC after RC.

Methods: We retrospectively evaluated clinicopathological data of 118 patients with non-metastatic urothelial BC after RC between 2008 and 2013 at a single center. The association between the De Ritis ratio and clinicopathological findings was assessed. The potential prognostic value of the De Ritis ratio was analyzed using the Kaplan-Meier method, and multivariate Cox analyses were performed to identify the independent predictors of metastasis-free survival, cancer-specific survival, and overall survival.

Results: According to the receiver operating curve of the De Ritis ratio for metastasis, we stratified the patients into 2 groups using a threshold of 1.3. A high De Ritis ratio was more likely to be associated with old age and the female sex. Kaplan-Meier estimates revealed that patients with a high De Ritis ratio had inferior metastasis-free survival, cancer-specific survival, and overall survival outcomes ($P = 0.012$, 0.024, and 0.022, respectively). Multivariate analysis revealed that a high De Ritis ratio was an independent prognostic factor for metastasis (hazard ratio [HR], 2.389; 95% confidence interval [CI], 1.161–4.914; $P = 0.018$), cancer-related death (HR, 2.755; 95% CI, 1.214–6.249; $P = 0.015$), and overall death (HR, 2.761; 95% CI, 1.257–6.067; $P = 0.011$).

Conclusions: An elevated De Ritis ratio was significantly associated with worse prognosis in patients who underwent RC for urothelial BC. This ratio might further improve the predictive accuracy for prognosis in BC.

Keywords: Bladder cancer, Prognosis, Survival, De Ritis ratio

* Correspondence: doctork@knu.ac.kr
[1]Department of Urology, School of Medicine, Kyungpook National University, Daegu, South Korea
[2]Department of Urology, School of Medicine, Kyungpook National University, Kyungpook National University Hospital, Daegu, South Korea
Full list of author information is available at the end of the article

Background

Urothelial carcinoma typically occurs in the urinary system: the kidney, urinary bladder, and accessory organs [1]. It is the most common type of bladder cancer (BC) and cancer of the ureters, urethra, and urachus. BC is the second most common malignancy of the genitourinary tract, and shows a male predominance in Korea; it has the seventh highest incidence in men [2]. An estimated total of 3824 new BC cases and 1412 BC-related deaths were expected to occur in Korea in 2016 [3]. Among newly diagnosed patients, approximately 70–80% present with non-muscle-invasive BC (NMIBC). NMIBC is typically managed by transurethral tumor resection, a minimally invasive surgical procedure. The prognosis of NMIBC patients can be favorable if the disease has not progressed to muscle-invasive BC (MIBC). However, NMIBC eventually progresses to MIBC in approximately 30% of patients. Radical cystectomy (RC) with pelvic lymph node dissection (PLND) is the customary treatment option for local MIBC. RC with PLND is sometimes used to treat NMIBC, including Bacille Calmette-Guerin (BCG)-refractory cases and high-grade tumors. Nonetheless, approximately 50% of patients experience a relapse within 2 years. The 3-year survival rate is less than 50% [4]. Neoadjuvant chemotherapy before RC has been recognized as a treatment to improve cancer-specific survival (CSS) rates. These results provided evidence for neoadjuvant chemotherapy [5, 6]. However, eligible patients are difficult to identify because of the poor prognostic value of the current clinical staging system, resulting in its underuse [7]. Therefore, a preoperative prognostic factor capable of adequately stratifying patients for optimal preoperative management is needed.

In most clinical fields, alanine aminotransferase (ALT) and aspartate aminotransferase (AST) are the most utilized liver enzymes. In 1957, the ratio of the serum activities of AST and ALT was initially described by De Ritis, and has been known as the De Ritis ratio (AST/ALT) [8]. Cancer and non-cancerous tissues generated these enzymes and they have been stated as important prognosticators in lots of malignant tumors. These include multiple myeloma, colonic, pancreatic, renal cell carcinoma (RCC), and upper tract urothelial cancer (UTUC) [9–13]. For example, Bezan et al. reported that the preoperative De Ritis ratio was an independent prognostic factor in patients with non-metastatic RCC [12]. The De Ritis ratio is hypothesized to be associated with increased anaerobic glycolysis, a process known as the Warburg effect. Due to the fact that urothelial carcinoma was also reported to be related to glucose metabolism, we hypothesized that the De Ritis ratio might also have a prognostic role in BC [14, 15]. To the best of our knowledge, the prognostic value of the De Ritis ratio has not been evaluated in patients with BC. Therefore, we aimed to evaluate the prognostic value of the De Ritis ratio in patients who underwent RC for BC.

Methods

Between August 2008 and May 2013, 118 patients with non-metastatic urothelial BC underwent RC at our hospital following Institutional Review Board approval (approval number: KNUMC 2016–05-021). Before RC, all the patients underwent transurethral resection of bladder tumors (TUR-BTs). After histopathological analyses and checking up the images, we carried out RC. The most of patients underwent RC were MIBC free of remote metastasis. Additionally, recurrent multifocal superficial refractory tumor, repeated transurethral resection, and BCG-resistant carcinoma in situ (CIS) are also indicators. We excluded the pateitns with previous pelvic radiation, clinical stage M1, prior combination surgery, and patients with chronic liver disease (hepatitis, liver cirrhosis, and severe fatty liver disease) including hepatitis B or C virus carriers. Open RC was performed through a midline incision in the typical manner [16, 17]. Robot-assisted RC was performed using the same surgical procedure, as reported by Menon et al. [18, 19]. The 2010 American Joint Committee on Cancer (AJCC) TNM staging system for BC was used for clinical T stage. [20]. Histologic grades were determined according to the 2004 World Health Organization (WHO) classification system [21]. Measurements of AST and ALT were routinely included in our preoperative workup and were performed before RC. Cisplastin-based chemotherapy was performed for at least 4 cycles in patients with good performance status among those with pT3, pT4, and node-positive disease. We used the published guidelines that apply to each patient for management and follow-up. [22].

To settle the ideal cutoff level, the receiver-operating characteristic (ROC) curve of the De Ritis ratio for metastasis (44 metastasis vs. 74 non-metastasis) was used. An optimal cutoff value of 1.3 was based on a maximal Youden index at this value. The area under the curve of the De Ritis ratio was 0.606 (Fig. 1). Subsequently, the high De Ritis ratio cohort was defined patients with De Ritis ratios ≥1.3 and the others (De Ritis ratio < 1.3) were allocated to the low De Ritis ratio cohort. Student's t-test and chi-square test were used to compare the clinicopathological features stratification according to De Ritis ratio. The survival spreads, including metastasis free survival (MFS), CSS and overall survival (OS), were assessed by the Kaplan-Meier method. Comparison of survival distributions was performed by a log-rank test between two cohorts. Factors independently associated with MFS, CSS, and OS were determined using a multivariate Cox proportional hazard regression model, with hazard ratios (HRs) and 95% confidence intervals (CIs) calculated for

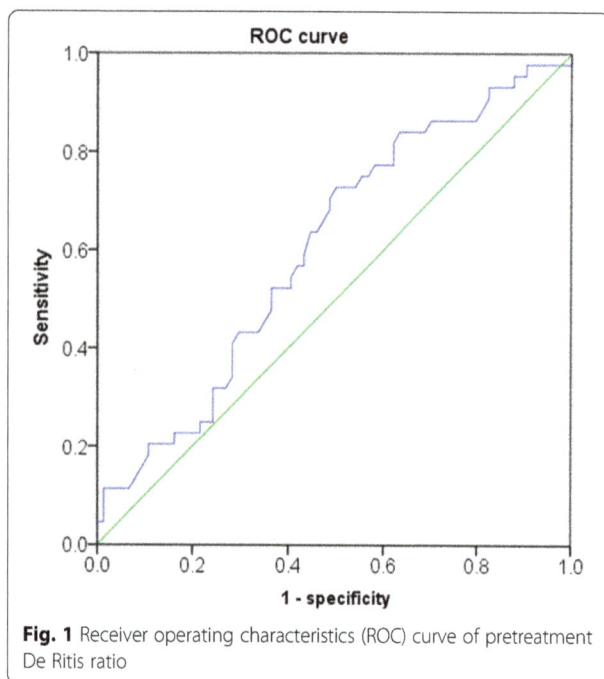

Fig. 1 Receiver operating characteristics (ROC) curve of pretreatment De Ritis ratio

each factor. Differences with p<0.05 were considered statistically significant. IBM SPSS ver. 18.0 (IBM Co., Armonk, NY, USA) was used for statistical analyses.

Results

Among the 118 patients, 49 had low De Ritis ratios and 69 had high De Ritis ratios. Their median age was 69 years (interquartile range, 60–74). Patients with high De Ritis ratios were significantly older and predominantly women, but were otherwise similar to patients with low De Ritis ratios with respect to body mass index, American Society of Anesthesiologists score, receipt of BCG instillation and neoadjuvant chemotherapy, clinical stage at the time of the latest TUR-BT, and presence of CIS at the time of the last TUR-BT (Table 1).

Comparisons of clinicopathological variables according to De Ritis ratios are summarized in Table 2. Most clinicopathological parameters, including pathological and histological grade, lymph node involvement, and lymphovascular invasion, did not differ significantly between the two groups.

The median follow-up duration was 34.1 months, during which 44 patients showed metastasis and 39 patients

Table 1 Patient demographics and preoperative characteristics

Parameters	Low De Ritis ratio (< 1.3, N = 49)	High De Ritis ratio (≥1.3, N = 69)	P
Age, y			0.029
< 70	32 (65.3)	31 (44.9)	
≥70	17 (34.7)	38 (55.1)	
Gender			0.032
Male	45 (91.8)	53 (76.8)	
Female	4 (8.2)	16 (23.2)	
BMI (kg/m^2, ±SD)	22.97 ± 3.28	22.16 ± 2.94	0.156
ASA classification			0.617
1	8 (16.3)	9 (13.0)	
≥2	41 (83.7)	60 (87.0)	
Clinical stage at latest TUR-BT			0.609
≤T1	19 (38.8)	30 (43.5)	
≥T2	30 (61.2)	39 (56.5)	
Presence of CIS at last TUR-BT			0.221
No	47 (95.9)	62 (89.9)	
Yes	2 (4.1)	7 (10.1)	
BCG instillation history			0.678
No	45 (91.8)	60 (89.6)	
Yes	4 (8.2)	7 (10.4)	
Neoadjuvant chemotherapy			0.92
No	40 (81.6)	56 (82.4)	
Yes	9 (18.4)	12 (17.6)	

BMI body mass index, *BCG* Bacille Calmette-Guerin, *ASA* American Society of Anesthesiologists, *TUR-BT* transurethral tumor resection of bladder tumor, *CIS* carcinoma in situ

Table 2 Comparison of clinicopathological variables according to De Ritis ratio in 118 patients who underwent radical cystectomy

Parameters	Low De Ritis ratio (< 1.3, N = 49)	High De Ritis ratio (≥1.3, N = 69)	P
Pathologic stage			0.75
T0, Tis, Ta	4 (8.2)	6 (8.7)	
T1	11 (22.4)	17 (24.6)	
T2	16 (32.7)	15 (21.7)	
T3	12 (24.5)	22 (31.9)	
T4	6 (12.2)	9 (13.0)	
Histologic grade			0.072
Low	4 (8.2)	1 (1.4)	
High	45 (91.8)	68 (98.6)	
Lymph node involvement			0.777
No	38 (77.6)	55 (79.7)	
Yes	11 (22.4)	14 (20.3)	
Lymphovascular invasion			0.465
No	41 (83.7)	54 (78.3)	
Yes	8 (16.3)	15 (21.7)	
Median follow-up periods (months, range)	40 (6.5–83.3)	31.8 (4.3–95.3)	0.089
Metastasis			0.015
No	37 (75.5)	37 (53.6)	
Yes	12 (24.5)	32 (46.4)	
Cancer-related death			0.045
No	39 (79.6)	43 (62.3)	
Yes	10 (20.4)	26 (37.7)	
Overall death			0.039
No	38 (77.6)	41 (59.4)	
Yes	11 (22.4)	28 (40.6)	

died, including 36 who died due to BC. Notably, patients with high De Ritis ratios had significantly inferior MFS (53.6% vs. 75.5%; $P = 0.015$), CSS (62.3% vs. 79.6%; $P = 0.045$), and OS (59.4% vs. 77.6%; $P = 0.039$) rates than those with low De Ritis ratios (Table 2). The Kaplan-Meier analyses showed significantly inferior survival outcomes for MFS ($P = 0.012$), CSS ($P = 0.024$), and OS ($P = 0.022$) in patients with high De Ritis ratios (Fig. 2). Moreover, the De Ritis ratio was found to be independently associated with metastasis (HR, 2.389; $P = 0.018$), cancer-related death (HR, 2.755; $P = 0.015$), and overall death (HR, 2.761; $P = 0.001$) on multivariable analysis (Table 3). To confirm these results, we performed additional analyses. The De Ritis ratio was tested as a continuous variable in another multivariate Cox regression model. The preoperative De Ritis ratio as a continuous variable ($P = 0.008$, $P = 0.003$, and $P = 0.002$, respectively) and pathological T stage ($P = 0.008$, $P < 0.001$, and $P < 0.001$, respectively) were independent predictors of metastasis, cancer-related death, and overall death (Table 3).

Discussion

BC most commonly affects elderly individuals and those with significant comorbidities and an impaired performance status [23]. RC remains the gold standard of treatment in patients with local MIBC and in some cases of NMIBC [18]. However, despite these aggressive local approaches, long-term prognosis remains poor due to disease recurrence accompanied by local and/or distant metastasis [24]. These poor outcomes suggest a need for ongoing risk stratification and appropriate selection of multimodal treatment approaches, such as chemotherapy in neoadjuvant or adjuvant settings. With recent advances in techniques, an extremely large number of new prognostic markers have been identified [25]. New biomarkers predictive of outcomes would help clinicians provide risk stratification for patients and serve as prognostic indicators for individual patients [26]. For clinical practice purposes, a potential prognosticator would generally have great potential if it could be easily and inexpensively determined by routine measures.

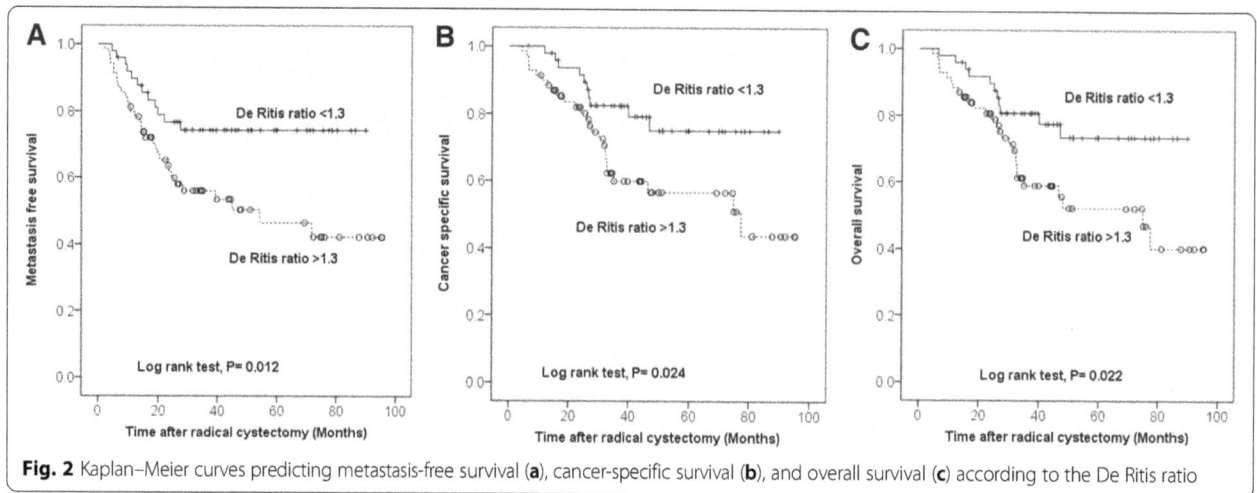

Fig. 2 Kaplan–Meier curves predicting metastasis-free survival (**a**), cancer-specific survival (**b**), and overall survival (**c**) according to the De Ritis ratio

In this study, we determined that an elevated De Ritis ratio showed a significant association with adverse outcomes in patients with BC who underwent RC. Patients with elevated De Ritis ratios showed significantly inferior survival outcomes in terms of MFS, CSS, and OS after RC in patients with BC. Moreover, elevated De Ritis ratios were found to be significant independent predictors of metastasis, cancer-related death, and overall death. To our knowledge, this study is the first to identify the De Ritis ratio as a novel significant prognostic biomarker in BC. Because the De Ritis ratio may be inexpensively and reproducibly measured, it might become a promising tool in the management of BC.

The amino transaminase enzymes (AST and ALT) which are strongly involved in cellular metabolism and cancer cell turnover, represent easily measurable potential blood-based biomarkers [12]. Amino transaminases are widely used to determine liver function in clinical care. Moreover, amino transaminases are used to identify liver diseases such as viral hepatitis and alcohol abuse. De Ritis et al. were the first to introduce the AST/ALT ratio as a useful indicator for differentiating the etiology of acute hepatitis [8]. Previous studies of certain types of cancer indicate that different levels of these enzymes are associated with patient prognoses [11–13, 27, 28].

For instance, the results from Tan et al. showed that AST/ALT ratio over 2.0 was an independent prognosticator of poor survival in patients with distal cholangiocarcinoma, [28], and Bezan et al. represented that preoperatively assessed De Ritis ratio (> 1.26) was significantly associated with the clinical course of patients with non-metastatic RCC [12]. Rawson and Peto retrospectively analyzed 3873 patients with small cell lung cancer and concluded that AST was a significant prognostic factor [27]. Lindmark et al. also reported that AST and ALT were significantly associated with patient survival after analyzing 212 patients with colorectal cancer [9].

Stocken et al. analyzed the data of 653 patients with advanced pancreatic cancer from 2 randomized studies. Stockon et al. also concluded that AST was independently related to CSS [11]. An additional study conducted by Kiba et al. reported that high AST and lactate dehydrogenase levels were significantly associated with inferior OS in patients who received bortezomib and dexamethasone chemotherapy for multiple myeloma [10]. Moreover, Nishikawa et al. first reported that the De Ritis ratio was a significant prognostic biomarker in UTUC [13]. They conducted a retrospective multivariate analysis of 109 patients and concluded that the De Ritis ratio, pathological stage, lymph node metastasis, and tumor grade were independent predictors of extravesical recurrence-free survival.

An enormous rise in glycolysis and glucose uptake was needed in tumorigenesis and cancer progression. Actually, the formation of abundant pyruvate and lactate is the common characteristics of tumor cells. Warburg discovered this event [29]. Although there is oxygen, the increase in the velocity of glucose delivery is accompanied by enhanced glycolysis. Increased glycolysis is known to be linked to several alterations in mitochondrial activity. Furthermore, increased glycolysis is also associated with nicotinamide adenine dinucleotide-related enzyme activity and glucose transporter activity [30].

Moreover, the malate-aspartate shuttle pathway has AST as a main component. Consequently, tumor metabolism might be associated with De Ritis ratio in several glucose using cancers. In addition, BC is noted as a glucose-reliant malignant tumor [14, 15, 30]. The uptake of glucose by BC cells via using fluorescence microscopy was explored by Whyard et al. [30]. They found that noteworthy changes in glucose consumption between normal urothelium and tumor cells. In this study, increased lactate production amplified the pyruvate synthesis and the concentration of glutamine was elevated.

Table 3 Multivariate Cox regression analysis of factors predictive of prognosis in bladder cancer after radical cystectomy

Parameters	HR	95% CI		P	HR	95% CI		P	Parameters	HR
Multivariate Cox proportional analysis to metastasis										
Age (< 70 vs. ≥70)	0.994	0.959	1.030	0.725	0.998	0.964	1.033	0.894		
Gender (male vs. female)	0.825	0.354	1.923	0.655	0.745	0.288	1.928	0.544		
BMI	0.972	0.867	1.088	0.618	0.957	0.854	1.073	0.450		
Pathologic T stage	1.667	1.234	2.251	0.001	1.776	1.296	2.434	< 0.001		
Lymph node involvement	1.727	0.895	3.335	0.103	1.816	0.942	3.501	0.075		
Grade	0.640	0.078	5.249	0.678	0.549	0.065	4.629	0.582		
De Ritis ratio (Low vs. high)	2.389	1.161	4.914	0.018						
De Ritis ratio (Continuous)					1.582	1.129	2.219	0.008		
Multivariate Cox proportional analysis of cancer-related death										
Age (< 70 vs. ≥70)	0.996	0.959	1.035	0.834	1.000	0.964	1.038	0.988		
Gender (male vs. female)	0.488	0.164	1.448	0.196	0.363	0.096	1.377	0.136		
BMI	0.941	0.825	1.073	0.361	0.919	0.807	1.046	0.200		
Pathologic T stage	1.841	1.297	2.612	0.001	1.933	1.342	2.784	< 0.001		
Lymph node involvement	1.613	0.775	3.358	0.201	1.708	0.823	3.546	0.151		
Grade	0.584	0.069	4.149	0.589	0.461	0.051	5.286	0.685		
De Ritis ratio (Low vs. high)	2.755	1.214	6.249	0.015						
De Ritis ratio (Continuous)					1.848	1.239	2.755	0.003		
Multivariate Cox proportional analysis of overall death										
Age (< 70 vs. ≥70)	0.999	0.963	1.037	0.956	1.004	0.969	1.041	0.807		
Gender (male vs. female)	0.471	0.161	1.377	0.169	0.337	0.088	1.285	0.111		
BMI	0.972	0.858	1.100	0.651	0.952	0.840	1.078	0.436		
Pathologic T stage	1.921	1.368	2.698	< 0.001	2.017	1.415	2.876	< 0.001		
Lymph node involvement	1.572	0.778	3.176	0.207	1.694	0.842	3.409	0.139		
Grade	0.326	0.065	5.372	0.538	0.556	0.064	4.718	0.538		
De Ritis ratio (Low vs. high)	2.761	1.257	6.067	0.011						
De Ritis ratio (Continuous)					1.860	1.262	2.743	0.002		

HR hazard ratio, *CI* confidence interval, *BMI* body mass index

The Warburg effect has all of these features. Based on these results and our data from the present study, it is likely that De Ritis ratio was linked to BC. However, the precise mechanism for revealing the relationship between increased De Ritis and poor prognosis of BC patients has not been established.

We would like to emphasize several drawbacks of this study. Initially, this was a retrospective study with a comparatively small number of patients, and the follow-up period was relatively short. Second, the existence of undetected liver pathologic conditions that can influence the serum levels of AST or ALT might distort the De Ritis ratio, although we excluded the patients with chronic liver disease (hepatitis, liver cirrhosis, and severe fatty liver disease) including hepatitis B or C virus carriers In addition, we did not evaluate the smoking history of the patients. Smoking is a significant risk factor for BC and plays an important role in BC progression; however, it was very difficult to obtain exact information on patient smoking. A self-completed questionnaire about smoking may have introduced recall bias. Some studies in Korea about the association between *BC* and smoking history showed discordant results. Lastly, we included only Korean population in our cohort. Additionally, studies of other ethnic groups are required before our results can be applied universally.

Conclusions

This study is the first of its kind to investigate the effect of a preoperative assessment of the De Ritis ratio. Our study was also the first to include the prognosis of patients with BC who underwent RC. An elevated De Ritis ratio was found to significantly increase the risk of metastasis, cancer-specific death, and general mortality after undergoing RC for BC. The De Ritis ratio should be regarded as an important tool to be used in counseling patients regarding expected outcomes.

Abbreviations

ALT: Alanine aminotransferase; AST: Aspartate aminotransferase; BC: Bladder cancer; BCG: Bacillus Calmette–Guérin; CI: Confidence interval; CSS: Cancer-specific survival; HR: Hazard ratio; MFS: Metastasis-free survival; MIBC: Muscle-invasive bladder cancer; NMIBC: Non-muscle-invasive bladder cancer; OS: Overall survival; RC: Radical cystectomy; RCC: Renal cell carcinoma; TUR-BT: Transurethral resection of bladder tumor; UTUC: Upper tract urothelial cancer

Acknowledgements

Not applicable.

Authors' contributions

YSH and THK were involved in project development, data collection, data analysis, manuscript writing, and manuscript editing. SHC, SWK, JWC, JNL, and BSK were involved in data collection and analysis. HTK, ESY, TGK, SYC and WTK were involved in data collection and manuscript editing. THK and WJK were involved in project development, data analysis, and manuscript editing. All authors read and approved the final manuscript.

Author details

[1]Department of Urology, School of Medicine, Kyungpook National University, Daegu, South Korea. [2]Department of Urology, School of Medicine, Kyungpook National University, Kyungpook National University Hospital, Daegu, South Korea. [3]Department of Urology, Chungbuk National University College of Medicine, Cheongju, South Korea.

References

1. Ha YS, Kim TH. Chemotherapy in advanced urothelial carcinoma. Korean J Urol Oncol. 2016;14(2):47–53.
2. Oh CM, Won YJ, Jung KW, Kong HJ, Cho H, Lee JK, Lee DH, Lee KH, Community of Population-Based Regional Cancer R. Cancer Statistics in Korea: Incidence, Mortality, Survival, and Prevalence in 2013. Cancer Res Treat. 2016;48(2):436–50.
3. Jung KW, Won YJ, Oh CM, Kong HJ, Cho H, Lee JK, Lee DH, Lee KH. Prediction of Cancer incidence and mortality in Korea, 2016. Cancer Res Treat. 2016;48(2):451–7.
4. Stein JP, Skinner DG. Radical cystectomy for invasive bladder cancer: long-term results of a standard procedure. World J Urol. 2006;24(3):296–304.
5. Grossman HB, Natale RB, Tangen CM, Speights VO, Vogelzang NJ, Trump DL, deVere White RW, Sarosdy MF, Wood DP Jr, Raghavan D, et al. Neoadjuvant chemotherapy plus cystectomy compared with cystectomy alone for locally advanced bladder cancer. N Engl J Med. 2003;349(9):859–66.
6. Advanced Bladder Cancer Meta-analysis C. Neoadjuvant chemotherapy in invasive bladder cancer: update of a systematic review and meta-analysis of individual patient data advanced bladder cancer (ABC) meta-analysis collaboration. Eur Urol. 2005;48(2):202–5 discussion 205–206.
7. Herr HW, Dotan Z, Donat SM, Bajorin DF. Defining optimal therapy for muscle invasive bladder cancer. J Urol. 2007;177(2):437–43.
8. De Ritis F, Coltorti M, Giusti G. An enzymic test for the diagnosis of viral hepatitis; the transaminase serum activities. Clin Chim Acta. 1957;2(1):70–4.
9. Lindmark G, Gerdin B, Pahlman L, Bergstrom R, Glimelius B. Prognostic predictors in colorectal cancer. Dis Colon Rectum. 1994;37(12):1219–27.
10. Kiba T, Ito T, Nakashima T, Okikawa Y, Kido M, Kimura A, Kameda K, Miyamae F, Tanaka S, Atsumi M, et al. Bortezomib and dexamethasone for multiple myeloma: higher AST and LDH levels associated with a worse prognosis on overall survival. BMC Cancer. 2014;14:462.
11. Stocken DD, Hassan AB, Altman DG, Billingham LJ, Bramhall SR, Johnson PJ, Freemantle N. Modelling prognostic factors in advanced pancreatic cancer. Br J Cancer. 2008;99(6):883–93.
12. Bezan A, Mrsic E, Krieger D, Stojakovic T, Pummer K, Zigeuner R, Hutterer GC, Pichler M. The preoperative AST/ALT (De Ritis) ratio represents a poor prognostic factor in a cohort of patients with nonmetastatic renal cell carcinoma. J Urol. 2015;194(1):30–5.
13. Nishikawa M, Miyake H, Fujisawa M. De Ritis (aspartate transaminase/alanine transaminase) ratio as a significant predictor of recurrence-free survival in patients with upper urinary tract urothelial carcinoma following nephroureterectomy. Urol Oncol. 2016;34(9):417 e419–5.
14. Yun SJ, Jo SW, Ha YS, Lee OJ, Kim WT, Kim YJ, Lee SC, Kim WJ. PFKFB4 as a prognostic marker in non-muscle-invasive bladder cancer. Urol Oncol. 2012; 30(6):893–9.
15. Chang SG, Lee JH, Hong DH, Lee HL, Chai SE, Hoffman RM. Comparison of glucose-consumption and thymidine-incorporation endpoints in histocultured human superficial bladder tumors. Anticancer Res. 1994;14(1A):77–83.
16. Stein JP, Quek ML, Skinner DG. Lymphadenectomy for invasive bladder cancer. II. Technical aspects and prognostic factors. BJU Int. 2006;97(2):232–7.
17. Stein JP, Skinner DG. Surgical atlas. Radical cystectomy. BJU Int. 2004; 94(1):197–221.
18. Bak DJ, Lee YJ, Woo MJ, Chung JW, Ha YS, Kim HT, Kim TH, Yoo ES, Kim BW, Kwon TG. Complications and oncologic outcomes following robot-assisted radical cystectomy: what is the real benefit? Investig Clin Urol. 2016;57(4):260–7.
19. Menon M, Hemal AK, Tewari A, Shrivastava A, Shoma AM, El-Tabey NA, Shaaban A, Abol-Enein H, Ghoneim MA. Nerve-sparing robot-assisted radical cystoprostatectomy and urinary diversion. BJU Int. 2003;92(3):232–6.
20. Osunkoya AO, Grignon DJ. Practical issues and pitfalls in staging tumors of the genitourinary tract. Semin Diagn Pathol. 2012;29(3):154–66.
21. Lopez-Beltran A, Bassi P, Pavone-Macaluso M, Montironi R. Handling and pathology reporting of specimens with carcinoma of the urinary bladder, ureter, and renal pelvis. Eur Urol. 2004;45(3):257–66.
22. Vrooman OP, Witjes JA. Follow-up of patients after curative bladder cancer treatment: guidelines vs. practice. Curr Opin Urol. 2010;20(5):437–42.
23. Prout GR Jr, Wesley MN, Yancik R, Ries LA, Havlik RJ, Edwards BK. Age and comorbidity impact surgical therapy in older bladder carcinoma patients: a population-based study. Cancer. 2005;104(8):1638–47.
24. Witjes JA, Comperat E, Cowan NC, De Santis M, Gakis G, Lebret T, Ribal MJ, Van der Heijden AG, Sherif A, European Association of U. EAU guidelines on muscle-invasive and metastatic bladder cancer: summary of the 2013 guidelines. Eur Urol. 2014;65(4):778–92.
25. Kim WJ. Changing landscape of diagnosis and treatment of bladder cancer. Investig Clin Urol. 2016;57(Suppl 1):S1–3.
26. Ha YS, Jeong P, Kim JS, Kwon WA, Kim IY, Yun SJ, Kim GY, Choi YH, Moon SK, Kim WJ. Tumorigenic and prognostic significance of RASSF1A expression in low-grade (WHO grade 1 and grade 2) nonmuscle-invasive bladder cancer. Urology. 2012;79(6):1411 e1411–6.
27. Rawson NS, Peto J. An overview of prognostic factors in small cell lung cancer. A report from the Subcommittee for the Management of lung Cancer of the United Kingdom coordinating committee on Cancer research. Br J Cancer. 1990;61(4):597–604.
28. Tan X, Xiao K, Liu W, Chang S, Zhang T, Tang H. Prognostic factors of distal cholangiocarcinoma after curative surgery: a series of 84 cases. Hepatogastroenterology. 2013;60(128):1892–5.
29. Warburg O. On the origin of cancer cells. Science. 1956;123(3191):309–14.
30. Whyard T, Waltzer WC, Waltzer D, Romanov V. Metabolic alterations in bladder cancer: applications for cancer imaging. Exp Cell Res. 2016; 341(1):77–83.

16

Clinical and morphological effects of hyperbaric oxygen therapy in patients with interstitial cystitis associated with fibromyalgia

Gerardo Bosco[1], Edoardo Ostardo[2], Alex Rizzato[1], Giacomo Garetto[3], Matteo Paganini[1]*[iD], Giorgio Melloni[4], Giampiero Giron[5], Lodovico Pietrosanti[5], Ivo Martinelli[5] and Enrico Camporesi[6]

Abstract

Background: Interstitial Cystitis (IC) is a debilitating disorder of the bladder, with a multifactorial and poorly understood origin dealing with microcirculation repeated damages. Also Fibromyalgia (FM) is a persistent disorder whose etiology is not completely explained, and its theorized alteration of pain processing can compromise the quality of life. Both these conditions have a high incidence of conventional therapeutic failure, but recent literature suggests a significant beneficial response to Hyperbaric Oxygen Therapy (HBOT). With this study, this study we evaluated the effects of HBOT on quality of life, symptoms, urodynamic parameters, and cystoscopic examination of patients suffering from both IC and FM.

Methods: We structured an observational clinical trial design with repeated measures (questionnaires, urodynamic test, and cystoscopy) conducted before and 6 months after a therapeutic protocol with hyperbaric oxygen for the treatment of patients suffering from both IC and FM. Patients were exposed to breathing 100% oxygen at 2 atm absolute (ATA) in a multiplace pressure chamber for 90 min using an oro-nasal mask. Patients undertook a cycle of 20 sessions for 5 days per week, and a second cycle of 20 sessions after 1 week of suspension.

Results: Twelve patients completed the protocol. Changes after HBOT were not significant, except for hydrodistension tolerance (mean pre-treatment: 409.2 ml; mean post-treatment: 489.2 ml; $p < 0.05$). A regression of petechiae and Hunner's ulcers was also noted 6 months after the completion of HBOT.

Conclusions: Our study showed no improvement of symptoms, quality of life, and urodynamic parameters, except for hydrodistension, and a slight improvement in cystoscopic pattern. However, to date, we could not demonstrate the significance of overall results to justify the use of HBOT alone in patients with IC and FM. This observation suggests that additional studies are needed to better understand if HBOT could treat this subset of patients.

Keywords: Hyperbaric medicine, Interstitial cystitis, Fibromyalgia

* Correspondence: paganini.mtt@gmail.com
[1]Environmental and Respiratory Physiology Laboratory, Department of Biomedical Sciences, University of Padova, Padova, Italy
Full list of author information is available at the end of the article

Background

Interstitial Cystitis (IC) is a rare, chronic, and disabling condition of the bladder that mainly affects females [1–3]. The specific etiology of IC is currently unknown but seems multifactorial, with interactions among autoimmune, neuroendocrine, allergic, and infectious pathways [4, 5]. Theories suggested that IC could derive from an abnormally increased number of mast cells, or could be related to an alteration of the glycosaminoglycan layer protecting urothelium from urine [6]. The activation of the inflammatory response induces alterations in the deep layers of bladder, such as fibrous substitution of the muscular tunic, thinning and discontinuity of the mucosa layer, capillary proliferation, and blood vessel degeneration [7].

Initial presentation of IC is subtle. The possible presence of infection (due to urothelium damage), an increase in void frequency, and a pain resistant to analgesia are early symptoms that make the diagnosis more challenging because of overlapping with those present in bacterial cystitis and several other diseases [8]. Unfortunately, patients spend about 5 to 10 years and a mean of 8 consults from different specialists before a correct diagnosis [9], while recurrent inflammation results in scar tissue development. The subsequent reduction of both bladder compliance and capacity, in conjunction with the gradual loss of functionality, determine chronic urinary tract symptoms [10], thus prompting cystoscopy and urometry that finally make the late diagnosis. Since the primary cause of IC is still hypothesized, conventional treatments – such as physical therapy, antidepressants, pentosan sulfate, immunosuppressants, intravescical therapy with lidocaine heparin and bicarbonate, and surgery [11] – mainly aim to alleviate symptoms. The effectiveness of most treatments does not exceed 60%, and symptoms return even after a period of improvement or recovery [9].

A pilot study showed that 76% of patients with histologically confirmed IC have another medical condition, such as Fibromyalgia Syndrome (FM), Chronic Fatigue Syndrome, and Irritable Bowel Syndrome [12]. FM is a persistent and debilitating disorder that compromises the quality of life, affecting 2–4% of the population with a 9:1 female to male ratio [13]. There is no agreement on the specific etiology of FM, even if some authors suggest that an abnormal brain activity regarding pain processing could be the leading cause [13]. Patients suffering from FM typically present with a triad of widespread chronic pain of long duration (> 3 months), sleep disturbance, and fatigue. Nonetheless, the possible association with other key symptoms such as allodynia, hyperalgesia, general muscular tension, nerve pain, cognitive impairment, and mood disturbance makes the diagnosis quite challenging because of several overlaps with other rheumatologic conditions [13, 14]. All these symptoms are included in the 2010 Fibromyalgia Diagnostic Criteria published by the American College of Rheumatology [15, 16].

Several integrated programs were proposed for FM, mainly targeting symptoms management using both pharmacological and physical exercise or behavioral therapy, but there is no consensus about these treatments, that have still limited effectiveness [13].

Recently, an increasing amount of literature suggested the efficacy of Hyperbaric Oxygen Therapy (HBOT) in patients with IC or FM. For instance, van Ophoven and colleagues reported an improvement of symptoms and bladder capacity in patients affected by IC and treated with HBOT [5], results confirmed also by Tanaka in patients with a form of IC resistant to conventional therapy [4]. On the other side, Yildiz and colleagues found a significant reduction of Visual Analogue Scale scores in patients affected by FM and a significant increase in pain threshold [17]. Moreover, the work of Efrati and colleagues demonstrated a decrease in symptoms of FM and positive changes in brain activity [13], concluding that HBOT plays an important role in FM management. However, no study has investigated the possible role of HBOT in patients affected from IC associated with FM (IC/FM) so far.

The aim of our study was to investigate the response of IC/FM patients subjected to HBOT. In detail, we evaluated the effectiveness of HBOT in IC/FM refractory to conventional therapy, focusing on changes in quality of life, pain modulation, modifications in bladder endoscopic and urometric patterns.

Methods

Subjects

Patients were enrolled and considered eligible for the study after a medical screening carried out at the ATiP Center of Hyperbaric Medicine (Padova, Italy), in order to exclude possible contraindications to HBOT (Fig. 1). No incentives were offered to increase the enrollment and compliance to the study. The inclusion criteria were: (a) pain in bladder filling that improves with urination; (b) pain (suprapubic, pelvic, urethral, vaginal, or perineal); (c) presence of glomerulation (grade II/III) (or bleeding +/– at the cystodistension) and positive histologic findings at biopsy [18]; (d) reduced capacity; (e) increased visceral sensitivity; (f) normal or reduced compliance; (g) symptoms refractory to conventional therapy; and (h) diagnosis of FM according to the 2010 American College of Rheumatology guidelines [15, 16]. These criteria were based on those of the European Society for the Study of Interstitial Cystitis (ESSIC), including patients with an ESSIC disease staging ≥2C [18].

The exclusion criteria were: (a) pregnancy (diagnosed or within the previous year); (b) age less than 18 years; (c) benign or malignant bladder tumors; (d) radiation cystitis; (e) symptomatic bladder diversions; (f) herpes in active phase; (g) bladder and urethral stones; (h) urinary frequency less than 10 times a day; (i) presence of symptoms

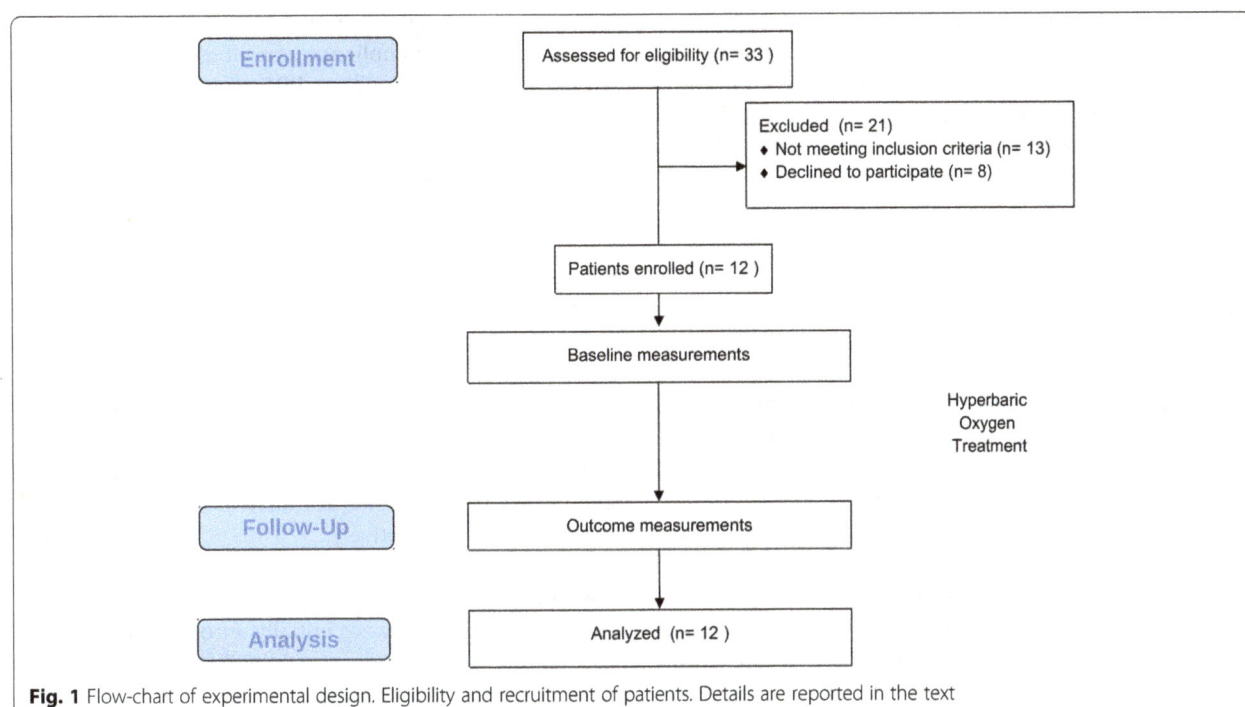

Fig. 1 Flow-chart of experimental design. Eligibility and recruitment of patients. Details are reported in the text

less than 12 months; and (l) bladder capacity > 400 ml with no sensitive urgency.

Experimental protocol

The experimental protocol received the approval by the local Human Ethical Committee (n° HEC-DSB 07/16) of the Department of Biomedical Science at University of Padova and adhered to the principles of the Declaration of Helsinki. Patients involved in the study read and signed an informed consent, were free to renounce the study at any time, and every precaution was taken to protect their privacy. All the patients were informed about the methods and aims of the study.

We structured an observational clinical trial design with repeated measures conducted before and 6 months after a therapeutic protocol with hyperbaric oxygen for the treatment of patients suffering from IC/FM. The authors confirmed that all ongoing and related trials for this intervention were retrospectively registered in the clinicaltrials.gov registry (NCT03693001). This study was not registered before enrollment of participants started because IC is an approved indication for HBOT in Italy and HBOT sessions were already planned in the therapeutic schedule of the enrolled patients. The whole study, comprehensive of recruitment and follow up after the experiment, took place between January and September 2018. This period seemed adequate for an evaluation over time of the treatment results on the most relevant symptoms of the pathology, i.e. pain, frequency of urination, urgency and evaluation of bladder capacity [1, 5]. Patients were exposed to breathing 100% oxygen at 2 atm absolute (ATA) in a multiplace

pressure chamber (Galeazzi, Zingonia, Italy) for 90 min using an overboard demand regulator while breathing through an oral-nasal mask. Each patient undertook a daily cycle of 20 sessions, 5 days a week. After 1 week of suspension, a second identical cycle of 20 sessions was performed.

The primary outcome was the modification in symptoms, assessed through several questionnaires that were administered to patients before (PRE) and 6 months after (POST) HBOT: (a) three-day voiding diary, (b) widespread pain index (WPI), (c) symptom severity scale (SSS), (d) Pelvic pain, Urgency and Frequency symptom scale (PUF), and (e) O'Leary-Sant questionnaire.

Questionnaires
Three-day voiding diary

It is a sheet for each 24-h period. Patients specified their bedtime and wake-up time directly in the upper part of the sheet. Later, they started recording all fluid intake (i.e., the total amount of fluids drank during a given time period) and urinary events (i.e., the amount of urine voided each time over a 24-h period). Moreover, the voiding diary presents specific fields to indicate either the amount of urine drained via catheter and/or each time the pad was changed. Patients write each time they had involuntary urine loss (even a small amount). As final outcomes, mean and maximum urine volume were considered.

Widespread pain index

WPI is a clinical diagnostic criterion proposed for patients with FM that do not rely on counting tender points [15]. It considers not only pain but also other

FM-related symptoms assessing their severity [15]. Physician asked the patient to indicate the location of any pain experienced during the week before the exam. As a result, WPI pointed out a total amount ranging from 0 to 19 points corresponding to the possibly-painful 19 body areas (i.e., areas of the shoulders, arms, hips, legs, jaws, chest, abdomen, back, and neck) [14].

Symptom severity scale

SSS focuses on 3 physical symptoms, as well as somatic symptoms in general [16]. In detail, symptoms are measured on the basis of a 0–3 severity scale considering fatigue, waking unrefreshed, and cognitive symptoms. The investigated period is the week before the questionnaire administration [14]. Later, the items are combined into a 0–12 scale assessing the somatic symptoms in general. The greater the amount, the more severe the symptomatology.

Pelvic pain, urgency and frequency symptom scale

Pelvic pain, Urgency and Frequency scale (PUF) is an eight-item questionnaire, largely used to evaluate symptoms of IC. It is organized in two subscales: symptom severity and level of bother. Total scores range from 0 to 35 (symptom subscale 0–23 and bother subscale 0–12). The higher the scores, the more severe the level of symptoms [19]. Scores > 12 indicate significant symptoms; scores of ≥15 have an 84% sensitivity in diagnosing IC based on positive potassium testing, which indicates abnormal permeability of bladder epithelium [1]. Also, the PUF was previously reported in persons with FM [20].

O'Leary-Sant index

The O'Leary-Sant index – also named Interstitial Cystitis Symptom Index (ICSI) – was proposed as a uniform outcome measure in IC [21]. The Interstitial Cystitis Problem Index (ICPI) was later developed from the ICSI as a corresponding problem index [22]. It measures the symptoms of the lower urinary tract and their influence on quality-of-life in subjects with IC. Test-retest reliability analysis and validation via administration to IC patients and asymptomatic controls resulted in a questionnaire with 8 items outlining two indexes: the symptom and the problem index [21, 23].

Cystoscopy, hydrodistension, and urodynamic evaluation

As secondary outcome, modifications in bladder endoscopic and urometric patterns were searched. Patients were assessed before (PRE) and 6 months after (POST) HBOT through cystoscopy, hydrodistension, and urodynamic examination. Hydrodistension was performed without sedation, applying a maximal filling pressure of 20–25 mmHg for 10 min. Petechiae were graded at PRE according to Nordling [24], and the improvement in lesions was defined as a downgrade found at POST.

Urodynamic testing allows recording of bladder sensitivity, capacity, and compliance as well as urethral and detrusor activity during filling. PRE and POST cystoscopy, hydrodistension, and urodynamic testing were performed by the same urologist, and urodynamic evaluation followed current International Continence Society standards.

Statistical analysis

Data were coded on a master sheet using a LibreOffice Calc spreadsheet (ver. 6.0.1.1, The Document Foundation, Berlin, Germany). A Two-tailed t-test for dependent means was used to analyze differences between pre and post-treatment means of questionnaires and quantitative data from Urodynamic testing, with a significance level of .05. Qualitative data from cystoscopy were analyzed descriptively.

Results

Thirty-three patients were initially enrolled for the study, and no contraindications to HBOT were found after medical screening. After application of inclusion and exclusion criteria, twenty patients were considered eligible for the study. However, 8 patients withdrew during the study (1 had problems with compensation maneuvers in the chamber; 3 because of the long travel needed to reach the hyperbaric facility; 4 did not provide a reason), and twelve patients concluded the study (M = 1; F = 11; mean age ± SD: 57 ± 10.57 years; mean duration of illness ± SD: 10,6 ± 9,33 years).

HBOT did not result in a statistically significant improvement both in questionnaires and in urodynamic testing, except for hydrodistension (mean pre-treatment: 409.167 ml; mean post-treatment: 489.167 ml; $p < .05$) (Table 1).

Cystoscopy performed after the treatment detected a reduction of petechiae and a regression of Hunner's ulcers (initially detected in only one patient), while glomerulations remained the same (Table 2).

Discussion

HBOT is emerging as a novel treatment in patients with IC and FM, as suggested by recent experiences in both the urologic and rheumatologic fields. In fact, hyperbaric oxygen is known to increase anti-inflammatory defenses over time and to promote neovascularization [25]. These mechanisms have been recently confirmed by Minami, who reported a reduction in H_2O_2-induced inflammation, edema, and fibrosis on the bladder of mice treated with HBOT [26]. On a molecular level, Thom demonstrated mobilization of bone marrow stem cells in response to hyperoxia, to hyperoxia and concluded that species that oxidative stress is the fundamental key mechanism of action of HBOT, exerting its effects on transcription through reactive oxygen and nitrogen species production

Table 1 Changes after hyperbaric oxygen treatment

	PRE	POST	P value
WPI	7.08 ± 5.14	5.75 ± 4.00	.46
SS	8.16 ± 2.88	7.50 ± 4.25	.60
PUF	22.83 ± 6.20	20.41 ± 6.69	.24
OS	13 ± 5.86	11.08 ± 5.17	.12
Mean urine volume (ml)	193.83 ± 89.61	201.27 ± 91.16	.75
Max urine volume (ml)	425.00 ± 257.30	383.33 ± 187.9	.47
Hydrodistension (ml)	409.16 ± 196.30	489.16 ± 149	.04
1st desire	103.50 ± 48.61	114.75 ± 37.33	.31
Strong desire	247.33 ± 99.79	245.41 ± 113.7	.91
Compliance	41.85 ± 27.06	44.18 ± 24.99	.74
Cystomanometric Capacity (ml)	318.10 ± 126.50	310.33 ± 133.5	.73
Urethral functioning (tension)	68.41 ± 25.69	75.33 ± 23.17	.47

After 20 HBO treatments, no statistically significant changes in assessed items were detected, except for hydrodistension ($p < .05$). *WPI* Widespread Pain Index, *SS* Symptom Severity score, *PUF* Pelvic Pain and Urinary Urgency Frequency, *OS* O'Leary Sant symptoms and problems index. Hydrodistension: derived from cystoscopy; 1st desire, voiding pain, compliance, cystomanometric capacity, and urethral functioning: derived from urodynamic testing

over several treatments [27]. Similarly, Minami and coll. demonstrated a decrease in mRNA expression of inflammatory biomarkers and an increase in endothelial nitric oxide synthase (eNOS) after HBOT [26]. Overall, HBOT results in enhanced perfusion and wound healing in ischemic tissues [25, 27].

HBOT is now widely used in urology for the treatment of radiation cystitis, cyclophosphamide-induced cystitis, emphysematous cystitis, or pelvic radiation disease, and the interest in treatment IC is currently growing [28]. The molecular mechanisms of IC development are still not well known, but current literature identifies a plausible cause in microcirculation. For instance, Tamaki and coll. suggested that an important pathophysiology way could result from a reduced blood flow in bladder's walls during its filling phase [29]. Concordantly, Lee J.D. and Lee M. verified that, in the bladder of IC patients, the expression of hypoxia-inducible factor-1α is increased both in muscle and urothelium of bladder, and Vascular Endothelial Growth Factor (VEGF) expression is higher in umbrella cells (apical cells) [6]. Both these studies could explain a hypoxic/ischemic damage, and therefore a possible useful role of HBOT in IC, as previously

demonstrated on an ischemia/reperfusion model on muscle mice by Bosco and coll. [30].

As hypothesized by Efrati and coll., HBOT induced an improvement of symptoms in patients with FM by increasing brain oxygenation, promoting neoangiogenesis and restoring normal patterns of pain processing [13].

Besides these recent evidences that favor HBOT in patients with IC and FM, no literature is available about such a treatment in patients with both the diseases, probably because of the rarity of this overlap in the general population.

Surprisingly, our results showed an isolated statistically significant improvement in hydrodistension, but no significant improvement in scores evaluating symptoms and life quality or other parameters at urodynamic testing (Table 1). These findings prompt several considerations, since no previous study has investigated the usefulness of HBOT in IC/FM patients.

With regard to FM, these findings do not support previous works that used HBOT to treat patients with FM alone [13, 17]. On the other hand, from the perspective of IC, our sample mostly included patients with non-ulcerative IC (11 out of 12) and our results are consistent with those of van Ophoven [5], Tanaka [4], and Wenzler [31] that demonstrated few effects on this subset of patients. Overall, this inconsistency may be due to the considerable delay in diagnosis of an IC/FM overlap and the conventional therapy administration, thus leading to resistance or failure to treatments. Another possible explanation for these results resides within the complicated medical management of these patients. In fact, since patients with FM have altered pathways of pain processing, an overlap with IC could probably worsen symptoms, and HBOT alone may be not sufficient to treat an overlap of both these diseases.

Table 2 Alterations observed in patients during cystoscopy before and 6 months after HBOT

	PRE	POST
Petechiae	11 patients	7 patients
Glomerulations	8 patients	8 patients
Hunner's ulcers	1 patient	no patients

After HBOT, there was a reduction of petechiae among treated patients, while no change was recorded regarding glomerulations. Of note, the only one patient presenting with Hunner's ulcers experienced a regression of the lesion.

In IC, urothelial alteration and deficiency of glycosaminoglycans may lead to a thinning of the mucosa up to the presence of Hunner's ulcers and/or fascicular fibrosis [29]. Cystoscopy usually documents these alterations by highlighting a bladder wall with inflamed areas, hemorrhagic areas, and fibrosis of the inner mucosal lining. If compared with non-ulcerative IC, Hunner's ulcers are characterized by histological findings of pancystitis, increase in plasma cells, expansion of clonal B-cells, and epithelial denudation [32]. According to our findings, glomerulations remained the same but there was a reduction of petechiae in most of the patients, thus suggesting possible improvement in oxygenation of apical tissues (Table 2). Expression of VEGF was not among the goals of our study but, according to literature, a reduction in petechiae could be linked with a reduction in VEGF expression in apical cells [6]. We also assisted to a regression of Hunner's ulcers after HBOT, a finding that matches those observed in recent studies by Tanaka [4] and by Wenzler [31] (Table 2).

The results of this study are promising but are subjected to a number of limitations. First, given the rarity of IC/FM overlap, we were able to enroll only 20 patients and 12 completed the study. Given the limited number of participants and the absence of a control group, results should be interpreted carefully. However, our sample size is greater than or similar to those of others previously cited studies, and a wider study – possibly multicentric – could help the scientific community to overcome this impasse. Second, since FM can overlap with several other conditions, the patients could have suffered from other diseases than IC and FM. In the future, a more precise stratification could be useful to draw conclusion on a larger sample of patients. Third, this study evaluated HBOT alone on patients, without tracking any other interventions such as education therapy, diet, or psychotherapy. Since the key of complex syndromes management resides in a multidisciplinary approach, we think that future trials should evaluate HBOT not alone but together with conventional treatments, in order to quantify its usefulness as an adjuvant therapy.

Conclusions

Patients with both IC and FM suffer from a complex and rare syndrome with a high level of therapeutic failure. According to literature, HBOT seems to be clinically effective in treating these two diseases when separated. Our study showed a statistically significant improvement of hydrodistension alone, but no significant improvement in symptoms, quality of life, and other urodynamic parameters in this subset of patients. Moreover, HBOT resulted in an improved cystoscopic pattern, with a healing of petechiae and Hunner's ulcers. Anyway, our results cannot justify HBOT alone in IC/FM patients. This is a spur to expand the sample and promote trials in the same field to better understand how HBOT could treat this rare subset of patients, especially as an adjuvant to conventional treatments.

Abbreviations

ATA: Atmospheres Absolute; FM: Fibromyalgia; HBOT: Hyperbaric Oxygen Therapy; IC: Interstitial cystitis; ICPI: Interstitial Cystitis Problem Index; ICSI: Interstitial Cystitis Symptoms Index; PUF: Pelvic pain, Urgency and Frequency scale; SSS: Symptom Severity Scale; VEGF: Vascular Endothelial Growth Factor; WPI: Widespread Pain Index

Acknowledgments

The authors wish to thank ATIP Centro di Medicina Iperbarica (Padova, Italy) and OTI Services (Marghera, Italy) for covering the cost for HBO treatments. Additionally, we are thankful to AICI (Associazione Italiana Cistite Interstiziale) that supported the recruitment of patients.

Authors' contributions

Conceived and designed the experiments: GB, EO, GpG, EC, and LP. Performed the experiments: GB, GG, EC, and IM. Analyzed the data: GM and MP. Contributed materials: IM and GG. Wrote the paper: MP, GB, AR, and EC. All authors approved the final version of the manuscript.

Author details

[1]Environmental and Respiratory Physiology Laboratory, Department of Biomedical Sciences, University of Padova, Padova, Italy. [2]Unità Operativa di Urologia, Azienda Ospedaliera Santa Maria degli Angeli, Pordenone, Italy. [3]ATIP Centro di Medicina Iperbarica, Padova, Italy. [4]Department of Statistics, Harvard School of Medicine, Boston, MA, USA. [5]OTI Services, Centro di Medicina Iperbarica, Venezia, Italy. [6]TEAMHealth Research Institute, TGH, Tampa, Florida, USA.

References

1. Parsons CL, Dell J, Stanford EJ, Bullen M, Kahn BS, Waxell T, et al. Increased prevalence of interstitial cystitis: previously unrecognized urologic and gynecologic cases identified using a new symptom questionnaire and intravesical potassium sensitivity. Urology. 2002;60:573–8.
2. Yang CC, Miller JL, Omidpanah A, Krieger JN. Physical examination for men and women with urologic chronic pelvic pain syndrome: a MAPP (multidisciplinary approach to the study of chronic pelvic pain) network study. Urology. 2018;116:23–9.
3. Clemens JQ, Meenan RT, Rosetti MC, et al. Prevalence and incidence of interstitial cystitis in a managed care population. J Urol. 2005;173:98.
4. Tanaka T, Nitta Y, Morimoto K, Nishikawa N, Nishihara C, Tamada S, et al. Hyperbaric oxygen therapy for painful bladder syndrome/interstitial cystitis resistant to conventional treatments: long-term results of a case series in Japan. BMC Urol. 2011;11:11.
5. van Ophoven A, Rossbach G, Oberpenning F, Hertle L. Hyperbaric oxygen for the treatment of interstitial cystitis: long-term results of a prospective pilot study. Eur Urol. 2004;46:108–13.
6. Lee J-D, Lee M-H. Increased expression of hypoxia-inducible factor-1α and vascular endothelial growth factor associated with glomerulation formation in patients with interstitial cystitis. Urology. 2011;78:971.e11–5.
7. Loran OB, Siniakova LA, Seregin AV, Mitrokhin AA, Plesovskiĭ AM, Vinarova NA. Hyperbaric oxygenation in the treatment of patients with interstitial cystitis: clinical and morphological rationale. Urologiia. 2011;3:3–5.
8. Mathers MJ, Lazica DA, Roth S. Non-bacterial cystitis: principles, diagnostics and etiogenic therapy options. Aktuelle Urol. 2010;41:361–8.
9. Binder I, Rossbach G, Van Ophoven A. Die komplexität chronischer beckenschmerzen am beispiel der interstitiellen zystitis. Teil 2: Therapie. Aktuelle Urologie. 2008;39:289–97.
10. Sutherland AM, Clarke HA, Katz J, Katznelson R. Hyperbaric oxygen therapy: a new treatment for chronic pain? Pain Pract. 2016;16:620–8.
11. He D-L. AB098. Progress in diagnosis and treatment of bladder pain syndrome/interstitial cystitis. Transl Androl Urol. 2015;4(Suppl 1). https://doi.org/10.3978/j.issn.2223-4683.2015.s098.

12. Nickel JC, Tripp DA, Pontari M, Moldwin R, Mayer R, Carr LK, et al. Interstitial cystitis/painful bladder syndrome and associated medical conditions with an emphasis on irritable bowel syndrome, fibromyalgia and chronic fatigue syndrome. J Urol. 2010;184:1358–63.

13. Efrati S, Golan H, Bechor Y, Faran Y, Daphna-Tekoah S, Sekler G, et al. Hyperbaric oxygen therapy can diminish fibromyalgia syndrome--prospective clinical trial. PLoS One. 2015;10:e0127012.

14. Arnold LM, Clauw DJ, McCarberg BH. FibroCollaborative. Improving the recognition and diagnosis of fibromyalgia. Mayo Clin Proc. 2011;86:457–64.

15. Wolfe F, Clauw DJ, Fitzcharles M-A, Goldenberg DL, Katz RS, Mease P, et al. The American College of Rheumatology Preliminary Diagnostic Criteria for fibromyalgia and measurement of symptom severity. Arthritis Care Res (Hoboken). 2010;62:600–10.

16. Wolfe F, Häuser W. Fibromyalgia diagnosis and diagnostic criteria. Ann Med. 2011;43:495–502.

17. Yildiz Ş, Kiralp M, Akin A, Keskin I, Ay H, Dursun H, et al. A new treatment modality for fibromyalgia syndrome: hyperbaric oxygen therapy. J Int Med Res. 2004;32:263–7.

18. van de Merwe JP, Nordling J, Bouchelouche P, Bouchelouche K, Cervigni M, Daha LK, et al. Diagnostic criteria, classification, and nomenclature for painful bladder syndrome/interstitial cystitis: an ESSIC proposal. Eur Urol. 2008;53:60–7.

19. Brewer ME, White WM, Klein FA, Klein LM, Waters WB. Validity of pelvic pain, urgency, and frequency questionnaire in patients with interstitial cystitis/painful bladder syndrome. Urology. 2007;70:646–9.

20. Jones KD, Maxwell C, Mist SD, King V, Denman MA, Gregory WT. Pelvic floor and urinary distress in women with fibromyalgia. Pain Manag Nurs. 2015;16:834–40.

21. O'Leary MP, Sant GR, Fowler FJ, Whitmore KE, Spolarich-Kroll J. The interstitial cystitis symptom index and problem index. Urology. 1997;49(5A Suppl):58–63.

22. Lubeck DP, Whitmore K, Sant GR, Alvarez-Horine S, Lai C. Psychometric validation of the O'leary-Sant interstitial cystitis symptom index in a clinical trial of pentosan polysulfate sodium. Urology. 2001;57(6 Suppl 1):62–6.

23. Ito T, Tomoe H, Ueda T, Yoshimura N, Sant G, Hanno P. Clinical symptoms scale for interstitial cystitis for diagnosis and for following the course of the disease. Int J Urol. 2003;10(Suppl):S24–6.

24. Nordling J, Anjum FH, Bade JJ, et al. Primary evaluation of patients suspected of having interstitial cystitis (IC). Eur Urol. 2004;45(5):662–9.

25. Camporesi EM, Bosco G. Mechanisms of action of hyperbaric oxygen therapy. Undersea Hyperb Med. 2014;41:247–52.

26. Minami A, Tanaka T, Otoshi T, Kuratsukuri K, Nakatani T. Hyperbaric oxygen significantly improves frequent urination, hyperalgesia, and tissue damage in a mouse long-lasting cystitis model induced by an intravesical instillation of hydrogen peroxide. Neurourol Urodyn. 2019;38(1):97–106.

27. Thom SR. Oxidative stress is fundamental to hyperbaric oxygen therapy. J Appl Physiol. 2009;106:988–95.

28. Gandhi J, Seyam O, Smith NL, Joshi G, Vatsia S, Khan SA. Clinical utility of hyperbaric oxygen therapy in genitourinary medicine. Med Gas Res. 2018;8:29–33.

29. Tamaki M, Saito R, Ogawa O, Yoshimura N, Ueda T. Possible mechanisms inducing glomerulations in interstitial cystitis: relationship between endoscopic findings and expression of angiogenic growth factors. J Urol. 2004;172:945–8.

30. Bosco G, Yang Z, Nandi J, Wang J, Chen C, Camporesi EM. Effects of hyperbaric oxygen on glucose, lactate, glycerol and anti-oxidant enzymes in the skeletal muscle of rats during ischaemia and reperfusion. Clin Exp Pharmacol Physiol. 2007;34:70–6.

31. Wenzler DL, Gulli F, Cooney M, Chancellor MB, Gilleran J, Peters KM. Treatment of ulcerative compared to non-ulcerative interstitial cystitis with hyperbaric oxygen: a pilot study. Ther Adv Urol. 2017;9:263–70.

32. Maeda D, Akiyama Y, Morikawa T, KunitaA OY, Katoh H, et al. Hunner-type (classic) interstitial cystitis: a distinct InflammatoryDisorder characterized by Pancystitis, with FrequentExpansion of clonal B-cells and EpithelialDenudation. PLoS One. 2015;10(11):e0143316. https://doi.org/10.1371/journal.pone.0143316.

17

Development of a high-precision bladder hyperthermic intracavitary chemotherapy device for bladder cancer and pharmacokinetic study

Mingchen Ba[1*], Shuzhong Cui[1*], Hui Long[2], Yuanfeng Gong[1], Yinbing Wu[1], Kunpeng Lin[1], Yinuo Tu[1], Bahuo Zhang[1] and Wanbo Wu[1]

Abstract

Background: Bladder hyperthermic intracavitary chemotherapy (HIVEC) has good effectiveness for bladder cancer, but conventional HIVEC systems lack precision and convenient application. To test the safety of a new HIVEC device (BR-TRG-II-type) in pigs and to perform a preliminary clinical trial in patients with bladder cancer.

Methods: This device was tested on six pigs to optimize the temperature and time parameters. Then, 165 patients (HIVEC after transurethral resection (TUR), $n = 128$; or HIVEC, $n = 37$) treated between December 2006 and December 2016 were recruited. Mitomycin C (MMC) was the chemotherapeutic agent. A serum pharmacokinetic study was performed. The primary endpoints were tumor recurrence, disease-free survival (DFS), and cumulative incidence rate (CIR) during follow-up. The adverse effects were graded.

Results: The animal experiment showed that 45 °C for 1 h was optimal. HIVEC was successful, with the infusion tube temperature stably controlled at about 45 °C, and outlet tube temperature of about 43 °C in all patients, for three sessions. Serum MMC levels gradually increased during HIVEC and decreased thereafter. The mean DFS was 39 ± 3.21 months (ranging from 8 to 78 months), and the DFS rate was 89.1% during follow-up. No adverse events occurred.

Conclusion: The use of the BR-TRG-II-type HIVEC device is feasible for the treatment of bladder cancer. Future clinical trials in patients with different stages of bladder cancer will further confirm the clinical usefulness of this device.

Keywords: Hyperthermic intracavitary chemotherapy, Bladder cancer, Survival, Animal model

Background

Bladder cancer ranks among the top five malignant tumors worldwide, with over 70,000 new patients diagnosed with bladder cancer each year in the United States [1]. The standard procedure for bladder cancer removal is still transurethral resection (TUR) or surgical resection [2], but recurrence is always a major concern. As

much as 80% of patients with bladder cancer confined to bladder epithelium will experience disease recurrence, and up to 45% of patients with invasion of lamina propria and 10% with carcinoma in situ will experience disease progression without treatment [3]. Intravesical Bacillus Calmette-Guerin (BCG) is recommended as adjuvant therapy [4], but recurrence and progression occurs in a substantial proportion of patients [5]. Mitomycin C (MMC) is also recommended as adjuvant treatment, but its efficacy is limited [6–9]. TUR or surgical resection alone cannot be performed microscopically, and systemic chemotherapy has only limited efficacy

* Correspondence: bamingchen@126.com; cuishuzhong@126.com
[1]Intracelom Hyperthermic Perfusion Therapy Center, Cancer Hospital of Guangzhou Medical University, No. 78 Hengzhigang Road, Guangzhou, Guangdong 510095, People's Republic of China
Full list of author information is available at the end of the article

against bladder cancer [3, 10]. Therefore, preventing recurrence of bladder cancer after TUR and preventing progression in patients unsuitable for TUR or surgical resection remain major problems in oncology [11, 12].

Bladder hyperthermic intracavitary chemotherapy (HIVEC) combines the advantages of local hyperthermia with intracavitary chemotherapy, which have a synergistic or at least additive effect in preventing bladder cancer recurrence post TUR or surgical resection [13–16]. However, available systems have issues in the precision of temperature control to the target site [6–9, 11–14, 16–19], limiting their efficacy and safety [3, 10, 13–18].

The BR-TRG-I-type hyperthermic intraperitoneal perfusion chemotherapy (HIPEC) device is a recent HIPEC device now approved by the Chinese Food & Drug Agency (license number 2009–3260924) and covered by two Chinese patents (ZL2006200613779 and ZL2006200613764). The BR-TRG-I-type HIPEC device has been shown to be safe and effective for the treatment of malignant ascites and peritoneal cancer [20]. The BR-TRG-I-type HIPEC device has been tested for hyperthermic intraperitoneal perfusion chemotherapy [21], but it is not suitable for bladder cancer. On the basis of the BR-TRG-I-type HIPEC device, we developed the BR-TRG-II-type HIVEC device, which has been shown to be safe and efficient in preventing the recurrence of non-muscle invasive bladder cancer (NMIBC) after TUR and prolonging disease-free survival (DFS) [12]. This device allows for a precise temperature ($\pm 0.2\,°C$) and flow ($\pm 5\%$) control [20]. Therefore, the aim of the present exploratory study was to test the safety of the device in pigs, and to perform a preliminary clinical trial in patients with bladder cancer treated.

Methods

Animals

Animal experiments with the BR-TRG-II-type HIVEC device were performed using six healthy female experimental pigs (*Sus scrofa domesticus*; 40–50 kg, median 52.6 kg; 4–6 months old, median 5 months) purchased from the Animal Experiments Center of Nanfang Medical University (Guangzhou, China). The experimental animals were sacrificed by intravenous air embolization after receiving general anesthesia with intravenous infusion of propofol (femoral vein, 3–8 ml/h, adjusted according to the condition of the animals). This study was approved by the Ethics Committee of Animal Experiments of Guangzhou Medical University (No. GZMU ECAE 20060326), Guangzhou, China. All animals were handled humanely, and all means were taken to minimize suffering. All experiments were carried out according to the animal experiment principles from the US National Institutes of Health and according to the regulations from the Chinese government.

Under endotracheal anesthesia, 24 F 3-way Foley catheters were introduced into the bladder cavity, and 5 ml

of warm saline were injected to inflate the sac and fix the catheter in the bladder cavity. The BR-TRG-II-type HIVEC device (Fig. 1) was connected to the catheter and loaded with a solution of 60 mg of MMC (Zhejiang Hisun pharmaceutical Limited by Share Ltd., Hangzhou, China) in 600 ml of sterile saline. The perfusion rate of the MMC solution was set as 150–200 ml/min. The experimental temperature and time (i.e., 44 °C, 46 °C, or 48 °C for 60 min) were set. The treatment temperature during HIVEC was measured by the device using temperature probes inserted in a blind pipe in an inflated water sac linked to an infusion tube near an infusion tube and in a blind pipe in an inflated water sac linked to an outlet tube near the 24 F 3-way Foley catheter (as shown in Fig. 2a b).

Based on the "resource equation" principle [22–24], on the results being observed, and on available resources, six pigs were randomized (random number table prepared by a third-party statistician) to the 44 °C, 46 °C, and 48 °C groups (2 pigs/group). Before HIVEC, the perfusion liquid was adjusted to the proper temperature. Any temperature change was monitored closely by the temperature probes. HIVEC was performed once a week for 3 weeks. The Foley catheter was pulled out after every session. The bladder mucosa changes after HIVEC were assessed by cystoscopic observation under endotracheal anesthesia [13, 19]. The observer was blind to grouping.

Clinical trial

Patients with bladder cancer were prospectively recruited from December 2006 to December 2016 at the Intracelom Hyperthermic Perfusion Therapy Center of the Cancer Hospital of Guangzhou Medical University. This study was retrospectively registered (chictr.org.cn: ChiCTR1900022099). The patients received TUR + HIVEC or HIVEC according to whether they were suitable or not for TUR [2]; there was no randomization for this part of the study, nor blinding. Bladder cancer was diagnosed and staged by cystoscopic observation, computerized tomography (CT), and/or magnetic resonance imaging (MRI) examination.

The inclusion criteria were: 1) ≥18 years of age; 2) diagnosis of bladder cancer by cystoscopic observation, CT, and/or MRI; 3) diagnosis confirmed by histopathological examination of a biopsy specimen; 4) no radiation therapy in the 4 weeks preceding enrollment; and 5) no chemotherapy in the 4 weeks preceding enrollment. The exclusion criteria were: 1) stage Ta bladder cancer; 2) known or possible bladder metastasis from other primary cancer; 3) known or possible bladder tumor expanding through the serosa, invading locally or metastasizing to other organs; 4) known or potential pregnancy; or 5) active inflammation or infection. Based on whether the patients were suitable for TUR or not,

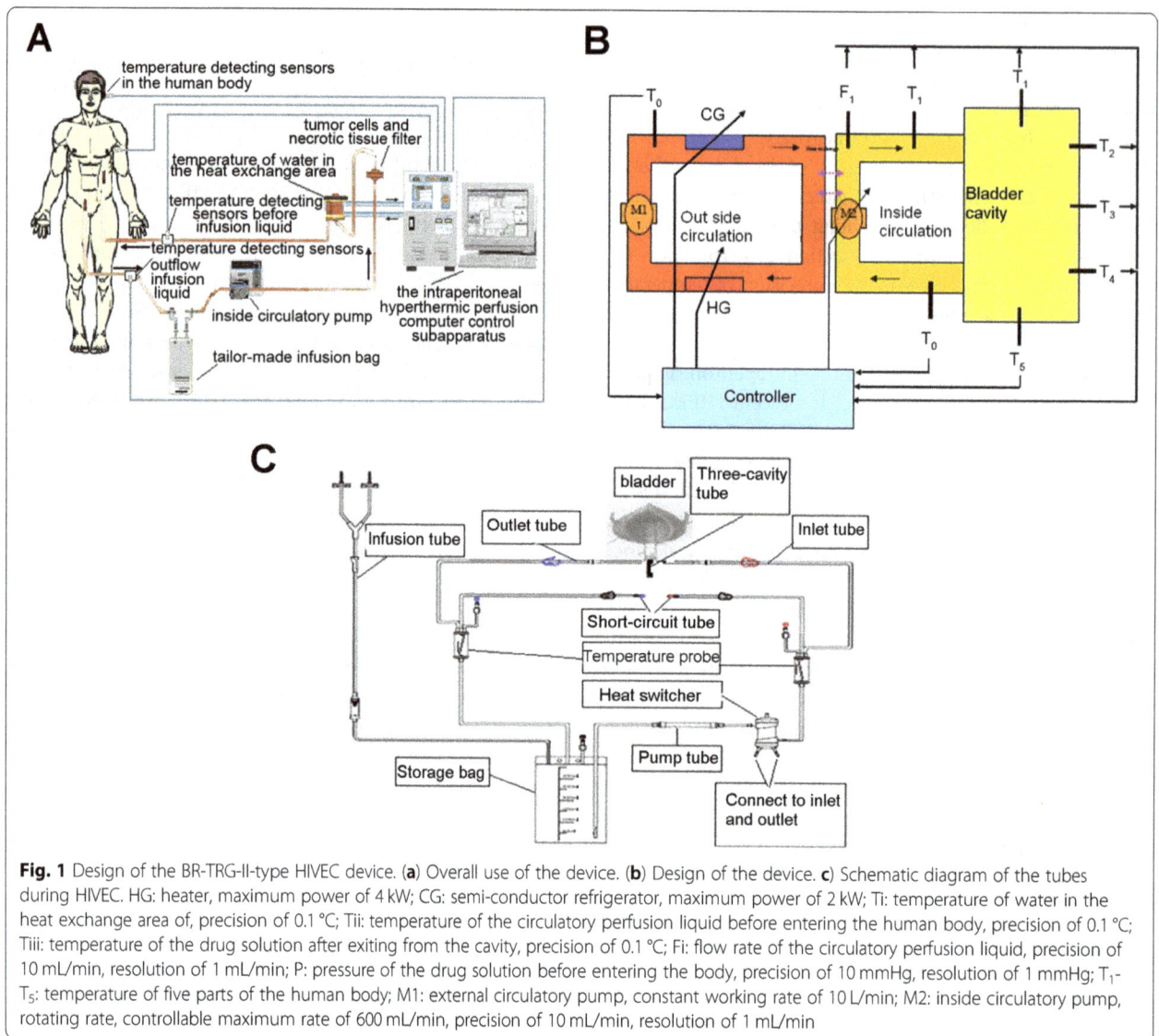

Fig. 1 Design of the BR-TRG-II-type HIVEC device. (**a**) Overall use of the device. (**b**) Design of the device. **c**) Schematic diagram of the tubes during HIVEC. HG: heater, maximum power of 4 kW; CG: semi-conductor refrigerator, maximum power of 2 kW; Ti: temperature of water in the heat exchange area of, precision of 0.1 °C; Tii: temperature of the circulatory perfusion liquid before entering the human body, precision of 0.1 °C; Tiii: temperature of the drug solution after exiting from the cavity, precision of 0.1 °C; Fi: flow rate of the circulatory perfusion liquid, precision of 10 mL/min, resolution of 1 mL/min; P: pressure of the drug solution before entering the body, precision of 10 mmHg, resolution of 1 mmHg; T_1-T_5: temperature of five parts of the human body; M1: external circulatory pump, constant working rate of 10 L/min; M2: inside circulatory pump, rotating rate, controllable maximum rate of 600 mL/min, precision of 10 mL/min, resolution of 1 mL/min

TUR + HIVEC or HIVEC was performed. TUR + HIVEC was performed for patients eligible for TUR but not for cystectomy and reconstruction because of comorbidities or incapacity to bear the surgical trauma. In patients unable to bear any surgery, HIVEC was performed.

All treatments were performed by our study team with clinical experience with TUR and HIVEC. This study was approved by the Medical Ethics Committee of the Cancer Hospital of Guangzhou Medical University (No. GZMU ECAE 20060326). Written informed consent was obtained from all patients. Some of the patients included in the present study were also included in a previous study by our group [12], but differences in the selection criteria resulted in different sample sizes and groups of patients between the two studies.

Transurethral resection

Cystoscopy was performed under epidural anesthesia. A 24-Fr monopolar resectoscope system (Karl Storz, Tuttlingen,

Germany) was used for TUR. Under cystoscopy, the profile and margins of the tumor were first defined. Resection was then performed carefully to avoid perforation and wall distention. The emptied bladder was manually manipulated on the pubic symphysis in cases of poorly located tumors. Small and flat lesions were positioned between the resection loop and the end portion of the resectoscope sheath. Hemostasis was carefully performed after tumor removal [13, 19].

HIVEC

HIVEC was directly performed for patients unsuitable for TUR, or 0–1 days after TUR. To do so, 24 F 3-way Foley catheters were introduced into the bladder cavity for HIVEC, and 5 ml of warm saline were injected to inflate the sac and fix the catheter in the bladder. The BR-TRG-II type high-precision HIVEC device was connected to tubes (Guangzhou Bright Medical Technology Co., Ltd.). A bag containing 60 mg of MMC in 500–700 ml (average

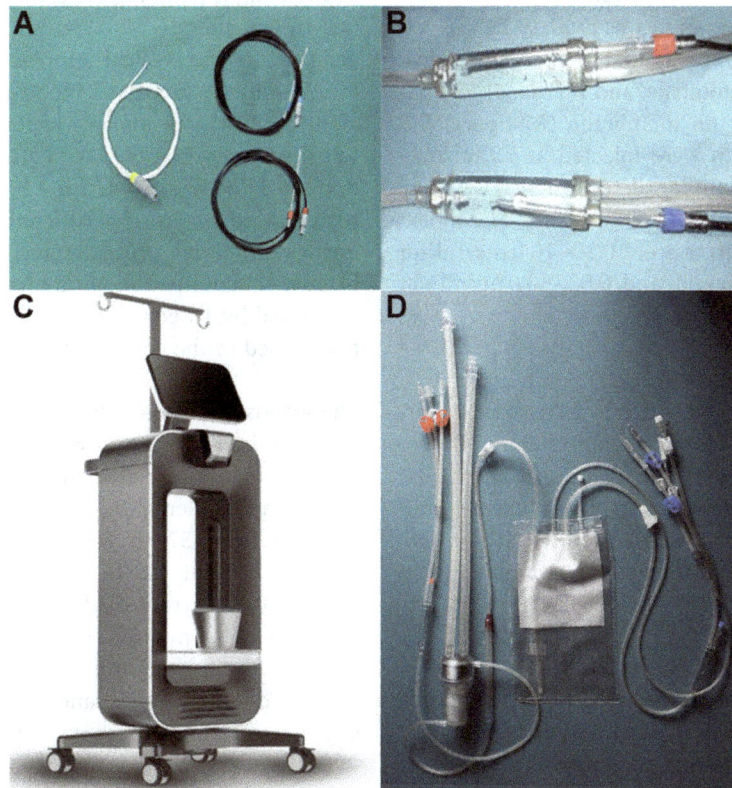

Fig. 2 Illustration of the BR-TRG-II-type HIVEC system for HIVEC. (**a**) Temperature-monitoring probes. One tip is placed into a fixed water sac linked to an infusion tube near an inlet (red cap) or outflow catheters (blue cap) at the top of a 24 F 3-way Foley catheter (yellow cap). (**b**) Temperature-monitoring probes location; red cap locates near the infusion catheters, and blue cap locates near the outflow catheters. (**c**) The device. **d**) The tubes

600 ml) of sterile saline, as previously reported [6, 7]. The liquid perfusion rate was set as 150–200 ml/min. The treatment temperature and time were set (i.e., 45 °C for 60 min) according to the patient's clinical data.

Before HIVEC, perfusion liquid was adjusted to 350–450 ml (average 400 ml) at 45 °C within the bladder according to the perfusion pressure and the patient's subjective experience. The amount of perfusion fluid within the bladder cavity could be increased or decreased according to the patient's subjective experience, and the temperature change was monitored closely by the temperature probe. The patient's vital signs (including blood pressure, heart rate, respiratory rate, and blood oxygen saturation) were monitored using a G3HJ20025 multi-parameter patient monitor (MINDRAY Bio-Medical Electronics Co. Ltd., Shenzhen, China). HIVEC treatment was terminated if any accidents happened, such as treatment temperature > 45 °C or bladder lumen pressure over patients' tolerance during HIVEC. HIVEC was performed once a week for 3 weeks. The 24 F 3-way Foley catheters were retained for 3–5 days for urine drainage after the first session for observing for eventual bleeding of the TUR wound.

Pathological examination

In all patients, the tumor tissues were taken before HIVEC or 4 weeks after HIVEC and were observed for histological changes by hematoxylin-eosin (H&E) staining, as described previously [13, 19]. Resected specimens were reviewed by an experienced pathologist blinded to grouping, as described previously [13, 19].

Pharmacokinetics of MMC

Venous blood (from the venous catheters at 0, 15, 30, 45, 60, 75, and 90 min) and perfusion liquid (from the short circuit outflow catheters of the perfusion system at 0, 15, 30, 45, 60, 75, and 90 min) samples were collected from 12 patients in the two groups. Perfusion liquid, serum, or MMC standard samples (degassed prior to use) (200 μl) were vortexed for 1 min with 200 μl of acetonitrile containing diazepam (20 μg; internal standard). The samples were separated by centrifugation at 15,000 rpm for 15 min. The supernatants (10 μl) were subjected to high-performance liquid chromatography (HPLC, aLC-20AB, Shimazdu, Kyoto, Japan). The stationary phase was Zorbax RP, and C_{18} (250 × 4.6 mm; particle size 5 μm) packed columns. The analysis was performed as previously reported [25], but with some modifications. The mobile phase was a 60:20:20 (%, volume) solution of 50 mM potassium dihydrogen phosphate buffer solution, acetonitrile, and methanol, pH 3.0, and filtered using a 0.22-μm membrane (Millipore, Billerica, MA, USA). Samples were injected at 1.2 ml/min. The absorption wavelength for detection was 210 nm. The column oven temperature was 35 °C. The linear ranges of the standard curves were 0.10–10.0 mg/ml for MMC in the perfusion liquid and 0.50–50.0 ng/ml for MMC in the serum [26, 27].

Follow-up

Follow-up was performed by urinary cystoscopic observation at 1 month after TUR and then each 3 months for 1 year. These patients underwent abdominal and pelvic CT scans at 3, 6, and 12 months, or when clinically indicated. After 1 year, follow-up was carried out at 6-month intervals or less frequently if the patients remained without evidence of disease.

Endpoints

The primary endpoints were tumor recurrence (diagnosed by cystoscopic observation, CT, or MRI), DFS, and cumulative incidence rate (CIR) during follow-up. The adverse effects of the anticancer drugs were graded according to the Common Toxicity Criteria of the National Cancer Institute for Adverse Events (CTCAE) [28].

Statistical analysis

In the animal part, a minimum of six animals was deemed necessary to reach any conclusion. For the human part, the sample size was not calculated because there was no randomization. This is a convenience sampling of all patients who met the criteria during the study period and agreed to participate in the study. All continuous data were tested for normal distribution using the Kolmogorov-Smirnov test, are presented as mean ± standard deviation, and were analyzed using the Student's t-test (intergroup comparisons) or repeated measure ANOVA with the LSD post hoc test (intragroup comparisons). Categorical data are presented as frequencies and were analyzed using the Fisher's exact test. CIR and DFS were analyzed using the Kaplan-Meier curve method with the log-rank test. Data were analyzed using SPSS 19.0 (IBM, Armonk, NY, USA). Two-sided P-values < 0.05 were considered statistically significant.

Results

Animal experimental data

The animal experiment showed that when using the device set at 44 °C for 1 h, a temperature of about 43 °C was achieved in the intravesical cavity without affecting the vital signs of the animals. The bladder mucosa showed slight pathological changes and returned to normal by 1 h after HIVEC. Setting HIVEC at 46 °C for 1 h achieved an intravesical temperature of about 45 °C and caused slightly increased blood pressure and heart rate, along with bladder mucosa hyperemia and edema, which returned to normal by 3 days after the final HIVEC. Setting the HIVEC at 48 °C for 1 h achieved an intravesical temperature of about 47 °C and caused significant increases in blood pressure and heart rate, along with bladder mucosa pathological changes that did not return to normal by 1 week after HIVEC. Therefore, 45 °C for 1 h was used in the clinical study.

Characteristics of the patients

One hundred and sixty-five patients with bladder cancer were eventually enrolled in this study. There were 108 males and 57 females, with a median age of 51 years (ranging from 37 to 76 years). Of these patients, 128 cases underwent HIVEC after TUR (including four patients with recurrent bladder cancers with a disease-free period of 3–6 months post-TUR), while 37 received HIVEC. There were no significant differences in age, gender, disease course, and tumor location, stage, and size between the two groups (all $P > 0.05$) (Table 1).

Gross outcomes of HIVEC

HIVEC was successful, with the infusion tube temperature stably controlled at about 45 °C, and an outlet tube temperature of about 43 °C (Fig. 3). All patients tolerated three sessions of HIVEC. For all patients in the HIVEC groups, gross hematuria stopped after 2 days after the first HIVEC, but slight hematuria lasted for up to one week following the first treatment.

Pharmacokinetics of MMC

The MMC concentration in the bladder perfusion fluid gradually decreased during treatment from 1 mg/ml to 0.967 mg/ml in the HIVEC + TUR group and 0.970 mg/ml in the HIVEC groups (P > 0.05) (Fig. 4a). The MMC concentration in the serum gradually increased during HIVEC treatment in both groups, to 4.32 ± 0.11, 7.86 ± 0.14, 10.08 ± 0.21, and 7.56 ± 0.16 ng/m at, 15, 30, 45, 60, and 75 min in the HIVEC + TUR group, which were significantly higher than in the HIVEC group (3.01 ± 0.09, 5.78 ± 0.11, 5.98 ± 0.12, and 5.66 ± 0.13 ng/ml, respectively) (Fig. 4b). The MMC concentration in serum decreased after HIVEC, being all below 3.28 ± 0.08 ng/ml at 90 min (Fig. 4b).

Cystoscopic and histological observation

In the HIVEC + TUR group, cystoscopy showed no viable tumor lesions, except in 12 patients who had T2 diseases; the lesions were showing as grey-white slough on the bladder mucosa around the lesions, accompanied by congestion and edema. In the HIVEC group, all patients showed

Table 1 Characteristics of the patients with bladder cancer

	HIVEC+TUR (n = 128)	HIVEC (n = 37)	P
Age (years)	50.7 ± 1.9 (37–66)	51.6 ± 2.3 (39–66)	0.07
Sex, n (%)			
Male	86 (67.2)	22 (59.5)	0.09
Female	42 (32.8)	15 (40.5)	0.07
Disease course (days)	11.4 ± 1.3	11.3 ± 1.6	0.07
Tumor location, n (%)			
Side wall	35 (27.3)	1 (2.7)	0.06
Posterior wall	27 (21.1)	2 (5.4)	0.08
Top area	19 (14.8)	1 (2.7)	0.08
Triangle area	10 (7.8)	17 (45.9)	0.06
≥ two tumors	37 (28.9)	16 (43.2)	0.07
Tumor size, n (%)			
≥ 0.5 cm	66 (51.6)	28 (75.6)	0.07
< 0.5 cm	62 (48.4)	9 (24.4)	0.09
Tumor stage, n (%)			
Tis	13 (10.2)	0	0.06
T_1	73 (57.0)	9 (24.3)	0.06
T_2	42 (32.8)	28 (75.7)	0.08
Tumor differentiation, n (%)			
G_1	41 (32.0)	11 (29.7)	0.08
G_2	54 (42.2)	14 (37.8)	0.08
G_3	33 (25.8)	12 (32.4)	0.75

HIVEC: bladder intracavitary hyperthermic perfusion chemotherapy

cystoscopic findings consistent with the findings observed in those with residual lesions in the HIVEC + TUR group. Pathological examination showed that the lesions presented degenerative necrosis and inflammatory cells such as eosinophils infiltrating the lamina propria (Fig. 5a) Complete necrosis accompanied by local vascular changes (such as necrosis and thrombosis) in the tumor small vessels were also observed, as well as stromal hemorrhage (Fig. 5b).

Follow-up

All patients were followed for at least 6 months. The median follow-up was 41.9 months (6.5 to 110 months) for the HIVEC + TUR group and 42.3 months (10.5 to 99.7 months) for the HIVEC group ($P > 0.05$). All patients were still alive at the moment of writing this paper. In the HIVEC + TUR group, cystoscopic observation showed tumor recurrence in 14 patients after HIVEC, which included nine patients with remaining tumor after HIVEC + TUR. The CIR was 10.9% (14 out of 128 patients). The mean DFS was 39 ± 3.21 months (ranging from 8 to 78 months), and the DFS rate was 89.1% during follow-up (Fig. 6a b). In the HIVEC group, bladder tumor numbers were decreased in 78.4% (29/37) patients or disappeared in 16.2% (6/37) patients; 51.35% (19/37) patients could undergo TUR 1–2 months after HIVEC.

Adverse effect

No gastrointestinal events or bone marrow suppression occurred. Laboratory tests showed no significant changes in blood, electrolytes, and liver and kidney functions

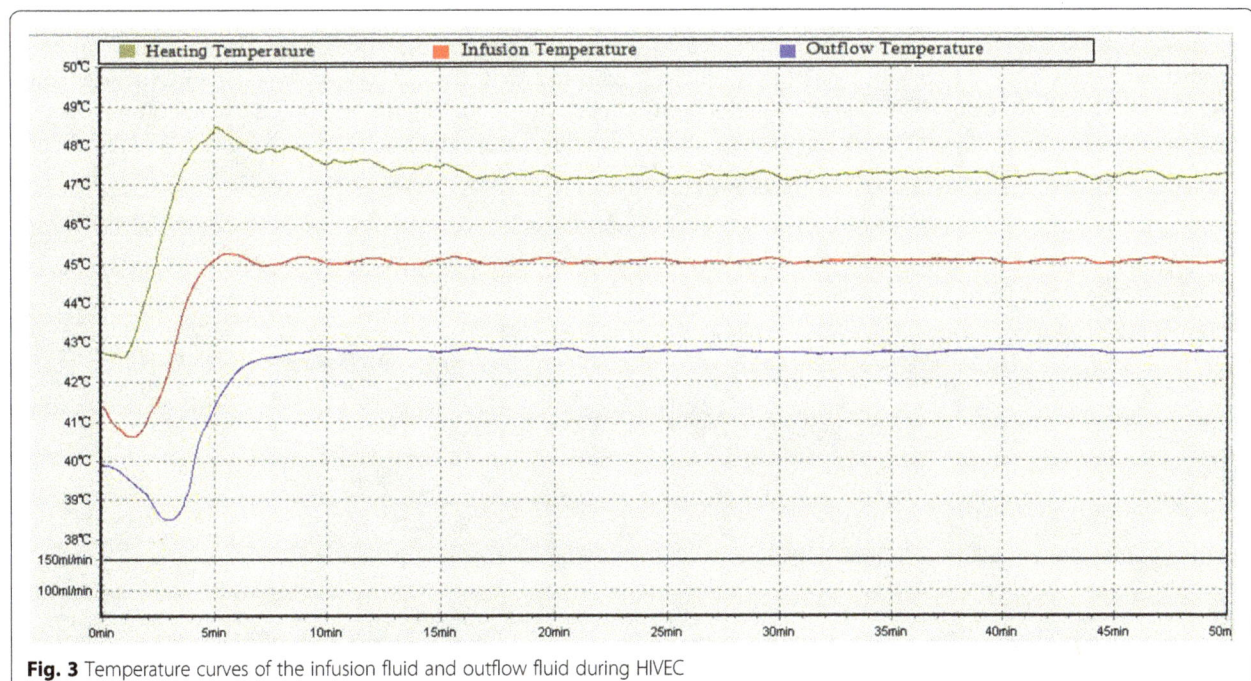

Fig. 3 Temperature curves of the infusion fluid and outflow fluid during HIVEC

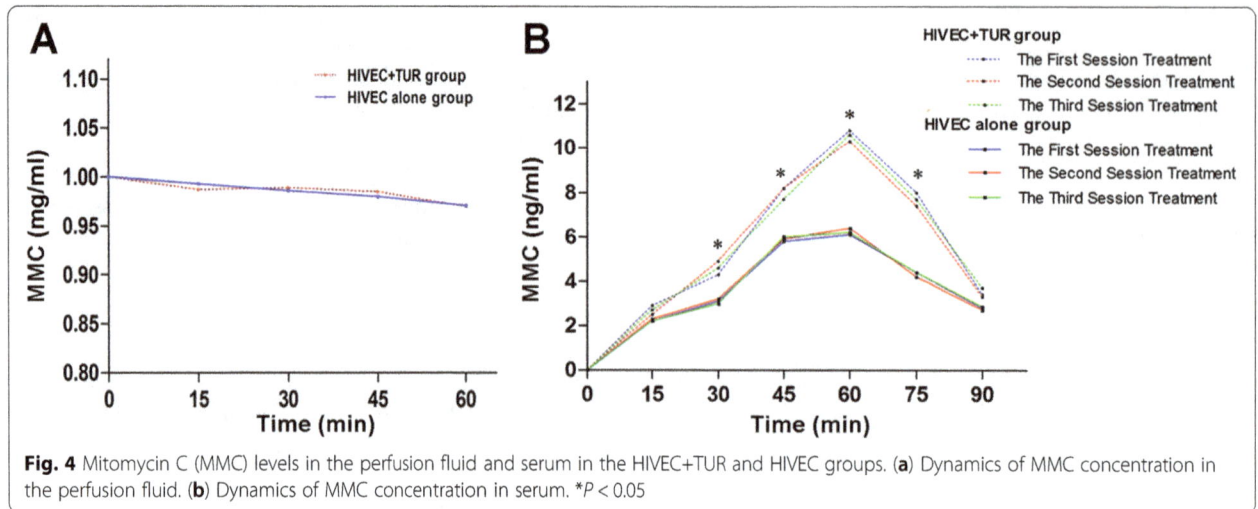

Fig. 4 Mitomycin C (MMC) levels in the perfusion fluid and serum in the HIVEC+TUR and HIVEC groups. (**a**) Dynamics of MMC concentration in the perfusion fluid. (**b**) Dynamics of MMC concentration in serum. *$P < 0.05$

after treatment in all patients. There were no genitourinary or dermatologic adverse reactions such as bladder spasms, chemical cystitis, or chemical irritation of scrotal skin in all patients.

Discussion

Bladder HIVEC has good effectiveness for bladder cancer [7–13, 19, 29], but the precision and convenient application of conventional HIVEC systems are unsatisfactory. Therefore, this study aimed first to examine the safety of a new HIVEC device (BR-TRG-II-type) in pigs, and then to perform a preliminary clinical trial in patients with bladder cancer. The results showed that the BR-TRG-II-type HIVEC device could be used for the treatment of bladder cancer. Nevertheless, the results need to be confirmed in patients with different cancer stages. Of note, HIVEC is an experimental treatment that is not currently included in any treatment guideline. Nevertheless, a number of studies using different, less accurate HIVEC systems have been performed [7–13, 19, 29], and this approach could

eventually be included in bladder cancer treatment guidelines. Since cystectomy cannot be performed in some patients [30], TUR combined with intravesical HIVEC could be a good option for these cases.

The most important physicians' concern during any treatment involving hyperthermia is setting an adequate temperature. Indeed, too high temperature will cause thermal damage, while too low temperature will not achieve the optimal therapeutic effects. Complicating the issue is the fact that in HIVEC, different body compartments will require different temperatures. In HIPEC, the intra-abdominal temperature generally does not exceed 43 °C because of the risk of intestinal adhesions and obstruction. On the other hand, for intravesical HIVEC, the temperature is usually set to 45 °C because bladder mucosa damage recovers fast [3, 9, 12, 14, 26, 31]. In the present paper, the preclinical experiments in pigs showed that the BR-TRG-II-type HIVEC device could meet the requirements for precise temperature control, heating, and cooling, hence ensuring stable, secure,

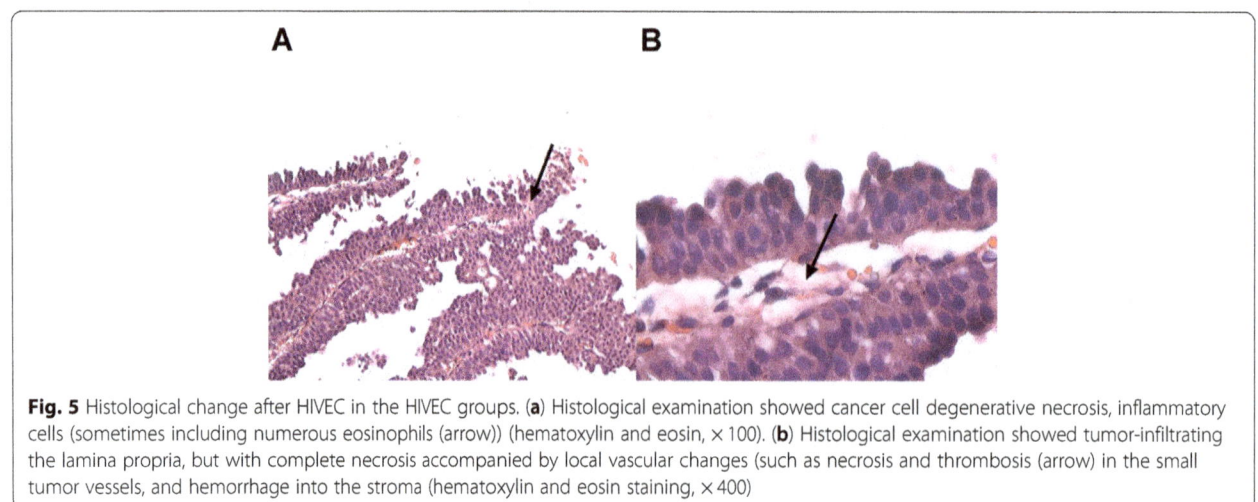

Fig. 5 Histological change after HIVEC in the HIVEC groups. (**a**) Histological examination showed cancer cell degenerative necrosis, inflammatory cells (sometimes including numerous eosinophils (arrow)) (hematoxylin and eosin, × 100). (**b**) Histological examination showed tumor-infiltrating the lamina propria, but with complete necrosis accompanied by local vascular changes (such as necrosis and thrombosis (arrow) in the small tumor vessels, and hemorrhage into the stroma (hematoxylin and eosin staining, × 400)

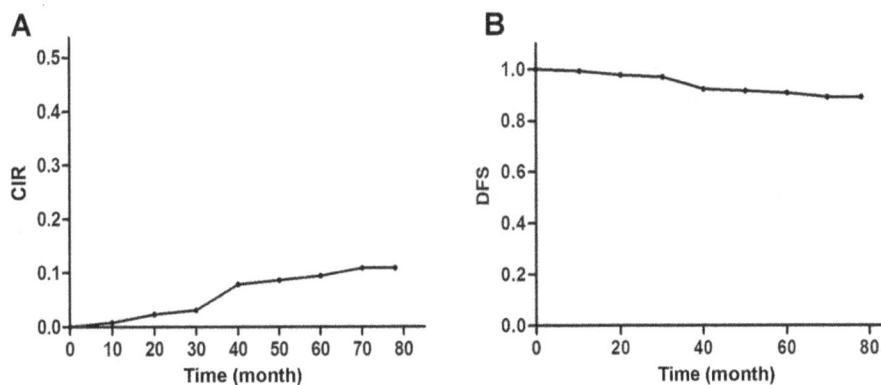

Fig. 6 Kaplan-Meier curves of cumulative incidence rate (CIR) and disease-free survival (DFS) for patients with bladder HIVEC after TUR. **a** Kaplan-Meier curves of cumulative incidence rate (CIR), and the CIR was 10.9% (14 out of 128 patients) for patients with bladder HIVEC after TUR. **b** Kaplan-Meier curves of disease-free survival (DFS), and the mean DFS was 39.0±1.2 months (ranging from 8 to 78 months), and the DFS rate was 89.1% during follow-up for patients with bladder HIVEC after TUR

reliable, and convenient application in the clinical setting. Furthermore, the experiments in pigs revealed that intravesical HIVEC at 45 °C for 1 h did not affect vital signs; the bladder mucosa showed only slight pathological changes, which returned to normal within 1 h after HIVEC completion.

Following the animal study, the preliminary clinical study and the results showed that HIVEC using the BR-TRG-II-type HIVEC device was feasible in a clinical setting, without any cases of postoperative deaths or serious complications. Gross hematuria disappeared after HIVEC in all patients, bladder lesions were smaller or even disappeared, and > 50% of the patients who were initially unsuitable for TUR got the chance to receive TUR after HIVEC, as supported by previous reports that revealed the advantages of HIVEC [4–9, 11–19, 32].

The use of intravesical MMC was tried in a number of previous studies [6–9, 11, 12]. Those studies used an MMC dose of at most 60 mg in 60 ml of saline (i.e., MMC at 1 mg/ml), which is considered safe and effective in clinical practice [6–9, 11, 12], but the knowledge of the vesical absorption rate of chemotherapeutic drugs is limited at best. In fact, high MMC concentrations has little relationship with the therapeutic effects [11, 15, 16, 18, 26]. In addition, the biological effects of cytotoxic drugs under high temperatures are poorly known. In the absence of concrete knowledge, we tested the use of continuous circulation of a fixed dose of chemotherapeutic drugs (60 mg) in a volume of 500–700 ml. In this preliminary trial, this dose was safe and effective. The absorption of MMC is related to damage to the bladder mucosa during intravesical HIVEC, and MMC concentration remains excessively high in the absence of mucosal damage, potentially leading to cystitis [6]. Taking those considerations into account, MMC concentration was 0.1 mg/ml in the present study, which is much higher than the 0.002 mg/ml (10

mg/5000 ml) used in HIPEC and systemic chemotherapy. In the preliminary studies, using different concentrations of MMC did not improve the therapeutic effects, but there were no adverse events either. Nevertheless, in the present study, intravesical HIVEC using high MMC concentration ensured a high, constant, and sustained local chemotherapeutic drug concentration thought to achieve the best chemotherapeutic efficacy. In the present study, the MMC concentration in the perfusion fluid was gradually decreased over HIVEC time, probably due to urine dilution or/and systemic absorption. Indeed, serum MMC levels increased during HIVEC and decreased after HIVEC, but previous studies in humans indicated that serum MMC concentrations after HIVEC do not reach a critical toxic threshold [8, 9]. In the present study, serum MMC concentrations peaked at 60 min, and the serum MMC levels stayed below the toxic value, and the half-life of MMC is 30–50 min [7, 8]. Accordingly with the higher absorption in the presence of mucosal damage, serum MMC concentrations in the TUR+ HIVEC group were significantly higher than those in the HIVEC group.

The effects of temperature on mucosal blood vessels could lead to plasma exudation and interstitial hemorrhage. There is also a risk that these vascular changes exacerbated the direct thermal injury to the lamina propria, sometimes resulting in necrosis with exfoliation of the epithelium [6, 7, 14, 18]. In the HIVEC group, complete necrosis accompanied by local vascular changes (such as necrosis and thrombosis) in the small tumor vessels and hemorrhage into the stroma was indeed observed. Because tumor vessels are more susceptible to thermal injury than normal tissue vessels, these changes may be responsible, at least in part, for inhibiting bladder cancer growth [7, 8].

It is recommended that HIVEC is performed for at least seven sessions, but there is no standard for intravesical HIVEC in China and worldwide. In the present study, only three HIVEC sessions were performed, mainly to study process and to prevent delays of further treatments. Additional treatments were performed for non-responsive patients after three sessions, which could include surgical resection, arterial embolization thermotherapy, intravesical chemotherapy plus immunotherapy, or intravesical HIVEC plus immunotherapy. Additional trials are necessary to determine the best treatment strategies for the treatment of bladder cancer and the exact place of intravesical HIVEC in those strategies.

This device is not without limitation. Since it is based on conductive heating, the temperature of the fluid can be accurately maintained, but the exact temperature of the bladder mucosa cannot be guaranteed due to heat loss by diffusion in adjacent tissues and blood circulation. Meanwhile, this study only tested the feasibility and safety of this device, as well as MMC pharmacokinetics. Because the incidence of bladder cancer is relatively low in China, the inclusion criteria of this study were relatively strict, leading to a relatively small sample size spanning over many years. Future studies with more patients will be performed to validate these results. A control group will also be included.

Conclusion

In conclusion, it is feasible to use the BR-TRG-II-type HIVEC device for patients with bladder cancers. This treatment tool has good prospects for widespread clinical application in patients with bladder cancer.

Abbreviations

BCG: Bacillus Calmette-Guerin; CIR: Cumulative incidence rate; CT: Computerized tomography; DFS: Disease-free survival; HIVEC: Hyperthermic intracavitary chemotherapy; MMC: Mitomycin C; MRI: Magnetic resonance imaging; TUR: Transurethral resection

Acknowledgments

None.

Authors' contributions

MC B and SZ C performed the development of the device, and the original literature search, and participated in drafting the manuscript. MC B and H L participated in the design of the study and performed the statistical analysis. MC B, SZ C, H L, YF G, YB W, KP L, YN T, BH Z, and WB W participated in by animal experiments and hyperthermic intraperitoneal perfusion chemotherapy (HIVEC). All authors read and approved the final manuscript.

Author details

[1]Intracelom Hyperthermic Perfusion Therapy Center, Cancer Hospital of Guangzhou Medical University, No. 78 Hengzhigang Road, Guangzhou, Guangdong 510095, People's Republic of China. [2]Department of Pharmacy, Guangzhou Dermatology Institute, Guangzhou, Guangdong, People's Republic of China.

References

1. Siegel R, Naishadham D, Jemal A. Cancer statistics, 2012. CA Cancer J Clin. 2012;62(1):10–29.
2. Penson DF. Re: effectiveness of adjuvant chemotherapy for locally advanced bladder Cancer. J Urol. 2016;196(2):352–4.
3. Douglass L, Schoenberg M. The future of Intravesical drug delivery for non-muscle invasive bladder Cancer. Bladder Cancer. 2016;2(3):285–92.
4. Veeratterapillay R, Heer R, Johnson MI, Persad R, Bach C. High-risk non-muscle-invasive bladder Cancer-therapy options during Intravesical BCG shortage. Curr Urol Rep. 2016;17(9):68.
5. Hayne D, Stockler M, McCombie SP, Chalasani V, Long A, Martin A, et al. BCG+MMC trial: adding mitomycin C to BCG as adjuvant intravesical therapy for high-risk, non-muscle-invasive bladder cancer: a randomised phase III trial (ANZUP 1301). BMC Cancer. 2015;15:432.
6. Inman BA, Stauffer PR, Craciunescu OA, Maccarini PF, Dewhirst MW, Vujaskovic Z. A pilot clinical trial of intravesical mitomycin-C and external deep pelvic hyperthermia for non-muscle-invasive bladder cancer. Int J Hyperth. 2014;30(3):171–5.
7. Colombo R, Salonia A, Leib Z, Pavone-Macaluso M, Engelstein D. Long-term outcomes of a randomized controlled trial comparing thermochemotherapy with mitomycin-C alone as adjuvant treatment for non-muscle-invasive bladder cancer (NMIBC). BJU Int. 2011;107(6):912–8.
8. Paroni R, Salonia A, Lev A, Da Pozzo LF, Cighetti G, Montorsi F, et al. Effect of local hyperthermia of the bladder on mitomycin C pharmacokinetics during intravesical chemotherapy for the treatment of superficial transitional cell carcinoma. Br J Clin Pharmacol. 2001;52(3):273–8.
9. Colombo R, Salonia A, Da Pozzo LF, Naspro R, Freschi M, Paroni R, et al. Combination of intravesical chemotherapy and hyperthermia for the treatment of superficial bladder cancer: preliminary clinical experience. Crit Rev Oncol Hematol. 2003;47(2):127–39.
10. Crezee H, Inman BA. The use of hyperthermia in the treatment of bladder cancer. Int J Hyperth. 2016;32(4):349–50.
11. Geijsen ED, de Reijke TM, Koning CC. Zum Vorde Sive Vording PJ, de la rosette JJ, Rasch CR, et al. combining Mitomycin C and regional 70 MHz hyperthermia in patients with nonmuscle invasive bladder Cancer: a pilot study. J Urol. 2015;194(5):1202–8.
12. Ba M, Cui S, Wang B, Long H, Yan Z, Wang S, et al. Bladder intracavitary hyperthermic perfusion chemotherapy for the prevention of recurrence of non-muscle invasive bladder cancer after transurethral resection. Oncol Rep. 2017;37(5):2761–70.
13. Soria F, Milla P, Fiorito C, Pisano F, Sogni F, Di Marco M, et al. Efficacy and safety of a new device for intravesical thermochemotherapy in non-grade 3 BCG recurrent NMIBC: a phase I-II study. World J Urol. 2016;34(2):189–95.
14. Owusu RA, Abern MR, Inman BA. Hyperthermia as adjunct to intravesical chemotherapy for bladder cancer. Biomed Res Int. 2013;2013:262313.
15. Ekin RG, Akarken I, Cakmak O, Tarhan H, Celik O, Ilbey YO, et al. Results of Intravesical chemo-hyperthermia in high-risk non-muscle invasive bladder Cancer. Asian Pac J Cancer Prev. 2015;16(8):3241–5.
16. Sousa A, Pineiro I, Rodriguez S, Aparici V, Monserrat V, Neira P, et al. Recirculant hyperthermic IntraVEsical chemotherapy (HIVEC) in intermediate-high-risk non-muscle-invasive bladder cancer. Int J Hyperth. 2016;32(4):374–80.
17. Rolevich AI, Zhegalik AG, Mokhort AA, Minich AA, Vasilevich VY, Polyakov SL, et al. Results of a prospective randomized study assessing the efficacy of fluorescent cystoscopy-assisted transurethral resection and single instillation of doxorubicin in patients with non-muscle-invasive bladder cancer. World J Urol. 2017;35(5):745–52.
18. Gofrit ON, Shapiro A, Pode D, Sidi A, Nativ O, Leib Z, et al. Combined local bladder hyperthermia and intravesical chemotherapy for the treatment of high-grade superficial bladder cancer. Urology. 2004;63(3):466–71.
19. Colombo R, Da Pozzo LF, Lev A, Freschi M, Gallus G, Rigatti P. Neoadjuvant combined microwave induced local hyperthermia and topical chemotherapy versus chemotherapy alone for superficial bladder cancer. J Urol. 1996;155(4):1227–32.
20. Ba MC, Cui SZ, Lin SQ, Tang YQ, Wu YB, Wang B, et al. Chemotherapy with laparoscope-assisted continuous circulatory hyperthermic intraperitoneal perfusion for malignant ascites. World J Gastroenterol. 2010;16(15):1901–7.
21. Cui S, Ba M, Tang Y, Liu J, Wu Y, Wang B, et al. B ultrasound-guided hyperthermic intraperitoneal perfusion chemotherapy for the treatment of malignant ascites. Oncol Rep. 2012;28(4):1325–31.
22. Charan J, Kantharia ND. How to calculate sample size in animal studies? J Pharmacol Pharmacother. 2013;4(4):303–6.
23. Festing MF, Altman DG. Guidelines for the design and statistical analysis of experiments using laboratory animals. ILAR J. 2002;43(4):244–58.
24. Festing MF. Design and statistical methods in studies using animal models of development. ILAR J. 2006;47(1):5–14.
25. Chen AP, Setser A, Anadkat MJ, Cotliar J, Olsen EA, Garden BC, et al. Grading dermatologic adverse events of cancer treatments: the common

terminology criteria for adverse events version 4.0. J Am Acad Dermatol. 2012;67(5):1025–39.

26. Milla P, Fiorito C, Soria F, Arpicco S, Cattel L, Gontero P. Intravesical thermo-chemotherapy based on conductive heat: a first pharmacokinetic study with mitomycin C in superficial transitional cell carcinoma patients. Cancer Chemother Pharmacol. 2014;73(3):503–9.

27. Abdelaleem EA, Naguib IA, Zaazaa HE, Hussein EA. Development and validation of HPLC and HPTLC methods for determination of Cefoperazone and its related impurities. J Chromatogr Sci. 2016;54(2):179–86.

28. Dwivedi R, Singh M, Kaleekal T, Gupta YK, Tripathi M. Concentration of antiepileptic drugs in persons with epilepsy: a comparative study in serum and saliva. Int J Neurosci. 2016;126(11):972–8.

29. Onishi T, Sugino Y, Shibahara T, Masui S, Yabana T, Sasaki T. Randomized controlled study of the efficacy and safety of continuous saline bladder irrigation after transurethral resection for the treatment of non-muscle-invasive bladder cancer. BJU Int. 2017;119(2):276–82.

30. NCCN. Clinical practice guidelines in oncology (NCCN guidelines). Bladder Cancer. Version 4.2019. National Comprehensive Cancer Network: Fort Washington; 2019.

31. van Valenberg H, Colombo R, Witjes F. Intravesical radiofrequency-induced hyperthermia combined with chemotherapy for non-muscle-invasive bladder cancer. Int J Hyperth. 2016;32(4):351–62.

32. Takai T, Inamoto T, Komura K, Yoshikawa Y, Uchimoto T, Saito K, et al. Feasibility of photodynamic diagnosis for challenging TUR- Bt cases including muscle invasive bladder cancer, BCG failure or 2nd-TUR. Asian Pac J Cancer Prev. 2015;16(6):2297–301.

18

Altered detrusor contractility and voiding patterns in mice lacking the mechanosensitive TREK-1 channel

Ricardo H. Pineda[1], Joseph Hypolite[1], Sanghee Lee[2], Alonso Carrasco Jr[3], Nao Iguchi[1], Randall B. Meacham[4] and Anna P. Malykhina[1*]

Abstract

Background: Previously published results from our laboratory identified a mechano-gated two-pore domain potassium channel, TREK-1, as a main mechanosensor in the smooth muscle of the human urinary bladder. One of the limitations of in vitro experiments on isolated human detrusor included inability to evaluate in vivo effects of TREK-1 on voiding function, as the channel is also expressed in the nervous system, and may modulate micturition via neural pathways. Therefore, in the present study, we aimed to assess the role of TREK-1 channel in bladder function and voiding patterns in vivo by using TREK-1 knockout (KO) mice.

Methods: Adult C57BL/6 J wild-type (WT, $N = 32$) and TREK-1 KO ($N = 33$) mice were used in this study. The overall phenotype and bladder function were evaluated by gene and protein expression of TREK-1 channel, in vitro contractile experiments using detrusor strips in response to stretch and pharmacological stimuli, and cystometry in unanesthetized animals.

Results: TREK-1 KO animals had an elevated basal muscle tone and enhanced spontaneous activity in the detrusor without detectable changes in bladder morphology/histology. Stretch applied to isolated detrusor strips increased the amplitude of spontaneous contractions by 109% in the TREK-1 KO group in contrast to a 61% increase in WT mice ($p \leq 0.05$ to respective baseline for each group). The detrusor strips from TREK-1 KO mice also generated more contractile force in response to electric field stimulation and high potassium concentration in comparison to WT group ($p \leq 0.05$ for both tests). However, cystometric recordings from TREK-1 KO mice revealed a significant increase in the duration of the intermicturition interval, enhanced bladder capacity and increased number of non-voiding contractions in comparison to WT mice.

Conclusions: Our results provide evidence that global down-regulation of TREK-1 channels has dual effects on detrusor contractility and micturition patterns in vivo. The observed differences are likely due to expression of TREK-1 channel not only in detrusor myocytes but also in afferent and efferent neural pathways involved in regulation of micturition which may underly the "mixed" voiding phenotype in TREK-1 KO mice.

Keywords: Urinary bladder, TREK-1 channel, Detrusor mechanosensitivity, Voiding, Micturition cycle

* Correspondence: Anna.Malykhina@ucdenver.edu
[1]Division of Urology, Department of Surgery, University of Colorado
Denver,Anschutz Medical Campus, 12700 E 19th Ave, M/S C317, Aurora, CO
80045, USA
Full list of author information is available at the end of the article

Background

The urinary bladder undergoes slow mechanical stretch during the storage phase of the micturition cycle without significant changes in intravesical pressure [5, 29]. Previous animal studies provided evidence that bladder stretch can activate mechanosensitive two-pore domain potassium (K_{2P}) channels [29, 46, 49]. The family of mechano-gated K_{2P} channels is highly expressed in the smooth muscle of visceral hollow organs where they regulate smooth muscle excitability by controlling the resting membrane potential [3, 4, 29, 52, 53]. Our previous studies confirmed that bladder capacity and detrusor relaxation in the human urinary bladder depends on the expression and function of TREK-1 channel, one of the members of the K_{2P} channel family [34]. TREK-1 has also been detected in the human myometrium, where it participates in the maintenance of uterine relaxation during pregnancy [3, 10, 55]. Further, expression of TREK-1 channels in vascular smooth muscle suggests a role in the regulation of the vascular tone and endothelial production of nitric oxide [44, 45].

A decrease in functional expression of TREK-1 channel in the bladder smooth muscle was shown to be associated with detrusor overactivity (DO) in the animal model of partial bladder outlet obstruction [4]. In humans, increased expression of TREK-1 was detected in pregnant women's myometrium. Interestingly, TREK-1 expression levels declined by the time of labor [3, 10, 55]. Experimental data obtained by our group in bladder specimens from patients with idiopathic DO confirmed a decreased expression of TREK-1 channels along with an altered response to pharmacological stimulation and diminished smooth muscle relaxation. Additionally, DO specimens had an increased basal tone and increased spontaneous contractile activity suggestive that TREK-1 channels affect bladder compliance during storage phase of the micturition cycle [48].

Limitations of in vitro experiments on isolated human bladders included the inability to assess the full spectrum of TREK-1 related effects on voiding function as the channel is also expressed in the nervous system and therefore, may indirectly participate in micturition modulation via a neural pathway. Members of the mechanosensitive K_{2P} channel family are abundantly expressed in the brain and sensory neurons of the dorsal root ganglia in humans [18, 20, 41]. However, the studies of functional changes in human neurons and nerve fibers have several ethical challenges making the use of animal models necessary for this type of investigations. Additionally, the absence of TREK-1 selective activators and inhibitors makes it difficult to isolate TREK-1 from other K_{2P} channels in primary cultured cells. Therefore, in the present study, we aimed to evaluate the effects of TREK-1 gene knockout on bladder contractile function

and voiding patterns by comparing wild-type (WT) and TREK-1 KO mice. We comprehensively assessed bladder phenotype in vivo and in vitro, measured detrusor basal tone, spontaneous activity, contractile function and relaxation in response to nerve and muscle-mediated stimulation of bladder smooth muscle (BSM), as well as determined bladder responses to different pharmacological stimuli.

Methods

Animals and experimental groups

Adult male and female C57BL/6 J wild-type (WT, $N = 32$) and TREK-1 knockout ($Kcnk2^{-/-}$, TREK-1 KO, $N = 33$) mice were used in this study. Wild type mice (10–12 weeks old) were obtained from Jackson Laboratories (Bar Harbor, ME, USA). TREK-1 KO mice, a generous gift from the laboratory of Dr. Min Zhou (Department of Neuroscience, The Ohio State University, Columbus, OH), were bred in the Breeding Core Barrier Facility at the University of Colorado Anschutz Medical Campus. Originally, the $Kcnk2^{-/-}$ mice were generated as described in [45]. Briefly, the TREK-1 gene, $Kcnk2$, spans approximately 136 kbp of the *M. musculus* genome and includes eight exons. The knockout mice were generated by replacing 4 kbp of the $Kcnk2$ gene including the second exon (excluding the first 23 bp), the second intron, the third exon and the first 23 bp of the third intron with a β-galactosidase/Neomycin selection cassette producing a truncated, nonfunctional protein.

All animals were housed in a regulated environment on a 12:12-h light/dark cycle with free access to food and water. There were no overt differences in feeding behavior, litter size, growth rate and body weight between the WT and TREK1 KO mice. All protocols were approved by the University of Colorado Institutional Animal Care and Use Committee.

RT-PCR for genotyping and PKC isoform expression

Genomic DNA was extracted using the REDExtract-N-Amp Tissue PCR Kit (Sigma-Aldrich, St Louis, MO. USA) from the urinary bladders of WT and TREK-1 KO mice. Genotyping was performed as previously described [45]. Briefly, the WT $Kcnk2$ allele was detected by using the following primer pairs: forward 5′-GCTG GGTGAAGTTCTTCAGC-3′, and reverse: 5′- CATT ACCTGGATGAGTTCGTC-3′. The $Kcnk2$ KO allele was detected using the primer pairs: forward 5′-GCAGCGCAT CGCCTTCTATC-3′ and reverse 5′-AGGAGATGAA-GACCTCTGCAAAGG-3′. End-point RT-PCR products from WT and TREK-1 KO specimens were subsequently run on 2% agarose gels. Gel images were taken and analyzed using the Doc-It LS Image Acquisition & Analysis System (UVP, LLC, Upland, CA, USA).

To compare the gene expression levels of several protein kinase C (PKC) isoforms expressed in the bladder, whole bladder tissues were removed from WT and TREK-1 KO mice, and snap-frozen in liquid nitrogen. Posteriorly, total RNA was extracted and purified using TRIzol® Plus RNA Purification Kit (Ambion, Thermo Fisher Sci. Waltham, MA, USA) according to the manufacturer's instructions. RNA concentrations and purity were determined spectrophotometrically on a Nanodrop device (Thermo Fisher Sci. Waltham, MA, USA). RNA integrity was evaluated by formaldehyde agarose gel electrophoresis, stained with ethidium bromide, and visualized under UV light. Isolated RNAs were stored at − 80 °C until use. First-strand complementary DNA (cDNA) was synthesized using the Qiagen OneStep RT-PCR kit (Qiagen, Valentia, CA. USA) by the manufacturer's guidelines. Products were stored at − 20 °C until the use. End-point PCR was performed using the Qiagen Multiplex PCR plus kit (Qiagen, Valentia, CA. USA) following the manufacturer's instructions. The following PKC isoforms were selected for comparison due to their significant level of expression in the urinary bladder: PKC-α (alpha), PKC-β (beta), PKC-γ (gamma), PKC- δ (delta), PKC-ε (epsilon), PKC-μ (mu) and PKC-τ (tau). Primer sequences for each isoform, gene accession numbers and predicted RT-PCR product sizes are listed in Table 1. Non-template control reactions were included in each reaction to test for possible RT-PCR contamination and were run in parallel with the experimental samples. End-point PCR products were analyzed by electrophoresis in 1.5% agarose gel, stained with ethidium bromide, and visualized under UV light.

Western blotting

Total protein was isolated from the urinary bladder by conventional tissue lysis with T-PER Tissue Protein Extraction Reagent (ThermoFisher Sci, Waltham, MA. USA) containing protease and phosphatase inhibitors (Sigma Aldrich, St Louis, MO. USA). Western blot experiments were performed with equal loads of the total protein per lane (20 μg). WT and KO samples were size fractionated by SDS-PAGE electrophoresis using 4–10% polyacrylamide Mini Protein gels (BioRad, Hercules, CA. USA). Proteins were then electrotransferred to polyvinylidene difluoride membranes (LICOR Biotechnology, Lincoln, NW. USA) and incubated for one hour at room temperature (RT) in Odyssey Blocking Buffer (TBS, LICOR Biotechnology, Lincoln, NW. USA). Membranes were subsequently washed three times in PBST for 10 min each and incubated with Anti-TREK-1 (F6, 1:1000, Santa Cruz Biotechnology, Dallas, TX. USA) and anti-Histone H3 as a house-keeping gene (1:2000, Abcam, Cambridge, MA. USA) in blocking buffer under constant agitation. We also tested other commercially available antibodies from the same company which included the C20, E-19, and H-75 anti-TREK-1 variants. The C20 and E19 anti-TREK-1 antibodies did not work for Western blotting, while H-75 antibody (aa352–426 within the C-terminus) showed two bands in WT animals and one band in TREK-1 KO (data not shown). Therefore, we used F6 anti-TREK-1 for Western blotting. The next day, membranes were rinsed three times with PBST for 10 min each time, and incubated with anti-mouse and anti-rabbit VRDye secondary antibodies (1:10000, LICOR Biotechnology, Lincoln, NW. USA) for 2 hrs at RT. Afterwards, membranes were rinsed three times with PBST for 10 min each and imaged using the Odyssey CLx imaging system (LICOR Biotechnology, Lincoln, NW. USA).

Table 1 Primers for PKC isoforms expressed in the urinary bladder

Name	Sequence	Fragment Size (bp)	Accession Number
PKCα-F	AGGAGCCACAAGCAGTATTC	93	NM_011101.3
PKCα-R	CCAGCTTCAGATCCCTGTAAAT		
PKCβ-F	GCAGAGCAAGGGCATTATTTAC	114	NM_001316672.1
PKCβ-R	CCATCCCAGATGTTCTCCTTAC		
PKCγ-F	GCACCTGAGATCATTGCCTATC	90	NM_011102.4
PKCγ-R	CTGTCCTGCCAACATCTCATAC		
PKCδ-F	TAGTGAGGAGGAGGCAAAGT	105	NM_001310682.1
PKCδ-R	CCGAAGAAGGTGGCGATAAA		
PKCε-F	GCTCGGAAACACCCTTATCT	100	NM_001310682.1
PKCε-R	ACATGAGGTCTCCACCATTTAC		
PKCμ-F	GCAGTGGAGTTAGAAGGAGAAG	123	XM_006515590.3
PKCμ-R	GGCTCACAGGAGACAGTAAAG		
PKCτ-F	CAGGGACCTGAAGCTTGATAAT	96	NM_008859.2
PKCτ-R	GCATCTCCTAGCATGTTCTCTT		

Tissue immunohistolabeling

WT and TREK-1 KO animals were anesthetized with isofluorane (2.5%) and perfused via the left cardiac ventricle with phosphate-buffered-saline (PBS, pH 7.4) followed by 4% paraformaldehyde in PBS (PFA) for 10 min. The colon, bladder, and kidneys were removed and placed in PFA for two hours at 4° C. Subsequently; the tissues were placed in 70% alcohol for at least 2 days before being dehydrated and embedded in paraffin. 4 μm -thick sections were cut and mounted on "frosted" slides (Fisher Scientific Co, Waltham, MA. USA) at the Morphology and Phenotypic Core of the University of Colorado Anschutz Medical Campus. Before immunolabeling, sections were washed in Xylene (Sigma-Aldrich, St Louis, MO. USA) to remove paraffin, re-hydrated in a graded ethanol series, washed with distilled water, and rinsed in 50 mM Tris-buffered saline (TBS, pH 7.4) for 5 min. Heat-induced epitope retrieval was performed by incubating the slides at $85-90^0$ C for 15 min in Target Retrieval Solution (DAKO, Agilent Pathology Solutions, Santa Clara, CA. USA). Once cold down to room temperature, the sections were washed twice in TBS containing 0.1% Tween 20 (TBST, Sigma-Aldrich, St Louis, MO. USA), and incubated for 30 min in casein blocking solution (CBS, DAKO, Agilent Pathology Solutions, Santa Clara, CA. USA). Slides were incubated overnight at 4^0 C (ON) in CBS with mouse monoclonal antibodies against the TREK-1 protein (F6, 1:300; Santa Cruz Biotechnology, Dallas, TX. USA). The next day, sections were rinsed three times with TBST for 5 min each time, and then incubated for 2 h at RT with a secondary antibody conjugated with Alexafluor 488-labeled anti-mouse IgG (1:500; Fisher Scientific Co, Waltham, MA. USA) in CBS. After incubation with secondary antibody, sections were washed three times with TBST for 5 min each, rinsed with TBS and counterstained with 200 nM 4′ 6-diamidino-2-phenylindoledihydrochloride (DAPI, Fisher Scientific Co, Waltham, MA. USA) in TBS for 3–5 min at RT and rinsed twice in TBS. Coverslips were mounted with Fluoromount-G (SoutherBiotech, Birmingham, AL. USA). Imaging was performed on an Olympus FV1000 confocal microscope with 40X plan-apo/1.4 numerical aperture objective and FV-viewer software (Olympus, Tokyo, JP). For visualization, three-dimensional z-stack images of x-y sections at 0.5 μm steps were collected. Two-dimensional average intensity projection images were generated for analysis in FIJI (Fiji Is Image J, [50]).

In vitro studies of bladder smooth muscle contractile function

Bladder smooth muscle (BSM) strips were isolated from WT ($N = 17$) and TREK-1 KO ($N = 17$) mice following the previously described procedures [23, 34]. Briefly, BSM strips (~8–10 mg each, 2–3 mm wide and 7–8 mm long) were placed in individual organ baths (Radnoti LLC, Monrovia, CA, USA), containing 7 ml of normal Tyrode Buffer (TB, in mM: NaCl 130.0, KCl 5.0, $CaCl_2$ 1.7, $MgCl_2$ 1.0, NaH_2PO_4 1.3, $NaHCO_3$ 17.0, Glucose, 10.0. pH 7.4) maintained at $37\,^\circ$C and equilibrated with a constant supply of 95% O_2–5% CO_2. Strips were subjected to 1 h equilibration followed by determination of the length of optimal force development (L_o). 1 μM of tetrodotoxin (TTX, Sigma-Aldrich) was added to fresh TB to minimize neural effects on BSM contractility. The strips were subjected to different pharmacological treatments including either arachidonic acid (AA; 10 μM), a TREK-1 channel agonist, or L-methionine (LM, 1 mM), a TREK-1 channel blocker [5, 34, 42]. Untreated muscle strips served as controls. At the end of the incubation period, in order to assess the effects of TREK-1 channels on stress-relaxation, all strips were subjected to an additional 30% stretch to the initially established L_o, and allowed for complete relaxation. Following the stretch protocol, a KCl test (bath solution was replaced with TB containing 125 mM KCl) was performed to ensure that the BSM could maintain the force after stretch [23, 24]. After KCl stimulation, muscle strips were washed three times (10 min each time) in fresh TB and allowed to recover for 30 min. After recovery, all strips were incubated with a non-specific PKC activator, Phorbol 12,13-Dibutyrate (PDBu, 1 μM: Sigma; Greenwood Village, CO), for 45 min.

A separate set of experiments was performed to evaluate the contribution of active and passive basal tone components in BSM from WT and TREK-1 KO bladders. After establishing L_0 in normal Ca^{2+} TB, the buffer was changed to Ca^{2+} free TB followed by 30 min incubation and measurements of the basal tone and spontaneous contractile activity of BSM strips. Some strips were subjected to an additional 30% stretch to evaluate stress-relaxation under Ca^2 free conditions. At the end of the testing protocol, all strips were treated with 2 μM of nifedipine, an L-type Ca^{2+} channel blocker, to assess the role of Ca^{2+} entry via voltage-gated Ca^{2+} channels on BSM tone and spontaneous activity.

All BSM experiments were recorded and analyzed using LabChart 8 Pro (AD Instruments, Colorado Springs, CO, USA), pClamp 10 (Molecular Devices, LLC. San Jose CA, USA) and Matlab R2014b (MathWorks, Natick, MA, USA). The following parameters were measured and analyzed: basal muscle tone (in g/g, g of force per g of muscle strip weight), amplitude of spontaneous contractions (g/g, measured as amplitude from the baseline level of each strip and normalized to its weight), peak force (PF; in g or g/g when normalized to the weight of the muscle strip), and integral force (IF) which reflects how long a muscle strip can maintain the contractile force before it starts relaxing [33].

Urodynamic evaluation of bladder function (awake cystometry)

Animals assigned for urodynamic evaluation of urinary bladder function (awake cystometry) underwent a survival surgical procedure to insert bladder catheters as previously described [35]. Briefly, the animals were anesthetized with isoflurane (VEDCO, St.. Albans, VT) and the bladder was exposed through a lower midline abdominal incision. A polyethylene tubing (PE-50, I.D. 0.58 mm, O.D. 0.96 mm; Intramedic, Becton Dickinson. Parsippany, NY) with a flared end was inserted through a puncture at the bladder dome, and sutured in place with purse string suture and 7.0 silk (Ethicon, Somerville, NJ). The catheter was then tunneled subcutaneously and exteriorized at the scapular region where it was sutured to the skin and filled with sterile saline solution. After confirming no leakage in the bladder, the catheter was plugged with a metal rod, and the muscle and skin layers were closed with a 5.0 silk suture (Ethicon, Somerville, NJ). Particular care was taken not to stretch the bladder during the procedure or to restrict the normal bladder movement once the catheter was in place.

Mice were allowed to recover from surgery (4–5 days) before the urodynamic study. Unanesthetized animals were placed in the cystometry cage, and allowed to acclimate for 30–40 min. Saline was slowly infused into the urinary bladder at a rate of 10 µl/min, and micturition cycles were recorded using the MED-CMG Small Animal Cystometry acquisition software (Catamount Research and Development). The following cystometric parameters were evaluated in this study: bladder capacity, pressure at the start of micturition, micturition rate, intravesical pressure, inter-micturition interval, and number of non-voiding contractions. Non-voiding contractions were defined as the increased values in detrusor pressure not associated with voiding, equal or larger than twice the mean value of baseline. The number of non-voiding contractions was measured for each micturition cycle, and then averaged per cycle based on the number of recorded cycles (e.g. voiding episodes) per animal. Normal voiding contractions had amplitudes of at least a third of maximal pressure recorded during a single micturition event.

Statistical analyses

The results are expressed as the mean ± standard error of the mean (SEM) with N reflecting the number of animals in each group and n being the number of recordings. Statistical significance between two groups was assessed by the Student two-way t-test followed by a comparison between groups using the Bonferroni's correction. When comparing more than two groups, one-way ANOVA with the post hoc Newman-Keuls test

was reported (Prism 7. GraphPad Software, La Jolla, CA. USA). Plots were made with OriginLab Data analysis software v 7.0 (OriginLab Co. Northampton, MA). Difference between the groups and treatments was considered statistically significant at $p \leq 0.05$.

Results

Genotyping of TREK-1 KO mice

In TREK-1 KO mice used for this study, the four transmembrane domains and two-pore forming regions were genetically truncated by replacing most of exon 2 and all exon 3 by a LacZ/Neo cassette [45]. We confirmed the deletions by performing end-point RT-PCR in mRNA extracted from TREK-1 KO and WT bladder tissue samples ($N = 5$ in each group). The WT primers were designed, as previously described, to include parts of intron 2 and exon 3 sequences, while the KO primers included part of the LacZ/Neo cassette and intron 3 [14]. The results of RT-PCR genotyping from TREK-1 KO and WT mice are shown in Fig. 1a. The sizes of the bands corresponding to TREK-1 KO and WT alleles were around ~ 200 and ~ 450 bp, respectively. Figure 1b represents a Western Blot image of the total protein isolated from WT, and TREK-1 KO mouse bladders probed with an anti-TREK-1 antibody showing one band ~ 50 kDa in WT but not in TREK-1 KO specimens (N = 5 in each group). As previously reported [14, 45], no significative changes were observed in fertility, number of the offspring or growth rate between the WT and TREK-1 KO groups.

Expression of TREK-1 in the visceral organs of WT and TREK-1 KO mice

Immunofluorescent tissue labeling was used to compare the presence and distribution of TREK-1 proteins in the visceral organs of WT and TREK-1 KO mice including the urinary bladder, colon, and kidneys. As shown in Fig. 2a (left panel), TREK-1 was expressed in the colon of WT animals with stronger labeling present in the colonic mucosa in comparison to the muscle staining. Intense TREK-1 immunoreactivity was also found in the muscularis mucosa layer. In contrast, TREK-1 KO animals showed a significantly reduced TREK-1 immunoreactivity across the colonic tissue (Fig. 2a, right panel). Confocal images of the bladder sections from WT group (Fig. 2b, left panel) displayed a homogeneous TREK-1 like staining across the detrusor with faint signal in the urothelium and serosa. In contrast, TREK-1 KO animals showed a significant reduction in TREK-1 immunofluorescence. Histologically, the urinary bladders showed no visible morphological alterations (Fig. 2d), and no significant differences were observed in bladder weight between WT and TREK-1 KO animals (9.3 ± 0.7 vs. 10.2 ± 0.6 mg, respectively). The body/bladder weight ratio (g/mg) in WT and TREK-1 KO

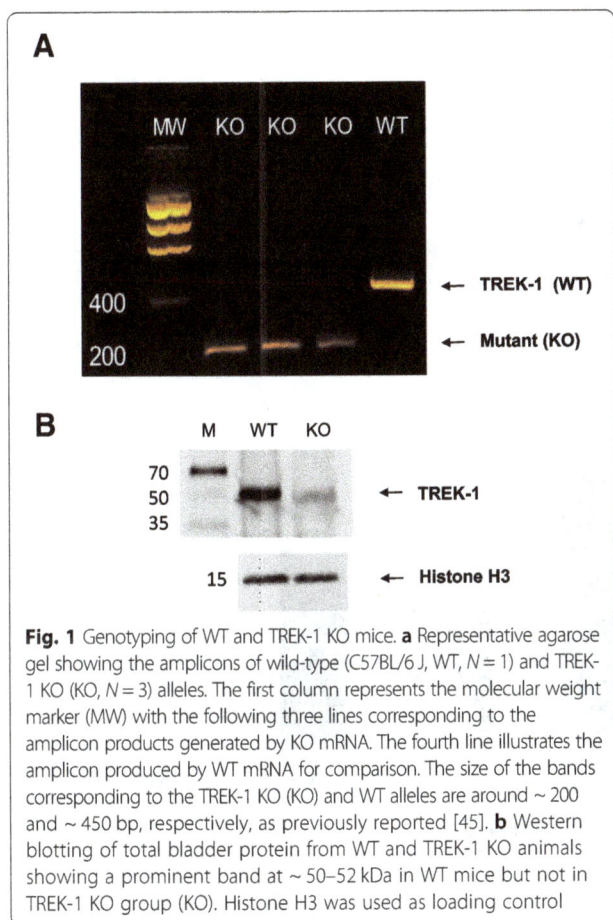

Fig. 1 Genotyping of WT and TREK-1 KO mice. **a** Representative agarose gel showing the amplicons of wild-type (C57BL/6 J, WT, $N = 1$) and TREK-1 KO (KO, $N = 3$) alleles. The first column represents the molecular weight marker (MW) with the following three lines corresponding to the amplicon products generated by KO mRNA. The fourth line illustrates the amplicon produced by WT mRNA for comparison. The size of the bands corresponding to the TREK-1 KO (KO) and WT alleles are around ~ 200 and ~ 450 bp, respectively, as previously reported [45]. **b** Western blotting of total bladder protein from WT and TREK-1 KO animals showing a prominent band at ~ 50–52 kDa in WT mice but not in TREK-1 KO group (KO). Histone H3 was used as loading control

mice was also similar between the groups (Fig. 2e). The kidneys were bean-shaped, ~ 1.0 cm in length and weighted individually 0.50 ± 0.1 g and 0.46 ± 0.1 g (WT and TREK-1 KO groups, respectively). Histological images taken at the cortex level showed no visible histological changes in TREK-1 KO mice compared with WT aminals. In WT mice, most of the tubules in the kidney nephrons were positively labeled with TREK-1 antibody (Fig. 2c, left panel) with very faint or no positive reaction at the glomerular level. A substantial reduction in TREK-1 immunoreactivity was observed in the kidneys from TREK-1 KO animals (Fig. 2c, right panel).

Deficiency of TREK-1 channel is associated with increased basal muscle tone and spontaneous contractions in the detrusor

We next evaluated the role of TREK-1 channels in the maintenance of the basal smooth muscle tone and spontaneous contractions in vitro. The weight of BSM strips isolated from WT and TREK-1 KO mice and used for contractile function studies was similar between the groups (8.0 ± 1.5 mg and 9.1 ± 2.1 mg, respectively, $N = 17$ and $n = 34$ in each group). The basal muscle tone of the strips at their optimal length (L0) was 50.7 ± 6.1 g/g in WT and

71.2 ± 8.5 g/g in TREK-1 KO mice (Fig. 3 a, $N = 17$; n = 34 in each group, $p \leq 0.01$). Application of AA caused 24% reduction in basal tone of WT muscle strips (from 50.7 ± 6.1 g/g to 38.5 ± 4.6 g/g, $p = 0.025$) whereas the strips from TREK-1 KO bladders had a similar tendency in response to AA, however, did not reach a level of statistical significance (Fig. 3a). In a different set of experiments, BSM strips underwent 30% stretch in addition to L_0 in order to evaluate stress-relaxation of the detrusor when the bladder undergoes a significant stretch upon reaching its maximal capacity. After the stretch protocol, BSM strips from WT mice experienced an increase in the basal tone up to 81.5 ± 7.3 g/g (58.3% to L_0 level, $p \leq 0.05$, Fig. 3b), whereas the strips from TREK-1 KO mice had an increase of 50% (from 71.2 ± 8.5 g/g to 107.2 ± 9.6 g/g, $p \leq 0.05$ to L_0 level). Application of LM did not significantly affect the basal muscle tone of the stretched strips in either group, however, incubation with AA led to 32% decrease in WT group ($N = 8$, $n = 8$, $p \leq 0.05$ to WT) without causing significant changes in TREK-1 KO group (N = 8, $n = 9$, Fig. 3 b). Analysis of spontaneous activity of BSM strips at L_0 revealed the presence of spontaneous contractions in TREK-1 KO group (2.2 ± 0.2 g/g, Fig. 3c, $p \leq 0.05$ to WT) in comparison to lower contractile activity in WT group (1.3 ± 0.1 g/g, Fig. 3 c, an insert shows representative raw traces of the spontaneous activity in both groups). Additional stretch increased the amplitude of spontaneous contractions by 61% in WT group (Fig. 3d, $p \leq 0.05$ to respective L_0 level) with the amplitude of spontaneous contractions in BSM strips being doubled in TREK-1 KO group (109% increase to respective L_0, Fig. 3d).

The differences observed in the basal muscle tone and frequency of spontaneous activity between WT and TREK-1 KO BSM strips were further tested in Ca^{2+} free TB to evaluate the role of active contractile processes due to Ca^{2+} influx into the cells. First, we incubated BSM from WT and TREK-1 KO animals in Ca-free solution for 30 min followed by either 30% additional stretch or incubation with nifedipine, a general L-type calcium channel blocker ($2 \mu M$, 30 min). Representitave recordings from WT and TREK-1 KO BSM strips are included in Fig. 4. Substitution of normal TB by Ca^{2+}-free TB reduced the basal muscle tone in both WT and TREK-1 KO BMS strips when compared to normal Ca^{2+} solution (Fig. 4a, middle traces). However, BSM from TREK-1 KO mice showed a ~ 2.0 fold increase in the amplitude of spontaneous contractions (from 2.2 ± 0.1 g/g in normal Ca^{2+} to 4.1 ± 0.1 g/g in Ca^{2+}-free TB, $N = 4$,$n = 8$ in each group, $p \leq 0.05$ to normal Ca TB). Application of additional stretch under Ca^{2+} free conditions showed decreased values of PF in both WT and TREK-1 KO groups by ~ 30–32% when compared to normal Ca^{2+} solution. The contractile reponses also had a significantly faster initial decline phase of stress-relaxation in both groups (Fig. 4b).

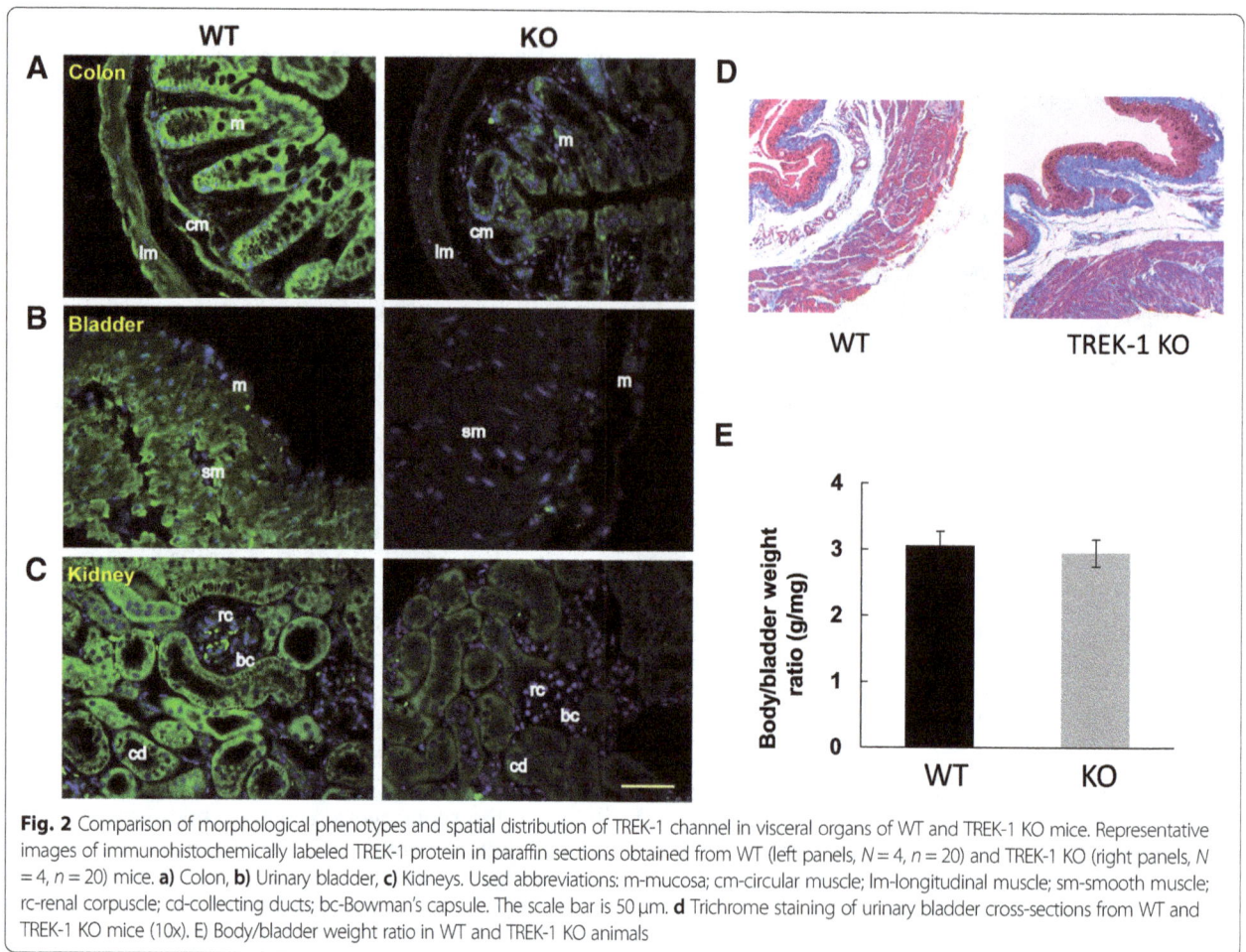

Fig. 2 Comparison of morphological phenotypes and spatial distribution of TREK-1 channel in visceral organs of WT and TREK-1 KO mice. Representative images of immunohistochemically labeled TREK-1 protein in paraffin sections obtained from WT (left panels, $N = 4$, $n = 20$) and TREK-1 KO (right panels, $N = 4$, $n = 20$) mice. **a)** Colon, **b)** Urinary bladder, **c)** Kidneys. Used abbreviations: m-mucosa; cm-circular muscle; lm-longitudinal muscle; sm-smooth muscle; rc-renal corpuscle; cd-collecting ducts; bc-Bowman's capsule. The scale bar is 50 μm. **d** Trichrome staining of urinary bladder cross-sections from WT and TREK-1 KO mice (10x). E) Body/bladder weight ratio in WT and TREK-1 KO animals

Enhanced force generation to electric field stimulation and high potassium in BSM strips from TREK-1 KO mice

Bladder smooth muscle strips from TREK-1 KO mice generated more contractile force in response to EFS (32 Hz) in comparison to WT group (222.2 ± 21.2 g/g and 162.2 ± 16.2 g/g, $p \leq 0.05$, Fig. 5a, middle panel). The IF calculated as ratio of the area under the curve (AUC) of a single contraction divided by its PF was also significantly higher for TREK-1 KO group in comparison to WT (250 ± 30.1 vs 163.1 ± 19.6, $p \leq 0.05$, Fig. 5a, right panel). Similar to the effects of EFS, TREK-1 KO strips also revealed an increased contractile response to high KCl stimulation (Fig. 5b). However, application of TREK-1 inhibitor (LM) and activator (AA) did not substantially change the contractile responses to high potassium in both WT and TREK-1 KO groups in comparison to baseline values (Fig. 5b).

Previous studies from our laboratory established that PKC activation with general agonist phorbol-12, 13-dibutyrate (PDBu) significantly reduced the amplitude and increased the frequency of spontaneous BSM contractions at low concentrations (10 nM) while causing an increase in muscle force generation at higher concentrations (1 μM). Although several previous studies

provided evidence that PKC mostly affects large conductance Ca^{2+}-activated potassium channels (BK), TREK-1 channels could also be modulated by PKC phosphorylation. Therefore, we tested the reponses to a PKC activator in TREK-1 KO bladders. Application of PDBu (1 μM) significantly increased PF (by 50%, $p \leq 0.05$, Fig. 6a) and the amplitude of spontaneous contractions in TREK-1 KO muscle strips when compared to WT group. Protein kinase C conveys both calcium-dependent, and calcium-independent effects on DSM contractility in vitro mediated via inhibition of myosine light chain phosphatase. However, it is still unknown if these separate effects are mediated by different PKC isoforms. Therefore, we aimed to test if elevated reponses to PKC stimulation in TREK-1 KO bladders may be due to compensatory changes in expression levels of the PKC isoforms present in the detrusor. The results of RT-PCR presented in Fig. 6b did not reveal any significant changes in the expression levels of 7 tested PKC isoforms including (PKC-α (alpha), PKC-β (beta), PKC-γ (gamma), PKC- δ (delta), PKC-ε (epsilon), PKC-μ (mu) and PKC-τ (tau)) between the WT and TREK-1 groups. This data suggests that the effects are

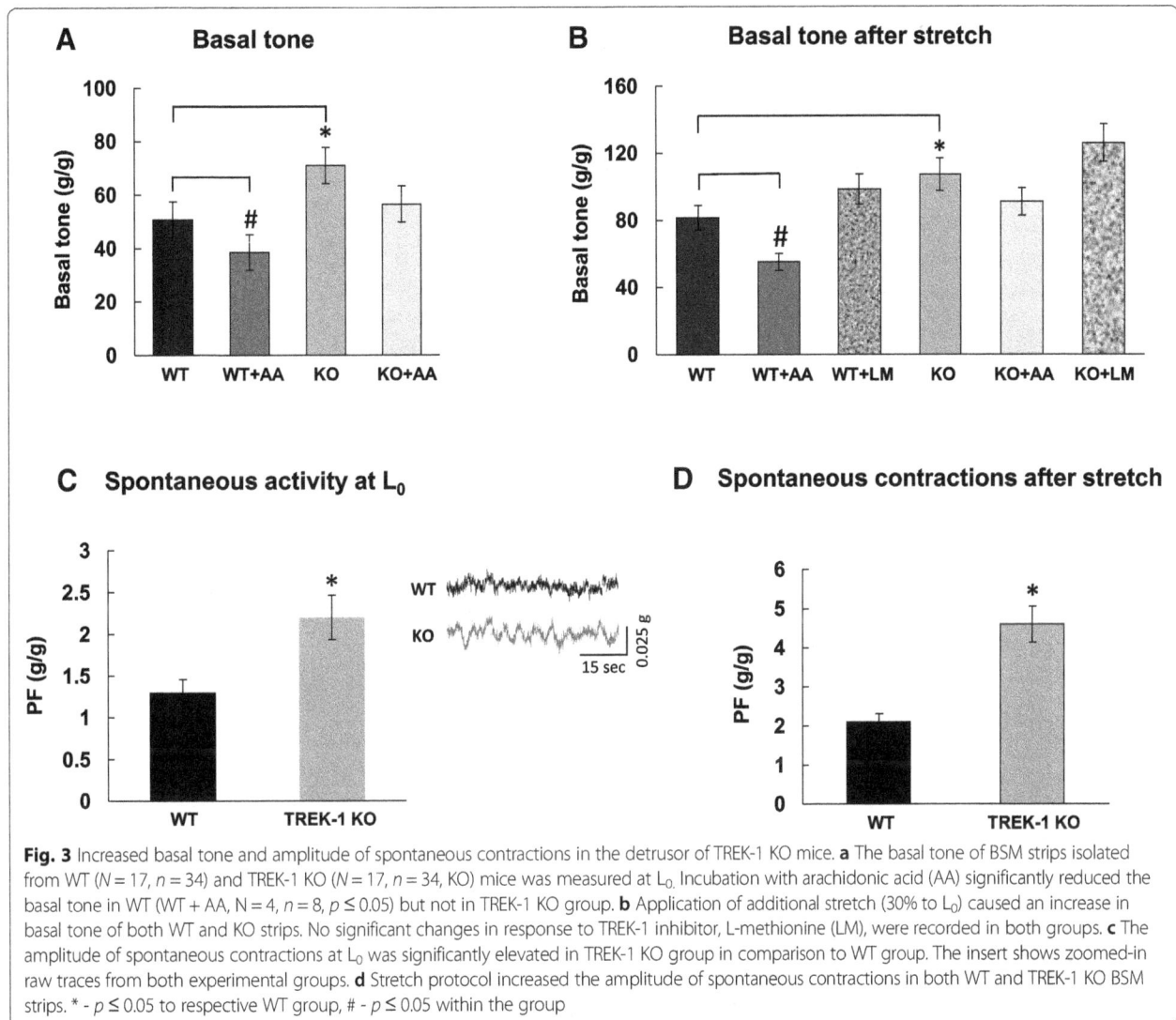

Fig. 3 Increased basal tone and amplitude of spontaneous contractions in the detrusor of TREK-1 KO mice. **a** The basal tone of BSM strips isolated from WT ($N = 17$, $n = 34$) and TREK-1 KO ($N = 17$, $n = 34$, KO) mice was measured at L_0. Incubation with arachidonic acid (AA) significantly reduced the basal tone in WT (WT + AA, N = 4, $n = 8$, $p \leq 0.05$) but not in TREK-1 KO group. **b** Application of additional stretch (30% to L_0) caused an increase in basal tone of both WT and KO strips. No significant changes in response to TREK-1 inhibitor, L-methionine (LM), were recorded in both groups. **c** The amplitude of spontaneous contractions at L_0 was significantly elevated in TREK-1 KO group in comparison to WT group. The insert shows zoomed-in raw traces from both experimental groups. **d** Stretch protocol increased the amplitude of spontaneous contractions in both WT and TREK-1 KO BSM strips. * - $p \leq 0.05$ to respective WT group, # - $p \leq 0.05$ within the group

likely due to the secondary regulatory changes in PKC–related signaling pathways.

Urodynamic analysis of bladder function in TREK-1 KO mice

The analysis of cystometrograms recorded under control conditions in WT ($N = 5$) and TREK-1 KO ($N = 6$) mice showed an approximately 2-fold increase in bladder capacity in TREK-1 KO animals in comparison to WT mice (210.0 ± 8.1 µl vs. 108.2 ± 8.0 µl, respectively.Figure 7 a, b and c. $p \leq 0.05$), and a significant prolongation of the intermicturition interval (540.0 ± 43.8 s vs 1188.4 ± 166.4 s, WT and KO mice, respectively. Figure 7d. $p \leq 0.05$). The substantially elevated volume of infused saline during storage phase, which is reflective of increased bladder capacity, with the prolonged duration of the voiding cycle point toward the development of an underactive phenotype in TREK-1 KO mice. However, although no differences were observed in bladder pressure at voiding

(32.1 ± 3.2 mmHg vs. 39.0 ± 2.7 mmHg, TREK-1 KO, and WT mice, respectively), BMS from TREK-1 KO animals showed a 2-fold increase in the number of non-voiding contractions (TREK-1 KO: 4.5 ± 0.6 vs WT: 2.0 ± 0.5, $p \leq 0.05$, Fig. 7e) per micturition cycle. Other urodynamic characteristics were not different between the WT and TREK-1 KO animals. Therefore, the overall TREK-1 KO bladder phenotype displays the characteristics of both bladder under- and overactivity.

Discussion

Evaluation of bladder phenotype in TREK-1 KO animals revealed significant differences in comparison to WT mice including elevated basal muscle tone, increased amplitude of basal spontaneous activity, limited pharmacological responses to TREK-1 activators and inhibitors, and elevated contractile responses to EFS and high potassium without significant changes in bladder morphology/histology. However, urodynamic study in TREK-1

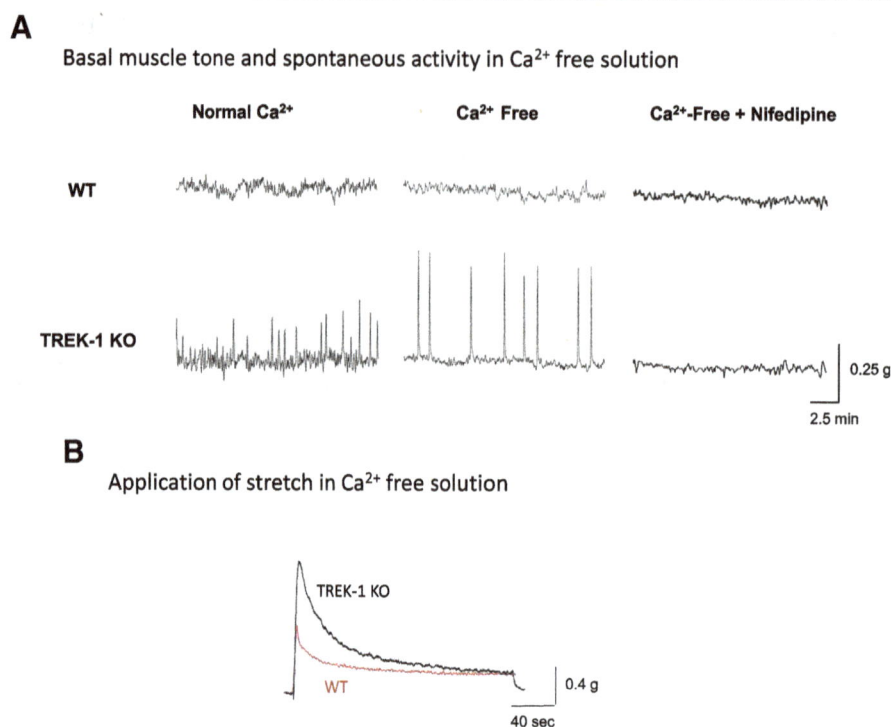

A

Basal muscle tone and spontaneous activity in Ca^{2+} free solution

| Normal Ca^{2+} | Ca^{2+} Free | Ca^{2+}-Free + Nifedipine |

WT

TREK-1 KO

0.25 g

2.5 min

B

Application of stretch in Ca^{2+} free solution

TREK-1 KO

WT

0.4 g

40 sec

Fig. 4 The effects of Ca^{2+} free solution and nifedipine on the basal muscle tone and spontaneous contractions in TREK-1 KO mice. **a** Representative traces of muscle tone and spontaneous activity in BSM strips from WT (upper panels) and TREK-1 KO (lower panels) animals. **b** Application of additional stretch under Ca^{2+} free conditions reduced the amplitude of the contractile response in both WT and TREK-1 KO animals

KO mice revealed a substantially longer inter-micturition interval, enhanced bladder capacity and increased number of non-voiding contractions in comparison to WT animals. Overall, the results of the combined in vivo and in vitro experiments provided evidence that global down-regulation of TREK-1 channel leads to "mixed" voiding phenotype in TREK-1 KO mice.

TREK-1 channel belongs to a family of mechanogated two-pore domain potassium channels (K_{2P}) that produce background conductances, and are regulated by a variety of stimuli (e.g., pH, temperature, stretch and lipids) to control resting membrane potential and cell excitability [7]. The TREK subfamily, encoded by the *KCNK2* gene, consists of three known members (TREK-1, TREK-2 and TRAAK) which participate in diverse transduction processes including mechano-sensitivity [6, 36, 38, 47], thermo-sensitivity [2, 26, 39], chemo-sensitivity [40], nociception, and neuroprotection [12, 15, 20, 31].

The results of Western blotting and IHC demonstrated that TREK-1 protein was substantially diminished in the urinary bladder of TREK-1 KO mice. The antibodies used for WB and IHC should detect any TREK-1 protein being translated, regardless of which one of the multiple start codons was used to initiate translation. Since we used the TREK-1 KO strain created by Namiranian et al. [45] in which both the second and

third exons of *Kcnk2* gene were deleted, all start codons present in both exons were deleted in this strain. Another group [17] created TREK-1 KO strain in which only the third exon was removed leaving an alternative start codon in exon 2, and, therefore, a truncated TREK-1 protein could be translated. In our study, we tested several TREK-1 antibodies. The anti-TREK-1 mouse monoclonal antibody from SantaCruz Biotechnology (F6, sc-398,449; mapped at aa354–380 near the C-terminus of hTREK-1) showed only one band ~ 50–52 kDa when used in WB (Fig. 1b). We also tested other commercially available antibodies from the same company which included the C20, E-19, and H-75 anti-TREK-1 variants. The C20 and E19 anti-TREK-1 antibodies did not work for Western blotting, while H-75 antibody (aa352–426 within the C-terminus) showed two bands in WT animals and one band in TREK-1 KO (data not shown) suggesting that it might be recognizing alternatively spliced variants or "off-target" proteins.

Increased basal muscle tone in the bladder of TREK-1 KO mice supports previous suggestions about the role of TREK-1 channel in maintaining the negative resting membrane potential in visceral smooth muscle [45]. Bladder muscle strips from TREK-1 KO mice also revealed the presence of spontaneous activity at both

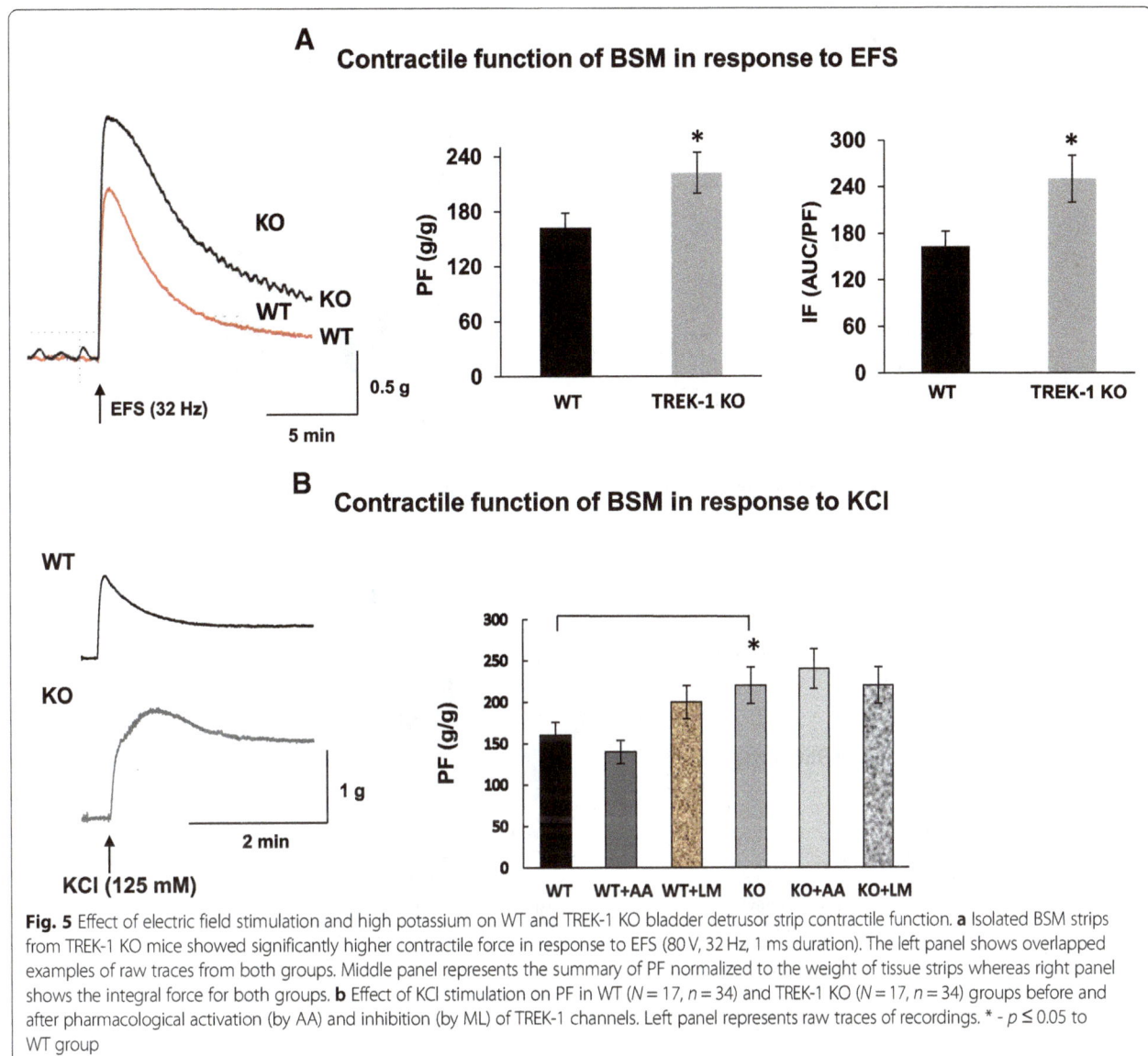

Fig. 5 Effect of electric field stimulation and high potassium on WT and TREK-1 KO bladder detrusor strip contractile function. **a** Isolated BSM strips from TREK-1 KO mice showed significantly higher contractile force in response to EFS (80 V, 32 Hz, 1 ms duration). The left panel shows overlapped examples of raw traces from both groups. Middle panel represents the summary of PF normalized to the weight of tissue strips whereas right panel shows the integral force for both groups. **b** Effect of KCl stimulation on PF in WT ($N = 17$, $n = 34$) and TREK-1 KO ($N = 17$, $n = 34$) groups before and after pharmacological activation (by AA) and inhibition (by ML) of TREK-1 channels. Left panel represents raw traces of recordings. * - $p \leq 0.05$ to WT group

resting level and after additional stretch. Spontaneous contractions have been previously recorded in a variety of bladder smooth muscle types including human [21, 58], rabbit [11, 24], rat [23], guinea pig [56], pig [25, 56], and mouse [28, 54]. It is possible that knockdown of TREK-1 may affect calcium mobilization and modify the threshold for smooth muscle excitability and/or contractility, thereby, increasing spontaneous activity, as observed in our study. To test this hypothesis, we incubated BMS strips in Ca^{2+}-free TB followed by the application of nifedipine, a L-type calcium channel blocker (Fig. 4). Incubation of TREK-1 KO strips in Ca^{2+}-free solution effectively reduced the basal tone to the levels similar to those observed in WT BMS strips. Interestingly, the reduced muscle tone observed in Ca^{2+}-free solution was associated with a 2-fold increase in the amplitude of spontanous contractions in TREK-1

KO group. The total elimination of spontaneous contractions and further reduction in basal tone by nifedipine suggests that TREK-1 channels participate in regulation of spontaneous contractions by stabilizing the membrane potential at voltages closer to the potassium resting potential. Overall, in addition to previously published data on human [3, 34] and animal [22, 42] visceral smooth muscle, our data provide additional evidence that TREK-1 channel plays a critical role in maintaining bladder basal tone, bladder compliance and modulates the response of the detrusor to stretch.

The contractile responses of BSM to EFS are mainly mediated by the release of neurotransmitters from intramural nerve terminals in the bladder wall causing detrusor contraction. We compared the responses of TREK-1 KO and WT muscle strips in their ability to generate force in response to EFS. The data showed

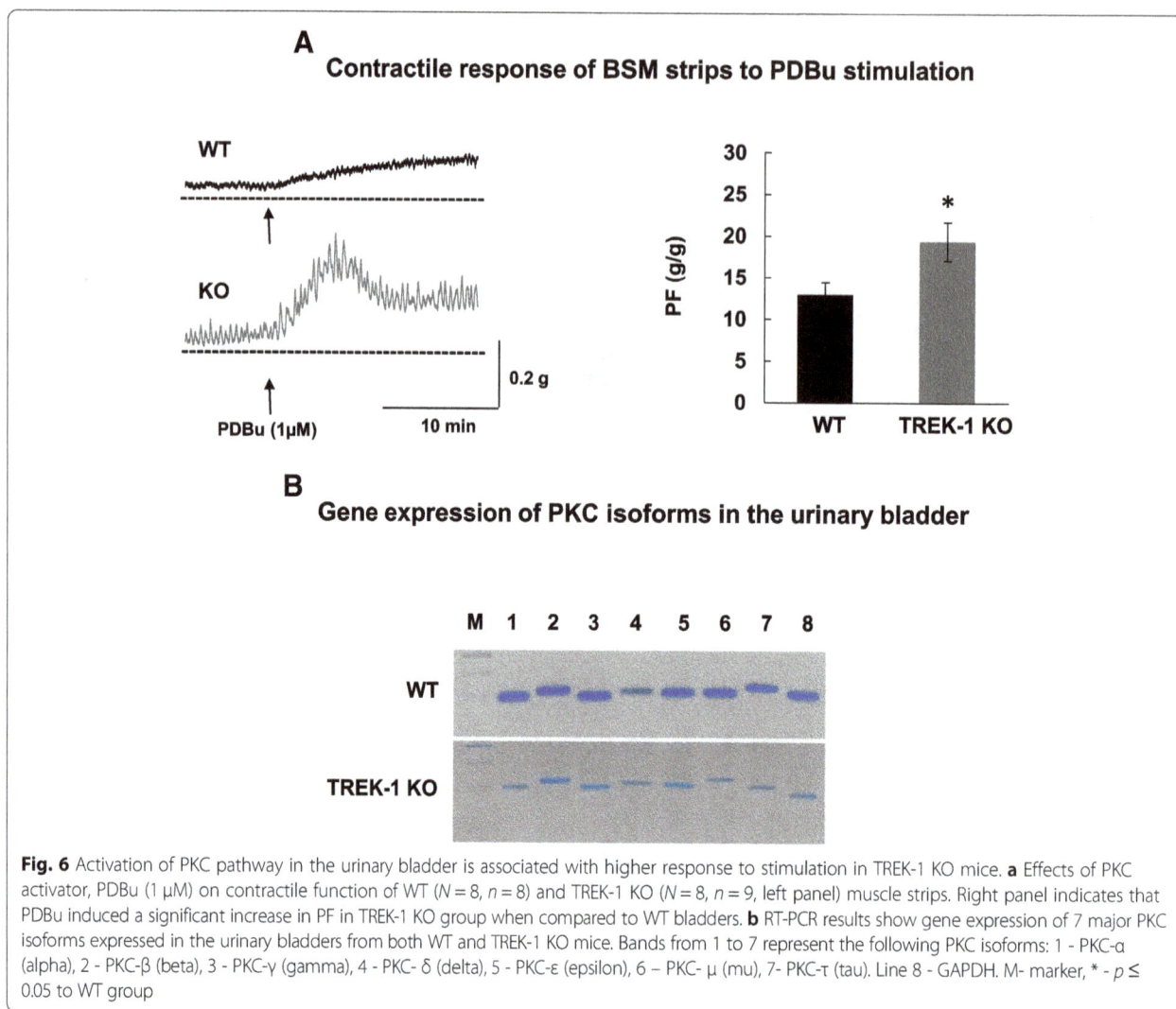

Fig. 6 Activation of PKC pathway in the urinary bladder is associated with higher response to stimulation in TREK-1 KO mice. **a** Effects of PKC activator, PDBu (1 μM) on contractile function of WT ($N = 8$, $n = 8$) and TREK-1 KO ($N = 8$, $n = 9$, left panel) muscle strips. Right panel indicates that PDBu induced a significant increase in PF in TREK-1 KO group when compared to WT bladders. **b** RT-PCR results show gene expression of 7 major PKC isoforms expressed in the urinary bladders from both WT and TREK-1 KO mice. Bands from 1 to 7 represent the following PKC isoforms: 1 - PKC-α (alpha), 2 - PKC-β (beta), 3 - PKC-γ (gamma), 4 - PKC- δ (delta), 5 - PKC-ε (epsilon), 6 – PKC- μ (mu), 7- PKC-τ (tau). Line 8 - GAPDH. M- marker, * - $p \leq$ 0.05 to WT group

that the loss of TREK-1 channels was associated with a significant increase in peak contractility in response to EFS (Fig. 5) while slowing the rate of relaxation in the TREK-1 KO muscle strips when compared to WT group. While EFS induces a contraction mainly via the release of acetylcholine from bladder nerves, KCl-induced contractions result from direct activation and depolarization of the detrusor muscle due to rapid membrane depolarization and the associated influx of Ca^{2+} via voltage-gated Ca^{2+} channels. Similar to EFS, high potassium solution also caused a significantly elevated amplitude of the contractile response in TREK-1 KO strips suggesting that increased contractility in the absence of TREK-1 channels is due to a partial membrane depolarization which shifts the resting membrane potential towards more positive values closer to the activation threshold of voltage-gated calcium channels.

Prior studies have reported that protein kinase C (PKC) may be able to phosphorylate TREK-1 channels in smooth muscle, thereby, modulating the contractile force [30, 37, 43]. We previously showed that activation of PKC by general PKC activator, PDBu, at low levels of stimulation could inhibit spontaneous contractions in rabbit [24] and rat [23] BSM while higher levels of PKC stimulation had the opposite effect. These data predict that upon down-regulation of TREK-1, the PKC activator, PDBu, should have a more positive contractile effect on KO muscle strips when compared to WT group. Our data are consistent with this analysis in that PDBu, indeed, increased both the PF and the amplitude of spontaneous contractions in TREK-1 KO muscle strips compared to the WT mice. Analysis of gene expression of different PKC isoforms expressed in the urinary bladder did not reveal significant differences between WT and TREK-1 KO mice. Therefore, additional studies will

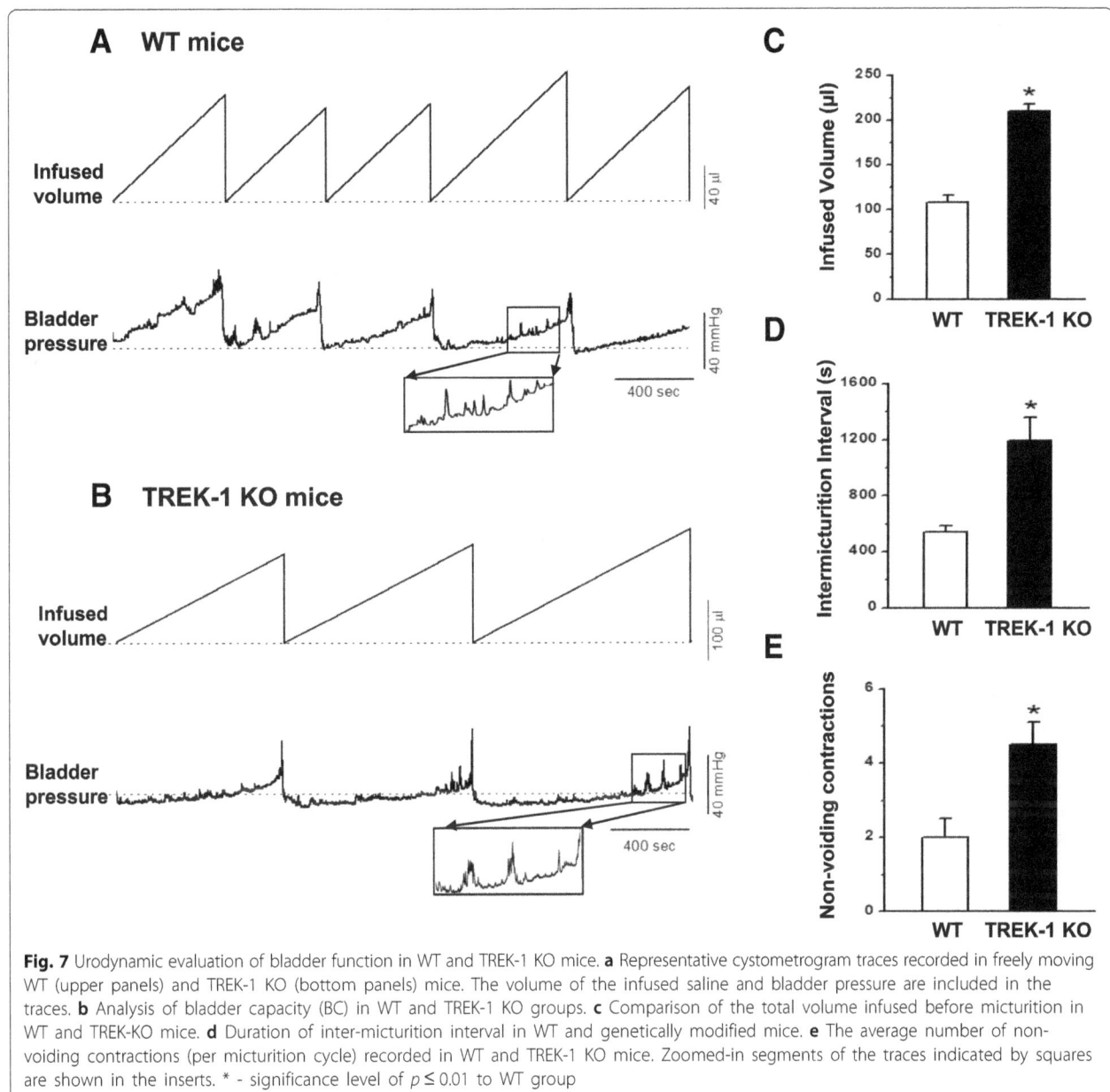

Fig. 7 Urodynamic evaluation of bladder function in WT and TREK-1 KO mice. **a** Representative cystometrogram traces recorded in freely moving WT (upper panels) and TREK-1 KO (bottom panels) mice. The volume of the infused saline and bladder pressure are included in the traces. **b** Analysis of bladder capacity (BC) in WT and TREK-1 KO groups. **c** Comparison of the total volume infused before micturition in WT and TREK-KO mice. **d** Duration of inter-micturition interval in WT and genetically modified mice. **e** The average number of non-voiding contractions (per micturition cycle) recorded in WT and TREK-1 KO mice. Zoomed-in segments of the traces indicated by squares are shown in the inserts. * - significance level of $p \leq 0.01$ to WT group

be required to evaluate if the elevated response to PKC activation in TREK-1 KO bladder is due to the changes in PKC phosphorylation or activation of different downstream signaling pathways.

In contrast to in vitro contractility results, the urodynamic evaluation of voiding function in vivo by awake cystometry revealed a significant increase in the duration of inter-micturition interval and enhanced bladder capacity, both of which usually define an underactive bladder phenotype. Despite these changes, the intravesical pressure during micturition was not affected by the TREK-1 knockdown, and the number of non-voiding contractions was almost 2-fold higher in these animals which is in line with the increased contractility of the detrusor observed during the in vitro studies discussed above. Taken together, these results suggest that knock-down of *Kcnk2* gene has dual or "mixed" effects on detrusor contractility and micturition patterns. One of the possible explanations could be associated with expression of the channel on vascular and visceral smooth muscle cells as well as on the fibers and neurons of the peripheral and central nervous system [19, 41]. The functional role of TREK-1 in smooth muscle cells is mainly to contribute to the "leak" current responsible for the maintenance of hyperpolarized resting membrane potential to keep the cells more relaxed during resting state [5, 10].

In the nervous system, TREK-1 was shown to control electrogenesis, differentiation, axonal migration, synaptogenesis, and neural response to temperature and mechanical stretch [1, 9, 13, 16, 19, 27, 31, 51]. In comparison to smooth muscle cells, where action potentials are driven by the influx of Ca^{2+} via L-type Ca^{2+} channels, excitability of neurons is regulated mainly by voltage-gated Na^+ channels. The lack of TREK-1 channel in neurons would shift the resting membrane potential towards more positive values (just like in smooth muscle cells) allowing for the rapid influx of Na^+ inside the cell, and, therefore, making both afferent and efferent neurons more excitable. The final result of this neuronal activity would depend on what neurons are more affected by these changes. An increase in afferent activity from the urinary bladder to the brain is usually associated with an increase in urgency and frequency of micturition associated with bladder overactivity. However, the efferent output from the brain to the bladder is mainly inhibitory to allow for the voluntary control of micturition. Therefore, increased excitability of efferent neurons would lead to increased inter-micturition interval and bladder underactivity, which we observed in our study in vivo. Future studies focused on manipulations of either afferent or efferent neural pathways are warranted to test this hypothesis.

Another possible explanation for the differences between in vitro and in vivo bladder phenotypes could be associated with some unknown alterations occurring during genetic modifications of the parental strain. TREK-1 was determined to mediate changes in the actin cytoskeleton independently of its channel activity in fetal neurons during development in a different strain of TREK-1 KO mice [32]. The same mouse strain showed an increased efficacy of 5-HT neurotransmission and resistance to depression [20]. Previous studies from our [35] and other [57] groups provided evidence that lower urinary tract function in mice varies in a consistent manner with strain and/or sex. For instance, voiding spot assay and cystometry performed in male and female C57BL/6 J, 129S1/SvImJ, NOD/ShiLtJ, and CAST/EiJ mice [8] to evaluate bladder function, established a significantly prolonged duration of the micturition cycle in genetically modified animals (129S1/SvImJ, NOD/ShiLtJ, and CAST/EiJ) in comparison to C57BL/6 J strain [8]. These results are in line with our cystometric recordings from TREK-1 KO mice. The differences between our study and the published results included the use of both sexes (males and females), the use of WT controls which were not littermates, and performance of cystometry without anesthesia in our experiments, as well as the absence of in vitro experiments in the previously published study.

The choice of the approach to create a genetically modified strain also seems to affect the function of different organs and tissues in genetically modified animals. For instance, the TREK-1 KO strain we adopted and used in our study, provided no evidence that TREK-1 is involved in the regulation of arterial diameter in cerebral arteries [45]. However, another TREK-1 KO strain [32] did present with the vascular phenotype. There is also a possibility that genetic knockdown of TREK-1 expression could trigger compensatory changes in other mechano-gated ion channels or related signaling cascades, thereby, affecting the final voiding phenotype as well as the response of the detrusor to stretch. Further studies are warranted to address these questions.

Conclusions

Our study provided evidence that global down-regulation of TREK-1 channels has dual effects on detrusor contractility and micturition patterns in vivo. The integrative effects of TREK-1, likely, depend on the expression and function of the channel not only in detrusor myocytes but also in afferent and efferent neural pathways regulating micturition. Future studies are warranted to identify the precise mechanisms of TREK-1 associated mechanotransduction between detrusor myocytes and afferent nerves in the bladder wall, as well as the role of TREK-1 in efferent fibers and central nervous system centers controlling voiding. This knowledge would provide a foundation for the development of novel therapeutic approaches to treat voiding dysfunction in patients with detrusor overactivity, overactive bladder, and bladder pain syndrome.

Abbreviations
AA: Arachidonic acid; AUC: Area under the curve; BK: Ca^{2+}-activated potassium channels; BSM: Bladder smooth muscle; DO: Detrusor overactivity; EFS: Electric field stimulation; IF: Integral force; IHC: Immunohistochemistry; KO: Knockout; L_0: The length of optimal force development; LM: L-methionine; PBS: Phosphate-buffered saline; PDBu: Phorbol 12,13-Dibutyrate; PF: Peak force; PFA: Paraformaldehyde; PKC: Protein kinase C; RT: Room temperature; TB: Tyrode Buffer; TBS: Tris-Buffered saline; TREK-1 channel: Two-pore domain potassium channel encoded by *Kcnk2* gene; TTX: Tetrodotoxin; WB: Western blotting; WT: Wild type

Acknowledgements
We thank Dr. Min Zhou and his lab members for providing the TREK-1 KO mice for our study, as well as Dr. John A Thompson from the Department of Neurosurgery, University of Colorado Denver for help with data analyses. Imaging experiments were performed in the University of Colorado Anschutz Medical Campus Advance Light Microscopy Core supported in part by Rocky Mountain Neurological Disorders Core (P30 NS048154) and by NIH/NCATS Colorado CTSI Grant (UL1 TR001082).

Authors' contributions
R.H.P. and A.P.M. conception and design of the research; R.H.P., J.H., S.L., A.C., and N.I. performed the experiments; R.H.P., J.H., S.L. and N.I. analyzed the data; R.H.P., R.B.M., J.H., S.L., N.I. and A.P.M interpreted the results of the experiments; R.H.P., J.H., S.L., and A.P.M prepared the figures; R.H.P. and A.P.M drafted the manuscript; R.H.P., R.B.M. and A.P.M edited and revised the manuscript; R.H.P., J.H., S.L., A.C., N.I., R.B.M., and A.P.M. approved the final version of the manuscript; all authors are accountable for all aspects of the work.

Author details
[1]Division of Urology, Department of Surgery, University of Colorado Denver,Anschutz Medical Campus, 12700 E 19th Ave, M/S C317, Aurora, CO

80045, USA. [2]Department of Urology, University of California San Diego, 3855 Health Science Drive, Room 4345, Bay 4LL, La Jolla, CA 92093, USA. [3]Children's Mercy Hospital, 2401 Gillham Rd, Kansas City, MO 64108, USA. [4]Division of Urology, Department of Surgery, University of Colorado Denver, Academic Office One Bldg., Rm 5602, 12631 East 17th Ave., M/S C319, Aurora, CO 80045, USA.

References

1. Afzali AM, Ruck T, Herrmann AM, Iking J, Sommer C, Kleinschnitz C, Preubetae C, Stenzel W, Budde T, Wiendl H, Bittner S, Meuth SG. The potassium channels TASK2 and TREK1 regulate functional differentiation of murine skeletal muscle cells. Am J Physiol Cell Physiol. 2016;311:C583–95.
2. Alloui A, Zimmermann K, Mamet J, Duprat F, Noel J, Chemin J, Guy N, Blondeau N, Voilley N, Rubat-Coudert C, Borsotto M, Romey G, Heurteaux C, Reeh P, Eschalier A, Lazdunski M. TREK-1, a K+ channel involved in polymodal pain perception. EMBO J. 2006;25:2368–76.
3. Bai X, Bugg GJ, Greenwood SL, Glazier JD, Sibley CP, Baker PN, Taggart MJ, Fyfe GK. Expression of TASK and TREK, two-pore domain K+ channels, in human myometrium. Reproduction. 2005;129:525–30.
4. Baker SA, Hatton WJ, Han J, Hennig GW, Britton FC, Koh SD. Role of TREK-1 potassium channel in bladder overactivity after partial bladder outlet obstruction in mouse. J Urol. 2010;183:793–800.
5. Baker SA, Hennig GW, Han J, Britton FC, Smith TK, Koh SD. Methionine and its derivatives increase bladder excitability by inhibiting stretch-dependent K(+) channels. Br J Pharmacol. 2008;153:1259–71.
6. Bang H, Kim Y, Kim D. TREK-2, a new member of the mechanosensitive tandem-pore K+ channel family. J Biol Chem. 2000;275:17412–9.
7. Bayliss DA, Barrett PQ. Emerging roles for two-pore-domain potassium channels and their potential therapeutic impact. Trends Pharmacol Sci. 2008;29:566–75.
8. Bjorling DE, Wang Z, Vezina CM, Ricke WA, Keil KP, Yu W, Guo L, Zeidel ML, Hill WG. Evaluation of voiding assays in mice: impact of genetic strains and sex. Am J Physiol Renal Physiol. 2015;308:F1369–78.
9. Bockenhauer D, Zilberberg N, Goldstein SA. KCNK2: reversible conversion of a hippocampal potassium leak into a voltage-dependent channel. Nat Neurosci. 2001;4:486–91.
10. Buxton IL, Singer CA, Tichenor JN. Expression of stretch-activated two-pore potassium channels in human myometrium in pregnancy and labor. PLoS One. 2010;5:e12372.
11. Chang S, Hypolite JA, Mohanan S, Zderic SA, Wein AJ, Chacko S. Alteration of the PKC-mediated signaling pathway for smooth muscle contraction in obstruction-induced hypertrophy of the urinary bladder. Lab Investig. 2009; 89:823–32.
12. Chemin J, Patel AJ, Duprat F, Lauritzen I, Lazdunski M, Honore E. A phospholipid sensor controls mechanogating of the K+ channel TREK-1. EMBO J. 2005;24:44–53.
13. Devader C, Khayachi A, Veyssiere J, Moha Ou Maati H, Roulot M, Moreno S, Borsotto M, Martin S, Heurteaux C, Mazella J. In vitro and in vivo regulation of synaptogenesis by the novel antidepressant spadin. Br J Pharmacol. 2015; 172:2604–17.
14. Du Y, Kiyoshi CM, Wang Q, Wang W, Ma B, Alford CC, Zhong S, Wan Q, Chen H, Lloyd EE, Bryan RM Jr, Zhou M. Genetic deletion of TREK-1 or TWIK-1/TREK-1 potassium channels does not Alter the basic electrophysiological properties of mature hippocampal astrocytes in situ. Front Cell Neurosci. 2016;10(13).
15. Duprat F, Lesage F, Patel AJ, Fink M, Romey G, Lazdunski M. The neuroprotective agent riluzole activates the two P domain K(+) channels TREK-1 and TRAAK. Mol Pharmacol. 2000;57:906–12.
16. Fink M, Duprat F, Lesage F, Reyes R, Romey G, Heurteaux C, Lazdunski M. Cloning, functional expression and brain localization of a novel unconventional outward rectifier K+ channel. EMBO J. 1996;15:6854–62.
17. Guyon A, Tardy MP, Rovere C, Nahon JL, Barhanin J, Lesage F. Glucose inhibition persists in hypothalamic neurons lacking tandem-pore K+ channels. J Neurosci. 2009;29:2528–33.
18. Hervieu GJ, Cluderay JE, Gray CW, Green PJ, Ranson JL, Randall AD, Meadows HJ. Distribution and expression of TREK-1, a two-pore-domain potassium channel, in the adult rat CNS. Neuroscience. 2001;103:899–919.
19. Heurteaux C, Guy N, Laigle C, Blondeau N, Duprat F, Mazzuca M, Lang-Lazdunski L, Widmann C, Zanzouri M, Romey G, Lazdunski M. TREK-1, a K+ channel involved in neuroprotection and general anesthesia. EMBO J. 2004; 23:2684–95.
20. Heurteaux C, Lucas G, Guy N, El Yacoubi M, Thummler S, Peng XD, Noble F, Blondeau N, Widmann C, Borsotto M, Gobbi G, Vaugeois JM, Debonnel G, Lazdunski M. Deletion of the background potassium channel TREK-1 results in a depression-resistant phenotype. Nat Neurosci. 2006;9:1134–41.
21. Hristov KL, Afeli SA, Parajuli SP, Cheng Q, Rovner ES, Petkov GV. Neurogenic detrusor overactivity is associated with decreased expression and function of the large conductance voltage- and ca(2+)-activated K(+) channels. PLoS One. 2013;8:e68052.
22. Hwang SJ, O'Kane N, Singer C, Ward SM, Sanders KM, Koh SD. Block of inhibitory junction potentials and TREK-1 channels in murine colon by Ca2+ store-active drugs. J Physiol. 2008;586:1169–84.
23. Hypolite JA, Chang S, Wein AJ, Chacko S, Malykhina AP. Protein kinase C modulates frequency of micturition and non-voiding contractions in the urinary bladder via neuronal and myogenic mechanisms. BMC Urol. 2015; 15(34).
24. Hypolite JA, Lei Q, Chang S, Zderic SA, Butler S, Wein AJ, Malykhina AP, Chacko S. Spontaneous and evoked contractions are regulated by PKC-mediated signaling in detrusor smooth muscle: involvement of BK channels. Am J Physiol Renal Physiol. 2013;304:F451–62.
25. Isogai A, Lee K, Mitsui R, Hashitani H. Functional coupling of TRPV4 channels and BK channels in regulating spontaneous contractions of the Guinea pig urinary bladder. Pflugers Arch. 2016;468:1573–85.
26. Kang D, Choe C, Kim D. Thermosensitivity of the two-pore domain K+ channels TREK-2 and TRAAK. J Physiol. 2005;564:103–16.
27. Kanjhan R, Anselme AM, Noakes PG, Bellingham MC. Postnatal changes in TASK-1 and TREK-1 expression in rat brain stem and cerebellum. Neuroreport. 2004;15:1321–4.
28. Kobayter S, Young JS, Brain KL. Prostaglandin E2 induces spontaneous rhythmic activity in mouse urinary bladder independently of efferent nerves. Br J Pharmacol. 2012;165:401–13.
29. Koh SD, Sanders KM. Stretch-dependent potassium channels in murine colonic smooth muscle cells. J Physiol. 2001;533:155–63.
30. Kreneisz O, Benoit JP, Bayliss DA, Mulkey DK. AMP-activated protein kinase inhibits TREK channels. J Physiol. 2009;587:5819–30.
31. Lauritzen I, Blondeau N, Heurteaux C, Widmann C, Romey G, Lazdunski M. Polyunsaturated fatty acids are potent neuroprotectors. EMBO J. 2000;19: 1784–93.
32. Lauritzen I, Chemin J, Honore E, Jodar M, Guy N, Lazdunski M, Jane Patel A. Cross-talk between the mechano-gated K2P channel TREK-1 and the actin cytoskeleton. EMBO Rep. 2005;6:642–8.
33. Lee H, Koh BH, Peri LE, Sanders KM, Koh SD. Purinergic inhibitory regulation of murine detrusor muscles mediated by PDGFRalpha+ interstitial cells. J Physiol. 2014;592:1283–93.
34. Lei Q, Pan XQ, Chang S, Malkowicz SB, Guzzo TJ, Malykhina AP. Response of the human detrusor to stretch is regulated by TREK-1, a two-pore-domain (K2P) mechano-gated potassium channel. J Physiol. 2014;592:3013–30.
35. Lei Q, Pan XQ, Villamor AN, Asfaw TS, Chang S, Zderic SA, Malykhina AP. Lack of transient receptor potential vanilloid 1 channel modulates the development of neurogenic bladder dysfunction induced by cross-sensitization in afferent pathways. J Neuroinflammation. 2013;10(3).
36. Lesage F, Terrenoire C, Romey G, Lazdunski M. Human TREK2, a 2P domain mechano-sensitive K+ channel with multiple regulations by polyunsaturated fatty acids, lysophospholipids, and Gs, Gi, and Gq protein-coupled receptors. J Biol Chem. 2000;275:28398–405.
37. Liu H, Enyeart JA, Enyeart JJ. Angiotensin II inhibits native bTREK-1 K+ channels through a PLC-, kinase C-, and PIP2-independent pathway requiring ATP hydrolysis. Am J Physiol Cell Physiol. 2007;293:C682–95.
38. Maingret F, Honore E, Lazdunski M, Patel AJ. Molecular basis of the voltage-dependent gating of TREK-1, a mechano-sensitive K(+) channel. Biochem Biophys Res Commun. 2002;292:339–46.
39. Maingret F, Lauritzen I, Patel AJ, Heurteaux C, Reyes R, Lesage F, Lazdunski M, Honore E. TREK-1 is a heat-activated background K(+) channel. EMBO J. 2000;19:2483–91.
40. Maingret F, Patel AJ, Lesage F, Lazdunski M, Honore E. Mechano- or acid stimulation, two interactive modes of activation of the TREK-1 potassium channel. J Biol Chem. 1999;274:26691–6.
41. Medhurst AD, Rennie G, Chapman CG, Meadows H, Duckworth MD, Kelsell RE, Gloger II, Pangalos MN. Distribution analysis of human two pore domain potassium channels in tissues of the central nervous system and periphery. Brain Res Mol Brain Res. 2001;86:101–14.

42. Monaghan K, Baker SA, Dwyer L, Hatton WC, Sik Park K, Sanders KM, Koh SD. The stretch-dependent potassium channel TREK-1 and its function in murine myometrium. J Physiol. 2011;589:1221–33.

43. Murbartian J, Lei Q, Sando JJ, Bayliss DA. Sequential phosphorylation mediates receptor- and kinase-induced inhibition of TREK-1 background potassium channels. J Biol Chem. 2005;280:30175–84.

44. Namiranian K, Brink CD, Goodman JC, Robertson CS, and Bryan RM, Jr. Traumatic brain injury in mice lacking the K channel, TREK-1. J Cereb Blood Flow Metab 31: e1–e6, 2011.

45. Namiranian K, Lloyd EE, Crossland RF, Marrelli SP, Taffet GE, Reddy AK, Hartley CJ, and Bryan RM, Jr. Cerebrovascular responses in mice deficient in the potassium channel, TREK-1. Am J Physiol Regul Integr Comp Physiol 299: R461–R469, 2010.

46. Patel AJ, Honore E. Properties and modulation of mammalian 2P domain K + channels. Trends Neurosci. 2001;24:339–46.

47. Patel AJ, Honore E, Maingret F, Lesage F, Fink M, Duprat F, Lazdunski M. A mammalian two pore domain mechano-gated S-like K+ channel. EMBO J. 1998;17:4283–90.

48. Pineda RH, Nedumaran B, Hypolite J, Pan XQ, Wilson S, Meacham RB, Malykhina AP. Altered expression and modulation of the two-pore-domain (K2P) mechanogated potassium channel TREK-1 in overactive human detrusor. Am J Physiol Renal Physiol. 2017;313:F535–46.

49. Sanders KM, Koh SD. Two-pore-domain potassium channels in smooth muscles: new components of myogenic regulation. J Physiol. 2006;570: 37–43.

50. Schindelin J, Arganda-Carreras I, Frise E, Kaynig V, Longair M, Pietzsch T, Preibisch S, Rueden C, Saalfeld S, Schmid B, Tinevez JY, White DJ, Hartenstein V, Eliceiri K, Tomancak P, Cardona A. Fiji: an open-source platform for biological-image analysis. Nat Methods. 2012;9:676–82.

51. Thomas D, Plant LD, Wilkens CM, McCrossan ZA, Goldstein SA. Alternative translation initiation in rat brain yields K2P2.1 potassium channels permeable to sodium. Neuron. 2008;58:859–70.

52. Tichenor JN, Hansen ET, Buxton IL. Expression of stretch-activated potassium channels in human myometrium. Proc West Pharmacol Soc. 2005;48:44–8.

53. Wellner MC, Isenberg G. Stretch effects on whole-cell currents of Guinea-pig urinary bladder myocytes. J Physiol. 1994;480 (Pt 3:439–48.

54. White RS, Zemen BG, Khan Z, Montgomery JR, Herrera GM, Meredith AL. Evaluation of mouse urinary bladder smooth muscle for diurnal differences in contractile properties. Front Pharmacol. 2014;5:293.

55. Wu YY, Singer CA, Buxton IL. Variants of stretch-activated two-pore potassium channel TREK-1 associated with preterm labor in humans. Biol Reprod. 2012;87:96.

56. Xin W, Li N, Fernandes VS, Petkov GV. Constitutively active PKA regulates neuronal acetylcholine release and contractility of Guinea pig urinary bladder smooth muscle. Am J Physiol Renal Physiol. 2016;310:F1377–84.

57. Yu W, Ackert-Bicknell C, Larigakis JD, MacIver B, Steers WD, Churchill GA, Hill WG, Zeidel ML. Spontaneous voiding by mice reveals strain-specific lower urinary tract function to be a quantitative genetic trait. Am J Physiol Renal Physiol. 2014;306:F1296–307.

58. Zagorodnyuk VP, Gregory S, Costa M, Brookes SJ, Tramontana M, Giuliani S, Maggi CA. Spontaneous release of acetylcholine from autonomic nerves in the bladder. Br J Pharmacol. 2009;157:607–19.

59. Pineda RH, Hypolite J, Lee S, Carrasco A, Iguchi N, Meacham RB, Malykhina AP. The lack of mechanosensitive K2P channel is associated with mixed voiding phenotype in mice. J Urology. 199(4S):e503–4.

19

Efficacy and safety of botulinum toxin a injection into urethral sphincter for underactive bladder

Guoqing Chen[1,2], Limin Liao[1,2]* and Fei Zhang[3]

Abstract

Background: The aim of this retrospective study was to evaluate the clinical efficacy and safety of botulinum toxin type A (BTX-A) injection into the urethral sphincter to treat patients with underactive bladder (UAB).

Methods: From September 2012 to December 2018, 35 patients with UAB who presented with dysuria were treated with BTX-A (Prosigne®, Lanzhou Biological Products, Lanzhou, China). All patients were evaluated using the International Continence Society standard for video-urodynamic examination before and 1 month after treatment. The index includes maximum urinary flow rate, detrusor leak point pressure, and maximum urethral pressure. Post-voiding residual urine volume was measured using ultrasound before, one and 3 months post injection.

Results: After 1 month of treatment, the maximum flow rate increased from 2.5 ± 1.1 ml/s to 6.6 ± 1.7 ml/s ($P < 0.05$). The maximum urethral pressure decreased from 73.5 ± 5.8 cmH$_2$o to 45.6 ± 4.3cmH$_2$O ($P < 0.05$). The detrusor leak point pressure decreased from 69.9 ± 20.7cmH$_2$O to 26.3 ± 7.4cmH$_2$O ($P < 0.01$). Post-voiding residual urine decreased from 282.8 ± 134.2 ml to 125.0 ± 92.1 ml ($P < 0.01$) but increased to 270.1 ± 129.0 ml 3 months post injection. Of the 35 patients, 57.1% (20/35) relied on clean intermittent catheterization (CIC) before injection, but 75.0% (15/20) of them could partly void 1 month after injection, and 25%(5/20) could void without CIC. Eight patients showed hydronephrosis before treatment; in three of them, hydronephrosis decreased slightly, while it resolved in two. All patients were followed for three to 6 months, and the effect lasted for about two to 3 months. No serious adverse events occurred in any patient.

Conclusions: The results suggest that Prosigne® injection into the urethral sphincter is an effective, safe, and inexpensive way to treat UAB.

Keywords: Urethral sphincter, Botulinum toxin type A, Underactive bladder, Residual urine volume

Background

Botulinum toxins (BTX) which derive from the Grampositive coccus *Clostridium botulinum* are the most potent known naturally occurring neurotoxins [1]. They can paralyze striated muscle by blocking acetylcholine release at the presynapse. U.S. Food and Drug Administration approved BTX for the treatment of strabismus, blepharospasm, and hemifacial spasm in 1989 [2]. BTX can be classified into seven different types: A, B, C, D, E, F, and G according to its different immune antigens [3]. The first licensed serotype in clinical use was BTX-A

with the trade name Botox® (Allergan Pharmaceuticals, Irvine, CA), but other brands also exist, including Dysport® (Ipsen Biopharm Ltd., Slough, UK), Xeomin® (Merz Pharmaceuticals UK Ltd., Hertfordshire, UK), Prosigne® (Lanzhou Biological Products, Lanzhou, China), and PurTox® (Mentor Corporation, Madison, WI) [4].

In recent years, BTX-A injection has been widely used in the treatment and research of lower urinary tract dysfunction [5]. The site of BTX-A injection is classified into simple detrusor injection for detrusor overactivity, simple sphincter injection, or detrusor-sphincter combined injection for sphincter spasm or detrusor sphincter dysfunction. Our department is the first in China to use BTX-A injection to treat lower urinary tract dysfunction. We used BTX-A (Prosigne®) injected into the

---

* Correspondence: lmliao@263.net
[1]Department of Urology, China Rehabilitation Research Center, Beijing 100068, China
[2]Department of Urology, Capital Medical University, Beijing, China
Full list of author information is available at the end of the article

detrusor for neurogenic detrusor overactivity [6] and interstitial cystitis [7] and achieved satisfactory results. We also used Prosigne® to inject into the urethral sphincter to treat underactive bladder (UAB). This retrospective study was to evaluate the efficacy and safety of Prosigne® in patients with UAB.

Methods

All subjects signed their informed consent for inclusion before they participated in the study. The study was conducted in accordance with the Declaration of Helsinki, and the protocol was approved by the Ethics Committee of China Rehabilitation Research Center (Project identification code: 2018–053-1). Before treatment, all patients underwent video-urodynamic examination according to the International Continence Society standard [8], and the maximum urinary flow rate, maximum urethral pressure, and detrusor leak point pressure were recorded. According to the classification of urodynamic diagnosis, 26 patients had detrusor underactivity, and nine had acontractile detrusor. There was no bladder-ureter reflux, and urinary ultrasound showed that eight patients had mild hydronephrosis. Twenty of the 35 patients had previously relied on clean intermittent catheterization (CIC). The above indicators were reviewed 1 month after treatment. Residual urine volume was measured by ultrasound before, one and 3 months post injection, and the mean of three measurements was taken.

BTX-A (Prosigne®) was used in treatment. The patients were treated in the lithotomy position with routine insertion of a 21F cystourethroscope. After identifying the circular external sphincter under the endoscope, a 6F bladder injection needle was inserted into the external sphincter using cystourethroscopy. One-hundred units of BTX-A were diluted with 8 ml saline and injected into the external sphincter. In the direction of the 3, 6, 9, and 12 points of the external sphincter, two needles were injected longitudinally near each point, a total of 8 needles. Each injection was 1 ml and 1 or 2 cm deep at the latent injection site. And after the operation, Foley catheter was indwelled.

Using GraphPad Prism 8 software, all measurement data were expressed by mean $\pm$ standard deviation; the paired t test and one-way ANOVA was used for group measurement data. $P < 0.05$ was considered to be statistically significant.

Results

From September 2012 to December 2018, 35 patients with UAB and dysuria underwent BTX-A (Prosigne®) injection into their urethral sphincter in our hospital, including 21 men and 14 women aged 19 to 77 (41.85 $\pm$ 15.80) years. Twenty-four patients had neurogenic bladder, and 11 had non-neurogenic, non-obstructive urinary retention. Specific etiologies are shown in Table 1. All patients were given a thorough explanation of the treatment and written informed consent before the injection.

The catheter was removed 7 days after injection with BTX-A. One month after treatment, all patients underwent video-urodynamic examination. The maximum urinary flow rate increased ($P < 0.05$), while the maximum urethral pressure and detrusor leak point pressure reduced by statistically significant amounts ($P < 0.05$) (Table 2). Residual urine decreased significantly 1 month post injection ($P < 0.05$) but increased to the same level as before treatment 3 months post injection (Fig. 1). Of the 35 patients, 57.1% (20/35) relied on CIC before injection, but 75.0% (15/20) of them could partly void 1 month after injection, and 25% (5/20) could void without CIC.

Urinary ultrasonography was conducted 1 month after treatment. Three patients had hydronephrosis without obvious relief, three had slight relief from hydronephrosis, and two had resolution of their hydronephrosis. The follow-up period was three to 6 months, and the relief lasted two to 3 months. No serious adverse reactions occurred in any patient. None of the patients had incontinence before the procedure, but mild urinary stress incontinence occurred in five patients after treatment and resolved two or 3 months later.

Discussion

UAB is a complicated clinical syndrome characterized by prolonged urination, with or without a sensation of incomplete bladder emptying, usually with hesitancy, a slow stream, and reduced sensation on filling [9]. According to possible mechanisms, UAB can be classified into three types: idiopathic, neurogenic, or myogenic [10]. In our study, 24 patients had neurogenic bladder, and 11 had non-neurogenic, non-obstructive urinary retention. Based on urodynamic examination, UAB can be classified into detrusor underactivity or acontractile detrusor [10]. In this study, 26 patients had detrusor underactivity, and nine had contractile detrusor.

Whether UAB was neurogenic or nonneurogenic, the main symptom of all patients was dysuria, which negatively affects quality of life-especially in patients with hydronephrosis due to ureteral reflux, in whom renal

Table 1 Patient's etiologies

Etiology	Number of patients
Neurogenic decease	24
Cone horsetail injury	10
Spina bifida and meningocele	8
Spinal surgery	6
Non-neurogenic, non-obstructive urinary retention	11
Total	35

Table 2 Comparison of urodynamic parameters in patients with underactive bladder before and after treatment

Urodynamic parameters	Baseline	One month
Pura.max (cmH$_2$O)	7 73.5 ± 5.8	45.6 ± 4.3*
DLPP (cmH$_2$O)	7 69.9 ± 20.7	26.3 ± 7.4*
Qmax (ml/s)	2. 2.5 ± 1.1	6.6 ± 1.7*

DLPP Detrusor leak point pressure, *Pura.max* Maximum urethral pressure, *Qmax* Maximum urinary flow rate. *:$p < 0.05$

dysfunction may occur at any time and be life-threatening. Reducing residual urine, avoiding overdistension, and preventing upper urinary tract damage are considered appropriate management for patients with UAB [9].

For these patients, the gold standard of treatment is intermittent catheterization [10]. However, some young patients do not accept intermittent catheterization but try to excrete urine through manual-assisted urination. Because manual-assisted urination (Crede and Valsalva urination) may cause bladder pressure to exceed the safe range, this method could induce or aggravate upper urinary tract damage and is not recommended [11]. For some patients in stable condition with no upper urinary tract damage and a strong willingness to urinate autonomously, BTX-A injection into the urethral sphincter combined with autonomous urination can be considered. However, long-term follow-up is necessary during the application period.

BTX-A is a pathogenic substance and the most powerful natural neurotoxin in nature. This neurotoxin infiltrates the nerve endings of presynaptic cholinergic neurons, enters neurons through receptor-mediated endocytosis, and catalyzes the decomposition of SNAP-25 protein, promoting the fusion of synaptic vesicles. This cleavage inhibits the secretion of acetylcholine, resulting in temporary chemical denervation and loss or weakening of nerve activity in target organs [3]. Usually, the chemical denervation is reversible. Dykstra et al. first injected 100 units of BTX-A into the external urethral

sphincter to treat patients with spinal cord injury in 1988 [12]. They concluded that the pressure of the urethra and bladder was reduced at the same time.

In this study, 35 patients with UAB underwent BTX-A injection into the urethral sphincter in our hospital. After treatment, the maximum urinary flow rate increased, while residual urine, maximum urethral pressure, and detrusor leak point pressure decreased.

The decrease of maximum urethral pressure and DLPP can effectively alleviate the effect of high bladder pressure on upper urinary tract. In this study, of eight patients with mild hydronephrosis before treatment, three had slight relief and two had resolution 1 month after injection. Fifteen patients still did not completely detach from CIC, but they can partially urinate autonomously and the frequency of CIC was reduced which improved the quality of life.

Although urethral BTX-A injection may increase the risk of urinary incontinence, this side effect gradually decreases as the BTX-A action is lost. The effect of BTX-A on the external urethral sphincter lasts for only three to 4 months, so patients require repeated injections; this negatively affects patient adherence. In this study, we used BTX-A (Prosigne®) to treat UAB. In clinical terms, Prosigne® can achieve satisfactory results in patients with detrusor overactivity, interstitial cystitis, or UAB. It is also inexpensive.

Unfortunately, the limitation of this study is that the sample size was small and heterogeneous. It is not clear how effective the BTX-A was in the subgroup of patients with neurogenic diseases. In the future, we need to increase the sample size to further clarify which subgroup BTX-A was better for.

Conclusions

Prosigne® urethral sphincter injection is a highly effective, minimally invasive, and inexpensive method for the treatment of UAB.

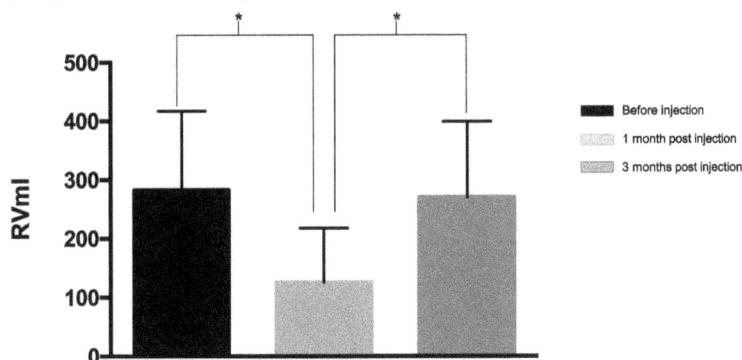

Fig. 1 Residual urine volume before, one and three months post injection. *: $P < 0.05$

Abbreviations

BTX-A: Botulinum toxin type A; DLPP: Detrusor leak point pressure; Pura.max: Maximum urethral pressure; Qmax: Maximum urinary flow rate; UAB: Underactive bladder

Acknowledgements

Not applicable.

Authors' contributions

GC participated in all procedures. He was responsible for data gathering and writing papers. FZ was responsible for data gathering and analyzing. LL was responsible for drafting and guiding work, as well as modifications to the thesis. All authors read and approved the final manuscript.

Author details

[1]Department of Urology, China Rehabilitation Research Center, Beijing 100068, China. [2]Department of Urology, Capital Medical University, Beijing, China. [3]Department of Urology, Baotou Central Hospital, Baotou 014040, China.

References

1. Rasetti-Escargueil C, Lemichez E, Popoff MR. Variability of botulinum toxins: challenges and opportunities for the future. Toxins (Basel). 2018;10:374–87.
2. Jankovic J. Botulinum toxin: state of the art. Mov Disord. 2017;32:1131–8.
3. Domenico T, Marco P. Novel botulinum neurotoxins: exploring underneath the iceberg tip. Toxins (Basel). 2018;10:190–207.
4. Gulamhusein A, Mangera A. OnabotulinumtoxinA in the treatment of neurogenic bladder. Biologics. 2012;6:299–306.
5. Jhang JF, Kuo HC. Botulinum Toxin A and lower urinary tract dysfunction: pathophysiology and mechanisms of action. Toxins (Basel). 2016;8:120–31.
6. Chen G, Liao L. Injections of Botulinum Toxin A into the detrusor to treat neurogenic detrusor overactivity secondary to spinal cord injury. Int Urol Nephrol. 2011;43:655–62.
7. Gao Y, Liao L. Intravesical injection of botulinum toxin A for treatment of interstitial cystitis/bladder pain syndrome: 10 years of experience at a single center in China. Int Urogynecol J. 2015;26:1021–6.
8. Rosier PFWM, Schaefer W, Lose G, Goldman HB, Guralnick M, Eustice S, et al. International Continence Society Good Urodynamic Practices and Terms 2016: Urodynamics, uroflowmetry, cystometry, and pressure-flow study. Neurourol Urodyn. 2017;36:1243–60.
9. Li X, Liao L. Updates of underactive bladder: a review of the recent literature. Int Urol Nephrol. 2016;48:919–30.
10. Li X, Liao L, Chen G, Wang ZX, Lu TJ, Deng H. Clinical and urodynamic characteristics of underactive bladder: Data analysis of 1726 cases from a single center. Medicine. 2018;97:9610–3.
11. Chang YH, Siu JJ, Hsiao PJ, Chang CH, Chou EC. Review of underactivebladder. J Formos Med Assoc. 2018;117:178–84.
12. Dykstra DD, Sidi AA, Scott AB, Pagel JM, Goldish GD. Effects of botulinum A toxin on detrusor-sphincter dyssynergia in spinal cord injury patients. J Urol. 1988;139:919–22.

20

A pilot study to assess the safety and usefulness of combined transurethral endoscopic mucosal resection and en-bloc resection for non-muscle invasive bladder cancer

Yasushi Hayashida[1], Yasuyoshi Miyata[2]*⬭, Tomohiro Matsuo[2], Kojiro Ohba[2], Hideki Sakai[2], Mitsuru Taba[3], Shinji Naito[3] and Keisuke Taniguchi[1]

Abstract

Background: Transurethral resection (TUR) is the standard operation used for non-muscle invasive bladder cancer (NMIBC). Although most solid tumors are principally removed via single block resection without incising the mass, disruption of the lesion is unavoidable in traditional TUR. Furthermore, pathological diagnosis is often difficult due to heat-related denaturation of tissues in TUR. Although transurethral en-bloc resection is useful for judging tumor invasion, it is associated with a prolonged operative duration. We attempted to show the safety and usefulness of combined endoscopic mucosal resection (EMR) and en-bloc resection in NMIBC patients.

Methods: We investigated 39 patients with clinical NMIBC who were treated using our original EMR + en-bloc resection technique, which involved removal of the tumor mass that protruded from the mucosa, using a polypectomy snare similar to that used for EMR. The residual lesion was removed using en-bloc resection. The operative period, duration of hospitalization, and recurrence rates were compared with those of conventional TUR ($n = 31$).

Results: The mean (standard deviation, range) time interval for EMR and total operative duration were 1.6 (1.1, 1–5) min and 18.3 (10.5, 3–48) min, respectively. The total operative duration was comparable to that of TUR (17.3 min, $p = 0.691$). The mean duration of catheterization in the EMR + en-bloc resection group (4.2 days) was also similar to that in the TUR group (3.7 days; $p = 0.285$). No severe complications were observed with EMR + en-bloc resection. The pathologists were able to determine tumor invasiveness with considerable certainty in all specimens obtained via the EMR + en-bloc procedure than via TUR, and the difference in the ease of diagnosis was statistically significant ($p = 0.016$). Recurrence rates were comparable ($p = 0.662$) between the EMR + en-bloc (15.4%) and TUR groups (19.4%).

Conclusions: Our results demonstrated that the EMR + en-bloc resection technique is feasible, safe, and useful for treating patients with NMIBC. Furthermore, this technique helps provide a more accurate pathological diagnosis.

Keywords: Endoscopic mucosal resection, En-bloc resection, Non-muscle invasive bladder cancer, Safety, Outcome

* Correspondence: int.doc.miya@m3.dion.ne.jp
[2]Department of Urology, Nagasaki University Graduate School of Biomedical Sciences, 1-7-1 Sakamoto, Nagasaki 852-8501, Japan
Full list of author information is available at the end of the article

Background

Bladder cancer (BC) is one of the most common urological malignancies in men [1]. Approximately 75–85% of newly diagnosed malignancies that are limited to the bladder mucosa or submucosa are classified as non-muscle invasive bladder cancers (NMIBCs) [2]. Transurethral resection (TUR) remains the gold standard for the treatment of NMIBC. The choice of a radical resection procedure is an important determinant of the outcome in patients with NMIBC. In addition, reaching an accurate diagnosis, especially in the pathologic stage (pT), is important to choose appropriate treatment strategies in these patients. Furthermore, an accurate histopathological diagnosis leads to reduction of overall treatment costs, because an unnecessary second TUR procedure or adjuvant intra-vesical therapy is avoided. Thus, the goal of TUR in early BC is to completely excise visible masses and obtain tissues for an accurate pathological diagnosis of the tumor.

Although TUR is an established and traditional treatment approach, it has various disadvantages. An accurate pathological diagnosis is often difficult because the tumor is removed piecemeal, and the extracted specimens often show morphological changes due to heat denaturation and tissue shrinkage caused by high energy of the resection loop [3, 4]. In addition, some specimens are rendered inadequate due to disorientation and absence of the detrusor muscle tissue. Moreover, although progression rate of NMIBC is relatively low, some researchers are of the opinion that the high number of exfoliated and scattered cancer cells produced during TUR, could lead to metastasis and recurrence due to subsequent seeding and re-implantation [5].

The oncological principle for almost all solid cancers the removal of the tumor via single block resection without incising and cutting into the mass. However, disturbing the tumor mass is unavoidable in traditional TUR. To solve these problems, an 'en-bloc' resection technique was suggested ~ 20 years ago [6]. Currently, there is a general agreement that en-bloc resection of bladder tumors is useful and safe for treating patients with NMIBC [7]. However, an international guideline on NMIBC recommends that only small-sized tumors (defined as those with a diameter < 1 cm) can be resected en-bloc [8]. In addition, en-bloc resection may require a prolonged operative duration, and an appropriate line of resection can be missed due to bleeding associated with large-sized tumors. Thus, en-bloc resection is not usually employed in patients with relatively large tumors.

Endoscopic mucosal resection (EMR) is a well-defined technique used for the operative removal of gastrointestinal masses. EMR has been used to extract precancerous polyps, early-stage malignant lesions in the esophagus and colon, and gastric cancer lesions. Recently, EMR has been reportedly utilized to remove large lesions in the gastrointestinal tract [9].

Therefore, we paid special attention to EMR for the operative treatment of BCs, especially the large-sized tumors. We hypothesized that performing EMR for the raised portion of a BC lesion can shorten the operative time required for subsequent en-bloc resection in patients with NMIBCs. To test this hypothesis, we investigated the operative time period and duration of both catheterization and hospitalization required, while using the EMR + en-bloc resection technique to treat patients with NMIBCs. In addition, we compared the measures of these variables to those associated with a conventional TUR procedure.

Methods
Patients

We received approval for the protocol (including the indication for patient selection), from the institutional review board of the National Hospital Organization Ureshino Medical Center to perform the EMR + en-bloc resection technique in selected patients, and to evaluate occurrence of complications, patient outcomes, and pathological diagnoses in those who were operated using either the combination technique or TUR. Written informed consent was obtained from all patients included in the study. In our hospital, while conventional TUR is performed as a standard procedure for the removal of all tumours diagnosed as NMIBC, en-bloc resection (without EMR) is utilized in patients with ≤3 lesions, each with diameter < 1.5 cm. In this study, we hypothesized that EMR may help reduce the operative duration required for the removal of relatively larger tumours. Therefore, we decided to include bladder tumour diameter ≥ 1.5 cm as the indication for our EMR + en-bloc method. The institutional review board permitted the employment of EMR + en-bloc operative method in patients with ≤3 tumours of diameters ≥1.5 cm, with prior detailed informed consent taken from the concerned patients. Therefore, we provided patients meeting the selection criteria, with in-depth information regarding both EMR + en-bloc and conventional TUR techniques including the surgical method, advantages, predictable complications, and cost of each technique. The combined surgical approach was finally chosen after exhaustive consultations with each selected patient and family, in accordance with the rules established by the institutional review board. Consequently, 39 patients finally underwent the EMR + en-bloc resection between January 2013 and December 2017.

However, for a comparative study of the clinicopathological features, we retrospectively collected and analyzed data of those bladder cancer patients, who underwent TUR and had > 3 tumors, with diameters < 1.5 cm or > 6 cm (the diameter of the largest mass operated using the combination technique). Finally, we included data of 80 patients, who underwent TUR for NMIBC without metastasis (diagnosed clinically), in this study. Those who received neo-adjuvant chemo- and radiotherapy were excluded. The baseline clinicopathological features of these patients at the time of the operation are shown in Table 1. Although this study is not a randomized clinical trial, we found no significant differences in the clinicopathological characteristics between the participants included in the EMR + en-bloc and the TUR groups (Table 1). Patients included in both groups received prophylactic antibiotics (e.g., cephalosporins) pre- and postoperatively.

Surgical technique

Sequential images describing the EMR + en-bloc resection are shown in Fig. 1. Firstly, a section of the target tumor mass protruding from the mucosa, was incised using a polypectomy snare (CAPTIVATOR II, Boston Scientific, Marlborough, MA, USA), similar to the one used in EMR [10]. Along with the polypectomy snare, we also used the monopolar ERBE VIO 300D (Endo Cut Effect 2, Tubingen, Germany) electrosurgical device to perform EMR. However, in this step, our method differed from that used for conventional EMR because, we did not inject a fluid or a gel into the submucosal layer, since pooling of the injected substance in the submucosal region is

difficult due to the anatomical characteristics of the bladder wall [11]. If the tumor was too large to be resected with a single application of the snare, it was used once more to flatten the residual tumor or mucosal tissue. Subsequently, a circular incision was created around the residual lesion using a T-shaped electrode needle TUR-in-saline system (Olympus®, Tokyo, Japan), while maintaining a distance of approximately 5–10 mm from the tumor edge, for subsequent en-bloc resection, similar to the technique employed for endoscopic submucosal dissection of superficial gastrointestinal tumors [12].

In the control group, conventional TUR was performed in 31 NMIBC patients, who were matched with those in the study group, based on factors including tumor diameter and clinical stage. An intravesical instillation of anthracycline antibiotics was performed in these patients in the immediate postoperative period, to prevent the tumor from spreading. Postoperative complications were assessed using the Clavien-Dindo classification [13]. Furthermore, two pathologists (MT and SN) determined the histopathological diagnoses (in all patients), which were used to prognosticate future outcomes. The pathological diagnosis made by each of the 2 observers were the same for each patient.

In this study, all operations were performed by a single surgeon (KT). He had experience in operating over 700 and 30 patients using TUR and en-bloc resection (for small masses) techniques, respectively. However, he had no special training in EMR. Therefore, he was verbally guided by a surgeon experienced in colonic EMR during the operative procedures for the first 3 patients.

Follow-up and outcomes

After TUR, we investigated all patients' cystoscopy and cytology results once every three months for 2 years and then every 3–6 months for 5 years depending on the pathological features. The mean (range) follow-up period of the study population was 26 (9–60) months.

Statistical analyses

The Mann-Whitney U test was used for comparisons involving continuous variables because of the relatively small number of patients. The chi-square test and Fisher's exact test were used to compare categorical data. All statistical analyses were two-sided and performed using StatView for Windows (version 5.0; Abacus Concepts, Inc., Berkeley, CA, USA) software. P values < 0.05 were considered representative of statistical significance.

Results

The tumors in all patients were successfully removed using en-bloc resection, and all extracted specimens were found to include detrusor muscle tissue. The information on the operative procedures is shown in Table 2.

Table 1 Clinicopathological features at operation

	EMR + en bloc	TUR	P value
	n = 39	n = 31	
Gender			0.591
Male	24 (61.5)	21 (67.7)	
Female	15 (38.5)	10 (32.3)	
Tumour			0.148
Primary	36 (92.3)	25 (80.6)	
Recurrent	3 (7.7)	6 (19.4)	
Location of main tumour			0.879
Lateral	14 (35.9)	13 (41.9)	
Posterior	13 (33.3)	9 (29.0)	
Dome	7 (17.9)	4 (12.9)	
Trigone	5 (12.8)	5 (16.1)	
Pathological grade			0.896
Grade 1	12 (30.8)	10 (32.3)	
Grade 2	19 (48.7)	16 (51.6)	
Grade 3	8 (20.5)	5 (16.1)	
Pathological T stage			0.915
Ta	19 (48.7)	16 (51.6)	
T1	18 (46.2)	14 (45.2)	
T2	2 (5.1)	1 (3.2)	

EMR endoscopic mucosal resection, TUR transurethral resection

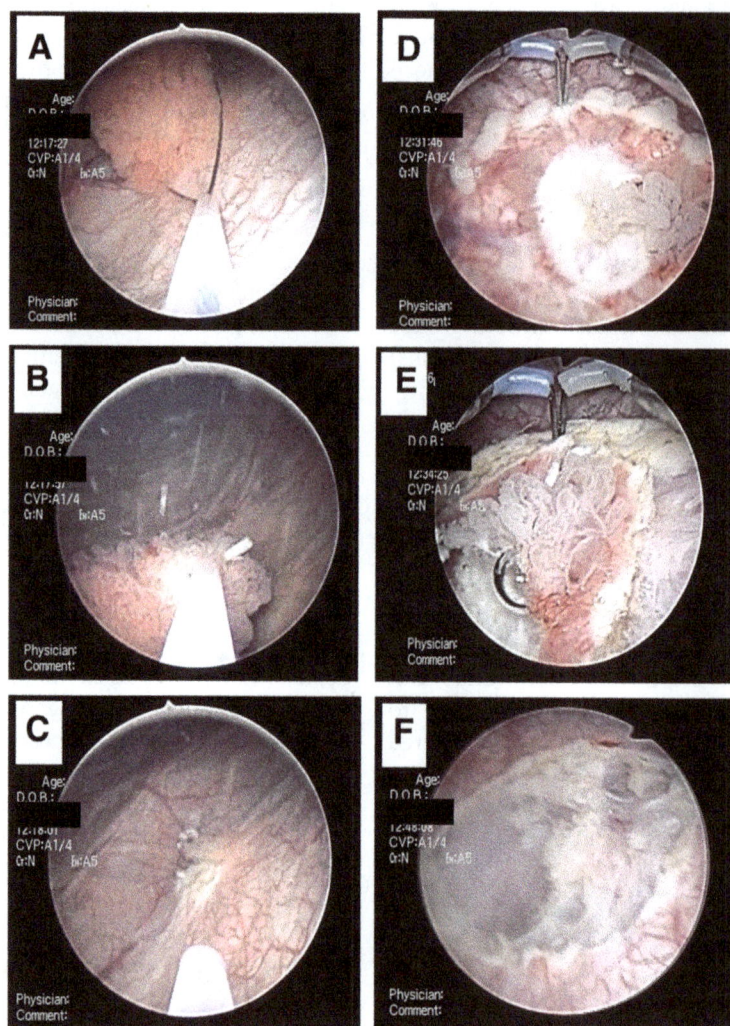

Fig. 1 A description of the surgical technique for performing EMR + en-bloc resection. **a** A snare is inserted at the base of the pedunculated tumor; **b** the snare is placed close to the bottom of the tumor, and EMR is performed; **c** a flat or residual tumor mass is shown; **d** a circular incision is created around the residual tumor, maintaining a distance of approximately 5–10 mm from the tumor edge; **e** en-bloc resection is performed, and **f** the tumor is completely resected. (EMR: endoscopic mucosal resection)

Table 2 Information on operation and hospitalization after operation

	EMR + En-bloc			Transurethral resection			P value
	Mean	SD	Range	Mean	SD	Range	
Age; years	69.7	7.7	55–86	70.5	6.6	53–80	0.635
Tumor number	1.3	0.6	1–3	1.4	0.6	1–3	0.458
Tumor size; cm	2.9	0.8	1.5–5.5	2.6	0.9	1.5–5.0	0.120
Operation time; min							
For EMR	1.6	1.1	1–5	–	–	–	
For en bloc	16.9	10.5	2–43	–	–	–	
Total	18.3	10.5	3–48	17.3	9.5	2–31	0.691
Catheterization: days	4.2	2.3	3–14	3.7	1.4	3–10	0.285
Clavien-Dindo score[a]	N	%		N	%		0.881
1	7	17.9		6	19.4		

[a]Overall postoperative complications postoperative day 0–90. EMR: endoscopic mucosal resection

There were no significant differences in the patients operated using either method, with respect to factors including age at the time of operation, number of tumors, or size of the main lesion. The mean (standard deviation [SD], range) operative periods for EMR and en-bloc resection were 1.6 (1.1, 1–5) min and 16.9 (10.5, 2–43) min, respectively. The total operative duration for the EMR + en-bloc resection and the TUR groups was 18.3 min (10.5, 3–48) and 17.3 min (9.5, 2–31), respectively, which was not significantly different between the two groups ($p = 0.691$). The operative time periods needed for the EMR + en-bloc resection of tumors with diameters $\geq$3.5 cm (28.3%; 11/39 patients) are shown in Table 3. While the total operative time for the removal of a 5.5-cm sized tumor was 41 min, the time interval required for EMR was only 2 min. Thus, EMR was completed within 3 min even for relatively large tumors.

Although the surgeon had no prior experience in EMR, he was able to perform it easily from the first operation, with only verbal guidance. In fact, the median time interval calculated for all EMRs in the 1st–5th, 6th–15th, 16th–30th, 31st–35th, and 36th–39th operated patients, was 2 min. We also show comparative data of the TUR group in Table 3. In the TUR group, 7

Table 3 Operation time in tumor $\geq$3.5 cm

Local of tumour	Tumour size; cm	Operation time; min		
		EMR	En-bloc	Total
EMR + en-bloc				
Lateral	3.5	1	21	22
Dome	4.0	1	21	22
Posterior	3.5	2	42	44
Lateral	4.0	3	10	13
Trigone	5.5	2	39	41
Dome	4.0	2	21	23
Lateral	3.5	1	16	17
Lateral	3.5	1	10	11
Dome	3.5	2	30	32
Lateral	3.5	1	9	10
Dome	4.0	2	5	7
TUR				
Dome	3.5	–	–	19
Lateral	4.5	–	–	39
Lateral	3.5	–	–	28
Posterior	5.0	–	–	31
Lateral	3.5	–	–	23
Lateral	3.5	–	–	20
Lateral	4.0	–	–	21
P value	0.826	–	–	0.470

EMR endosopic mucosal resection, TUR transurethral resection

patients (22.5%) had tumors with diameters $\geq$3.5 cm, and there were no significant differences in the total operative time periods ($p = 0.470$) required for these patients.

With regard to safety assessment, no severe complications, e.g., acute bleeding, occurred during or after the operation in both the EMR + en-bloc and the TUR groups. None of the patients required a blood transfusion. In the EMR + en-bloc resection group, no patient required conversion to conventional TUR. Although a minor perforation (visible fat tissue) occurred in one patient in the EMR + en-bloc resection group, surgical treatment or peritoneal drainage was unnecessary. Total 7 (17.9%) and 6 patients (19.4%) in the EMR + en-bloc and TUR groups, respectively, experienced grade 1 complications as per the Clavien-Dindo scale. However, no patient had $\geq$grade 2 complications. The risk of occurrence of complications was found to be similar across both groups ($p = 0.881$, Table 2). The mean duration of urinary catheterization in the EMR + en-bloc resection group (mean, 4.2 days; SD, 2.3 days) was also similar to that in the TUR group (mean, 3.7 days; SD, 1.4 days; $p = 0.285$).

The pathologists were able to determine the invasive status with considerable certainty in all specimens of patients in the EMR + en-bloc resection group. However, both pathologists commented that determining malignant invasion into the bladder submucosal connective tissues was difficult in 6 of the 31 specimens (19.4%) of the patients in the TUR group, due to heat denaturation. Statistical analysis showed that this difference in ease of diagnosis between both groups was statistically significant ($p = 0.016$). These 6 patients further underwent a second TUR procedure because their tumors were judged as high grade, with or without pT1 (invasion of lamina propria) disease, though residual cancer cells were not detected in such specimens.

After a mean follow-up of 12 months, 6/39 (15.4%) and 6/31 (19.4%) patients in the EMR + en-bloc resection and the TUR groups, respectively, experienced recurrence of the bladder mucosal cancer. Thus, the recurrence rate of NMIBCs was found to be similar across both groups ($p = 0.662$).

Discussion

We demonstrated that the novel EMR + en-bloc resection technique is safe and useful and enables an accurate pathological diagnosis in BCs, though the operative time period and duration of hospitalization required are similar to those observed with conventional TUR. While en-bloc resection has various advantages with respect to diagnosis and treatment of BCs, as compared to those achieved with conventional TUR, it also has its disadvantages, e.g., prolonged surgical duration. Our novel combined approach aimed to solve this main disadvantage of en-bloc resection.

There are various opinions on the suitable tumor size and number of lesions that indicate the need for en-bloc resection. Hurle et al. suggested that patients with a single tumor with diameter < 30 mm and/or those with < 4 lesions are eligible for en-bloc resection [14]. In another study, tumors > 40 mm in diameter were excluded [15]. A tumor diameter > 25 mm has been suggested as a clear contraindication for en-bloc resection [16]. The European Association of Urology guidelines mentioned that small tumors (defined as those with a diameter < 10 mm) can be resected en-bloc [8]. Reports within the past 5 years have shown that the mean diameter of tumors operated using en-bloc resection, was between 1.58–2.63 cm, and the operative duration was between 21.46–58.2 min (Table 4). However, the mean tumor size and operative period for our EMR + en-bloc resection technique were 2.90 mm and 20.0 min, respectively. Based on these results, we suggest that this method can be used to resect tumors more efficiently, as compared with previous en-bloc resection techniques.

Electrical and laser devices have been mainly utilized for en-bloc resection in BCs. After Saito described the utility and safety of laser en-bloc resection of bladder tumors in 2001 [26], other reports have indicated the effectiveness of Ho:YAG or Tm:YAG laser treatment [17–22, 25]. The advantages of en-bloc laser resection include absence of the obturator reflex, minimal intraoperative bleeding, reduced hospitalization period, and lower complications, as compared to conventional TUR [21, 27, 28]. However, laser resection is inferior to electrical resection in terms of availability and medical economics, because, not every hospital has access to laser devices, which also render the treatment expensive. We emphasize that our EMR + en-bloc resection method has a relatively low cost and can be used commonly, as it does not require a special device. Therefore, our EMR + en-bloc method can be employed worldwide, even in developing countries.

A metanalysis showed that en-bloc resection can provide high-quality specimens for the pathological diagnosis of BC [29]. Our study supports this finding because the extracted specimens of the EMR + en-bloc resection group were clearly suitable for the pathological diagnosis. The histopathological diagnosis is one of the strongest determinants of treatment alternatives in further management of BCs, e.g., second TUR procedure or intra-vesical therapy. It is also used to determine the post-treatment follow-up schedule. An accurate pathological diagnosis leads to suppression of the overall treatment costs and reduces the mental and physical burden on the affected patient. The novel EMR + en-bloc resection approach can therefore be included, while planning an optimal strategy for the treatment and observation of patients with NMIBC.

To perform en-bloc resection of large, malignant bladder tumors, several investigators have used various modified methods and employed new devices. Naselli et al. retrieved tumors with diameters ≤45 mm using Collins loop and laparoscopic forceps [30], while Frische et al. reported performing en-bloc resection of tumors ≤75 mm in diameter, using a water jet dissector and needle knife for transurethral dissection [31]. Unfortunately, up to 45 min were needed for tumor resection in the former procedure,

Table 4 A review of literature on en-bloc resection within recent 5 years

Author: device	N	Tumour size; cm	Tumour number	Operation time; min	Reference/Year
E-ERBT					
Kramer: Monopolar	91	2.13 (0.71)	1.48 (0.74)	27.19 (11.96)	[17]/2015
Kramer: Bipolar	65	2.25 (0.71)	1.62 (0.86)		
Hurle	74	1.98 (0.59)[a]	1 (1–4)	–	[14]/2016
L-ERBT					
Liu: Thulium YAG	64	1.31 (0.23)	2.8 (1.2)	48.2 (15.8)	[18]/2013
He: Green-light KTP	45	1.8 (0.8–3.0)	–	21 (12–38)	[19]/2014
Chen: Thulium YAG	71	2.6 (1.4)	1.8 (1.5)	56.5 (37.4)	[20]/2015
Muto: Thulium YAG	55	2.36 (1.47)		33 (14)	[21]/2015
Kramer; Holmium YAG	50	2.63 (0.79)	1.36 (0.56)	29.65 (12.46)	[17]/2015
Kramer: Thulium YAG	15	1.66 (0.73)	2.60 (0.73)		
Migliari: Thulium	58	2.5 (0.5–4.5)	–	25 (12–30)	[22]/2015
Chen: Green-light LBO	83	1.85 (1.07)	1.76 (0.81)	21.46 (10.42)	[23]/2016
Zhang: Vela	38	2.1 (0.8–3.0)	–	23 (15–43)	[24]/2017
D'souza: Holmium YAG	27	1.58 (0.31)	2.5 (1.5)	58.2 (15.8)	[25]/2017

Data were showed as mean (SD or range)

[a]Among 74 patients, 6 underwent a combination of ERBT and TURBT *E-ERBT* electrical en-bloc resection of bladder tumor, *L-ERBT* laser en-bloc resection of bladder tumor, *YAG* Yttrium Aluminum Garnet, *KTP* potassium-titanyl-phosphate, *LBO* lithium triborate

while the authors did not describe the precise operative duration for the latter method. Furthermore, one study evaluated the combined use of electrical en-bloc resection of the tumor (E-EBRT) and TUR to treat patients with NMIBC [13]. In that study, although E-EBRT was performed for single tumor masses ≤3 cm and for those BCs with ≤4 lesions, the en-bloc resection was limited to tumors with ≤3 lesions, and those with diameters ≥4 cm were removed via TUR. However, as shown in Table 3, our EMR + en-bloc resection technique was useful for extracting tumors with diameters ≥3.5 cm. Furthermore, with regard to safety and adverse events, no patient operated using our combined approach required conversion to conventional TUR, blood transfusion, or additional surgical procedures, in this study. Thus, we emphasize that our EMR + en-bloc method has some advantages for resection of relatively larger tumors.

A randomized study of 142 patients showed that there was no significant difference in recurrence rates achieved with en-bloc resection and conventional TUR ($p = 0.383$) [20]. In addition, a multicenter European study of 221 patients, supported this finding [17]. Although our study population is relatively small as compared to those in other studies, we also found a comparable rate of recurrence between patients in the EMR + en-bloc resection and the conventional TUR groups. Furthermore, a previous report showed that the recurrence rates after 12 months were 24.5 and 18.5% for E-EBRT and laser en-bloc resection of the tumor (L-EBRT), respectively [17]. Comparatively, in our study, the recurrence rate observed in the EMR + en-bloc resection group was 15.4% after 12 months. Thus, the recurrence rate of BC observed with our en-bloc resection method was similar to, or even better than that achieved with the L-EBRT technique.

The major limitations of this study include its non-randomized design and the relatively small study-population (which also affected collection of follow-up data). However, we believe that our findings are significant as those of a preliminary study, because this is the first report of the utilization of an original, easily adopted, and cost-effective EMR + en-bloc resection technique that may be used effectively in patients with NMIBC. In addition, this operation was performed by a single surgeon in a single institution, and clinicopathological features were matched between the EMR + en-bloc and TUR groups. Therefore, biases occurring due to surgical technique and patient background were kept to a minimum. However, another limitation was that the pathologists could not be blinded, as they were able to determine the surgical method employed, from the histopathological characteristics of resected tissues. However, this was a retrospective study and the two pathologists were not made aware of the design and significance of the study when they made the histopathological diagnosis.

Furthermore, another limitation is that the health insurance system in Japan differs from those in other countries. Consequently, certain data, including duration of catheterization, were influenced because their costs were covered by this system, which should be considered during data analysis. However, we believe that the influence of such differences is not that significant on our discussion because they were comparable across both treatment groups. Finally, we recommend that further detailed, large-scale research based on the results of this preliminary study are necessary to determine the safety and usefulness of the EMR + en-bloc resection technique in patients with BC. Long-term clinical studies with inclusion of patients with larger-sized tumors are important to determine and improve upon the efficacy and safety of this original operative approach.

Conclusions

Our results showed that the novel EMR + en-bloc resection technique is feasible, useful, and safe for treating patients with NMIBC. In addition, an accurate pathological diagnosis can be reached, using this technique. Further large-scale, multicenter, randomized controlled trials with long-term follow-up, are needed to validate our findings and to improve the long-term outcomes in patients with NMIBC.

Abbreviations
BC: Bladder cancer; E-EBRT: Electrical en-bloc resection of the tumor; EMR: Endoscopic mucosal resection; NMIBC: Non-muscle invasive bladder cancer; TUR: Transurethral resection

Acknowledgements
None.

Authors' contributions
Y-H handled project development, participated in the data collection, and undertook writing of the manuscript. Y-M analyzed data and handled project development. T-M, K-O, and H-S participated in data collection. M-T and S-N handled the pathological analysis. K-T performed the procedures and participated in data collection. All authors have read and approved the final manuscript.

Author details
¹Department of Urology, National Hospital Organization Ureshino Medical Center, 2436 Shimosyuku, Ureshino 843-0393, Japan. ²Department of Urology, Nagasaki University Graduate School of Biomedical Sciences, 1-7-1 Sakamoto, Nagasaki 852-8501, Japan. ³Department of Pathology, National Hospital Organization Ureshino Medical Center, 2436 Shimosyuku, Ureshino 843-0393, Japan.

References
1. Siegel RL, Miller KD, Jemal A. Cancer statistics, 2017. CA Cancer J Clin. 2017; 67(1):7–30. https://doi.org/10.3322/caac.21387.
2. Babjuk M1, Oosterlinck W, Sylvester R, et al. EAU guidelines on non-muscle-invasive urothelial carcinoma of the bladder, the 2011 update. Eur Urol. 2011;59(6):997–1008. https://doi.org/10.1016/j.eururo.2011.03.017.
3. Herr HW, Donat SM. Quality control in transurethral resection of bladder tumours. BJU Int. 2008;102(9 Pt B):1242–6. https://doi.org/10.1111/j.1464-410X.2008.07966.x.
4. Zhang KY, Xing JC, Li W, Wu Z, Chen B, Bai DY. A novel transurethral resection technique for superficial bladder tumor: retrograde en bloc resection. World J Surg Oncol. 2017;15(1):125. https://doi.org/10.1186/s12957-017-1192-6.

5. Engilbertsson H, Aaltonen KE. Björnsson et al. transurethral bladder tumor resection can cause seeding of cancer cells into the bloodstream. J Urol. 2015;193(1):53–7. https://doi.org/10.1016/j.juro.2014.06.083.

6. Kawada T, Ebihara K, Suzuki T, et al. A new technique for transurethral resection of bladder tumors: rotational tumor resection using a new arched electrode. J Urol. 1997;157(6):2225–6.

7. Ukai R, Hashimoto K, Iwasa T, et al. Transurethral resection in one piece (TURBO) is an accurate tool for pathological staging of bladder tumor. Int J Urol. 2010;17(8):708–14. https://doi.org/10.1111/j.1442-2042.2010.02571.x.

8. Babjuk M, Böhle A, Burger M, et al. EAU guidelines on non-muscle-invasive urothelial carcinoma of the bladder: update 2016. Eur Urol. 2017;71(3):447–61. https://doi.org/10.1016/j.eururo.2016.05.041.

9. Heitman SJ, Tate DJ, Bourke MJ. Optimizing resection of large colorectal polyps. Curr Treat Options Gastroenterol. 2017;15(1):213–29. https://doi.org/10.1007/s11938-017-0131-5.

10. Ono H, Yao K, Fujishiro M, et al. Guidelines for endoscopic submucosal dissection and endoscopic mucosal resection for early gastric cancer. Dig Endosc. 2016;28(1):3–15. https://doi.org/10.1111/den.12518.

11. Ro JY, Ayala AG, el-Naggar A. Muscularis mucosa of urinary bladder. Importance for staging and treatment. Am J Surg Pathol. 1987;11(9):668–73.

12. Tanaka S, Kashida H, Saito Y, et al. JGES guidelines for colorectal endoscopic submucosal dissection/endoscopic mucosal resection. Dig Endosc. 2015; 27(4):417–34. https://doi.org/10.1111/den.12456.

13. Clavien PA, Barkun J, de Oliveira ML, et al. The Clavien-Dindo classification of surgical complications: five-year experience. Ann Surg. 2009;250(2):187–96. https://doi.org/10.1097/SLA.0b013e3181b13ca2.

14. Hurle R, Lazzeri M, Colombo P, et al. "En bloc" resection of nonmuscle invasive bladder Cancer: a prospective single-center study. Urology. 2016; 90(4):126–30. https://doi.org/10.1016/j.urology.2016.01.004.

15. Sureka SK, Agarwal V, Agnihotri S, et al. Is en-bloc transurethral resection of bladder tumor for non-muscle invasive bladder carcinoma better than conventional technique in terms of recurrence and progression?: a prospective study. Indian J Urol. 2014;30(2):144–9. https://doi.org/10.4103/0970-1591.126887.

16. Lodde M, Lusuardi L, Palermo S, et al. En bloc transurethral resection of bladder tumors: use and limits. Urology. 2003;62(6):1089–91.

17. Kramer MW, Rassweiler JJ, Klein J, et al. En bloc resection of urothelium carcinoma of the bladder (EBRUC): a European multicenter study to compare safety, efficacy, and outcome of laser and electrical en bloc transurethral resection of bladder tumor. World J Urol. 2015;33(12):1937–43. https://doi.org/10.1007/s00345-015-1568-6.

18. Liu H, Wu J, Xue S, et al. Comparison of the safety and efficacy of conventional monopolar and 2-micron laser transurethral resection in the management of multiple nonmuscle-invasive bladder cancer. J Int Med Res. 2013;41(4):984–92. https://doi.org/10.1177/0300060513477001.

19. He D, Fan J, Wu K, et al. Novel green-light KTP laser en bloc enucleation for nonmuscle-invasive bladder cancer: technique and initial clinical experience. J Endourol. 2014;28(8):975–9. https://doi.org/10.1089/end.2013.0740.

20. Chen X, Liao J, Chen L, et al. En bloc transurethral resection with 2-micron continuous-wave laser for primary non-muscle-invasive bladder cancer: a randomized controlled trial. World J Urol. 2015;33(7):989–95. https://doi.org/10.1007/s00345-014-1342-1.

21. Muto G, Collura D, Giacobbe A, et al. Thulium:yttrium-aluminum-garnet laser for en bloc resection of bladder cancer: clinical and histopathologic advantages. Urology. 2014;83(4):851–5. https://doi.org/10.1016/j.urology.2013.12.022.

22. Migliari R, Buffardi A, Ghabin H. Thulium laser endoscopic En bloc enucleation of nonmuscle-invasive bladder Cancer. J Endourol. 2015;29(11): 1258–62. https://doi.org/10.1089/end.2015.0336.

23. Chen J, Zhao Y, Wang S, et al. Green-light laser en bloc resection for primary non-muscle-invasive bladder tumor versus transurethral electroresection: a prospective, nonrandomized two-center trial with 36-month follow-up. Lasers Surg Med. 2016;48(9):859. https://doi.org/10.1002/lsm.22565.

24. Zhang Z, Zeng S, Zhao J, et al. A pilot study of vela laser for en bloc resection of papillary bladder cancer. Clin Genitourin Cancer. 2017;15(3): e311–4. https://doi.org/10.1016/j.clgc.2016.06.004.

25. D'souza N, Verma A. Holmium laser transurethral resection of bladder tumor: our experience. Urol Ann. 2016;8(4):439. https://doi.org/10.4103/0974-7796.190815.

26. Saito S. Transurethral en bloc resection of bladder tumors. J Urol. 2001; 166(6):2148–50.

27. Zhu Y, Jiang X, Zhang J, et al. Safety and efficacy of holmium laser resection for primary nonmuscle-invasive bladder cancer versus transurethral electroresection: single-center experience. Urology. 2008;72(3):608–12. https://doi.org/10.1016/j.urology.2008.05.028.

28. Kramer MW, Bach T, Wolters M. Current evidence for transurethral laser therapy of non-muscle invasive bladder cancer. World J Urol. 2011;29(4): 433–42. https://doi.org/10.1007/s00345-011-0680-5.

29. Wu YP, Lin TT, Chen SH, et al. Comparison of the efficacy and feasibility of en bloc transurethral resection of bladder tumor versus conventional transurethral resection of bladder tumor: a meta-analysis. Medicine (Baltimore). 2016;95(45):e5372.

30. Naselli A, Introini C, Germinale F, et al. En bloc transurethral resection of bladder lesions: a trick to retrieve specimens up to 4.5 cm. BJU Int. 2012; 109(6):960–3. https://doi.org/10.1111/j.1464-410X.2012.10982.x.

31. Fritsche HM, Otto W, Eder F, et al. Water-jet-aided transurethral dissection of urothelial carcinoma: a prospective clinical study. J Endourol. 2011;25(10): 1599–603. https://doi.org/10.1089/end.2011.0042.

21

Preoperative neutrophil to lymphocyte ratio improves recurrence prediction of non-muscle invasive bladder cancer

Itamar Getzler[1*†] (iD), Zaher Bahouth[1†], Ofer Nativ[1], Jacob Rubinstein[2] and Sarel Halachmi[1]

Abstract

Background: This study aims to prospectively evaluate the ability of Neutrophil-to-Lymphocyte ratio (NLR) to forecast recurrence in patients with non-muscle invasive bladder cancer (NMIBC). This is a continuation of our two previous retrospective studies that indicated the NLR > 2.5 criterion as a predictor of recurrence in patients with NMIBC.

Methods: Since December 2013, all patients admitted to our department for TUR-BT and agreed to participate, had a blood drawn for cell count and differential 24 h prior to surgery. Patients with pathological NMIBC were followed prospectively for disease recurrence. The end-point of the follow up was either a cancer recurrence or the termination of the study. Univariate and multivariate Cox regressions were performed to assess the NLR > 2.5 predictive capability for recurrence, versus and in conjunction to the pathologically based EORTC score, among additional statistical analyses.

Results: The study cohort included 96 men and 17 women with a median age of 72 years. Sixty-four patients (56.6%) have had a recurrence during the study occurring at the median time of 9 months (IQR 6, 13), while the median follow-up time for patients without recurrence was 18 months (IQR 10, 29). Univariate Cox regressions for recurrence demonstrated significance for NLR > 2.5 for the whole cohort ($p = 0.011$, HR 2.015, CI 1.175–3.454) and for the BCG sub-group ($p = 0.023$, HR 3.7, CI 1.2–11.9), while the EORTC score demonstrated significance for the 'No Treatment' subgroup ($p = 0.024$, HR 1.278, CI 1.03–1.58). When analyzed together as a multivariate Cox model, the NLR > 2.5 and EORTC score retained their significance for the aforementioned groups, while also improving the EORTC score significance for the whole cohort.

Conclusion: NLR > 2.5 was found to be a significant predictor of disease recurrence and demonstrated high hazard ratio and worse recurrence-free survival in patients with NMIBC, especially in those treated with BCG. Additionally, our data demonstrated statistical evidence that NLR > 2.5 might have an improving effect on the EORTC score's prediction when analyzed together.

Keywords: Neutrophil-lymphocyte ratio, NLR, NMIBC, urothelial carcinoma, Recurrence, Bladder cancer

Background

Bladder cancer is the most common malignancy of the urinary tract, and the 4th most common cancer in males in developed countries [1]. Upon diagnosis, the majority (~ 75%) of patients with bladder cancer present with non-muscle invasive disease (NMIBC), which by definition includes the Tis, Ta and T1 pathologic stages [2].

As such, NMIBC represents a heterogeneous group of tumors with different rates of recurrence, progression and disease-related mortality. Consequently, each subgroup of NMIBC should be followed up and treated differently [3]. The main concern during treatment of NMIBC is progression to a muscle invasive stage (T2), which dramatically worsens prognosis [4]. To prevent this scenario, clinical and pathological factors are commonly used to categorize patients into different risk groups. These methods, such as the EORTC (European Organization for Research and Treatment of Cancer)

* Correspondence: itamargetzler@gmail.com
†Itamar Getzler and Zaher Bahouth contributed equally to this work.
[1]Department of Urology, Bnai Zion Medical Center, Faculty of Medicine, Technion - Israel Institute of Technology, Golomb 47, 31048 Haifa, Israel
Full list of author information is available at the end of the article

Risk Tables, help physicians predict the probability of progression and recurrence, and ultimately – help decide the most appropriate treatment [3, 5].

However, these grouping systems are far from optimal: would a probability of recurrence of 35% per year justify an aggressive treatment? Is a 15% chance of progression per 1 year a sufficient reason to perform a cystectomy? [5]. Thus, we still lack a strong prognostic factor that could help predict patient-specific risk rather than group-specific risk of recurrence and progression.

According to recent studies cited below, the systemic inflammatory response state triggered by the tumor micro-environment alters acute phase reactants and hematologic components - including changes in serum neutrophil and lymphocyte counts that leads to relative neutrophilia and lymphocytopenia. This state of elevated Neutrophil-Lymphocyte ratio (NLR) is associated with worse disease-free and overall survival in a variety of different malignancies [6–8].

Among patients with bladder cancer, an elevated NLR was associated with advanced stage, increased mortality, and decreased overall survival in patients with muscle-invasive disease [9–11], along with higher risk of recurrence and progression in non-muscle invasive disease [12, 13]. Specifically, in both our retrospective studies which employed different methods of analysis, NLR > 2.5 was found to be a significant predictor of recurrence [12, 13]. Following these results, and in addition to the fact that prospective data regarding the role of NLR in predicting disease recurrence and progression in NMIBC have never been published, the aim of the current study was to prospectively evaluate the role of NLR > 2.5 as a predictor of disease recurrence in patients with primary NMIBC.

Methods

Study design & procedures

This was a single center, prospective cohort study. Recruited patients were pathologically confirmed to have non-invasive BC stages – Ta, T1 and Tis, after undergoing trans-urethral resection of bladder tumor (TUR-BT). Tumors were graded and staged according to the 2004 WHO grading system [14]. Pre-operative NLR was recorded using the admission's (usually 24 h prior to surgery) complete blood count (CBC) with differential. Follow up invitations were sent out every 3 months for urine cytology, upper tract imaging, cystoscopy and treatment based on the American Urological Association (AUA) guidelines [15]. We point out that given the nature of a prospective study design, an intervention that might affect the variables is not desirable, and hence the treatment was chosen according to best practice guidelines and not according to our assumption that NLR may play a role. The end-point of the follow up was

either a cancer recurrence or the termination of the study. Some degree of non-compliance to the follow up and treatment was expected, and so the last date of follow-up was recorded for missing and deceased patients. This study was based on the principles of Helsinki and was approved by the institutional review board.

Objectives

A primary objective of the study was to evaluate the effect of NLR > 2.5 on NMIBC recurrence after trans-urethral resection of bladder tumor (TUR-BT). This effect on recurrence was to be evaluated against the current standard means to predict recurrence, which is the EORTC's prediction table. Secondary objectives were to evaluate the effect of NLR > 2.5 on recurrence, when stratified by different variables including the pathologic grade, stage and the intra-vesical treatment. These objectives were set in advance, and were meant to test the hypothesis that a prediction of recurrence by NLR > 2.5 can be produced prospectively, and not only retrospectively [12, 13].

Participants

Eligible Patients were ≥ 18 years with pathologically confirmed NMIBC who underwent trans-urethral resection of bladder tumor (TUR-BT) since December 2013. An Inclusive approach was taken in order to examine broad and general effect of NLR, not only on some naïve or carefully chosen groups. Key exclusion criteria were: T2 Stage, hematologic malignancies, acute infections, and patients without preoperative NLR. All pathological grades were included.

Statistical analysis

Clinical features between groups were evaluated using Student t-test or chi-square test. Recurrence-free survival was evaluated using Kaplan-Meier survival plots and Log Rank was used to compare between groups. Univariate and multivariate Cox regressions were performed to assess the NLR2.5 predictive capability for recurrence, versus and in conjunction to the EORTC score. The analysis was first performed for the whole cohort, and next stratified by the 'Treatment Type' Groups: 'No Treatment', 'Mitomycin C (MMC)' or 'Bacillus Calmette–Guérin (BCG)', as the treatment choice should affect the recurrence in a meaningful way.

The EORTC Score was calculated in accordance to Sylvester et al. [5]. The tumors' pathological variables are inherently included in the EORTC score, in a way that is already established to be statistically significant. As such, further statistical analysis of the pathological variables is redundant. The results are presented as hazard ratios along with their 95% confidence intervals. A 2-sided P value of < 0.05 was considered statistically significant. Data was analyzed using IBM SPSS v23.0.

Results

Between December 2013 and October 2016, 113 patients were recruited to the study. The cohort included 96 men and 17 women with a median age of 72 years (IQR 63, 81) with a confirmed pathological diagnosis of NMIBC. Sixty-four patients (56.6%) have had a recurrence during the study, occurring at the median time of 9 months (IQR 6, 13), while the median follow-up time for patients without recurrence was 18 months (IQR 14, 30). The median NLR was 2.69 (IQR 1.9, 4.35) including 69 patients (58%) who have had NLR > 2.5. Table 1 shows an analysis of differences in clinical features between groups divided by recurrence. Table 2 shows an analysis of differences in clinical features between groups divided by NLR-2.5.

Similar to our retrospective study, NLR (> 2.5) was correlated significantly with recurrence ($p = 0.003$) but also with age (68 vs 78 years, $P = 0.0001$) and stage ($p = 0.01$). The significant p-value correlation with CIS is irrelevant as only 3 patients had CIS.

Whole cohort Kaplan-Meier survival plot factored by NLR2.5 was then performed and showed a significant difference ($p = 0.007$) in mean recurrence-free survival - (18.6 months vs 26.7 months, Fig. 1). Mean recurrence-free survival of NLR > 2.5 stratified by stage, grade and treatment type (sub-group analysis), showed statistical significance for the Ta Stage ($p = 0.022$, 18.7 vs 27 months), G1 Grade ($p = 0.031$, 17.1 vs 23 months) and the BCG sub-group ($p = 0.013$, 21.3 vs 34.1 months) of 37 patients, Figs. 2, 3 and 4. Sub-group breakdown (i.e Ta stage and T1 stage) is presented as lettered graphs ("A", "B" etc) under each figure. A persistent trend albeit without statistical significance was seen for the other stratifications (T1 Stage, G3 Grade and the other treatment types) in that the NLR > 2.5 groups always fared worse than the NLR < 2.5 groups.

In the univariate, whole cohort NLR2.5 Cox regression for recurrence, NLR2.5 was found significant ($p = 0.01$) with Hazard ratio of 2.029 (CI 1.185–3.472), indicating

Table 1 Patient and tumor characteristics of the study cohort stratified by recurrence

		Patient Groups						P-Value
		No Recurrence			Recurrence			
		Count	Row N %	Median (IQR)	Count	Row N %	Median (IQR)	
Age		49	43.4%	70 (62, 78)	64	56.6%	75 (65, 83)	0.290
Sex	Female	6	35.3%		11	64.7%		0.466
	Male	43	44.8%		53	55.2%		
Grade	1	35	45.5%		42	54.5%		0.765
	2	1	50.0%		1	50.0%		
	3	13	38.2%		21	61.8%		
Stage	Ta	38	46.3%		44	53.7%		0.299
	T1	11	35.5%		20	64.5%		
CIS	No	47	42.7%		63	57.3%		0.409
	Yes	2	66.7%		1	33.3%		
Number Of Tumors	Single Tumor	14	40.0%		21	60.0%		0.885
	2–7 Tumors	29	44.6%		36	55.4%		
	8 or More	6	46.2%		7	53.8%		
Tumor Diameter	< 30 mm	36	47.4%		40	52.6%		0.218
	30 mm or more	13	35.1%		24	64.9%		
Past TCC	No	33	41.3%		47	58.8%		0.480
	Yes	16	48.5%		17	51.5%		
WBC		49	43.4%	7.9 (7.05, 9.66)	64	56.6%	7.71 (6.17, 10)	0.373
NLR		49	43.4%	2.35 (1.7, 3.43)	64	56.6%	2.87 (2.29, 4.65)	0.287
NLR-2.5	Below 2.5	28	59.6%		19	40.4%		0.004
	Above 2.5	21	31.8%		45	68.2%		
Treatment Type	No Treatment	15	34.1%		29	65.9%		0.053
	MMC	12	37.5%		20	62.5%		
	BCG	22	59.5%		15	40.5%		

Table 2 Patient and tumor characteristics of the study cohort stratified by neutrophil-to-lymphocyte ratio (NLR)

		Patient Groups						P-Value
		Below 2.5			Above 2.5			
		Count	Row N %	Median (IQR)	Count	Row N %	Median (IQR)	
Age		47	41.6%	69 (59, 75)	66	58.4%	77 (70, 83)	
Status	No Recurrence	28	57.1%		21	42.9%		0.003
	Recurrence	19	29.7%		45	70.3%		
Sex	Female	6	35.3%		11	64.7%		0.568
	Male	41	42.7%		55	57.3%		
Grade	1	35	45.5%		42	54.5%		0.293
	2	0	0.0%		2	100.0%		
	3	12	35.3%		22	64.7%		
Stage	Ta	40	48.8%		42	51.2%		0.012
	T1	7	22.6%		24	77.4%		
CIS	No	44	40.0%		66	60.0%		0.037
	Yes	3	100.0%		0	0.0%		
Number Of Tumors	Single Tumor	14	40.0%		21	60.0%		0.635
	2–7 Tumors	26	40.0%		39	60.0%		
	8 or More	7	53.8%		6	46.2%		
Tumor Diameter	< 30 mm	30	39.5%		46	60.5%		0.512
	30 mm or mo re	17	45.9%		20	54.1%		
Past TCC	No	32	40.0%		48	60.0%		0.593
	Yes	15	45.5%		18	54.5%		
WBC		47	41.6%	7.58 (6.17, 8.6)	66	58.4%	8.91 (7.05, 10.5)	0.007
Treatment Type	No Treatment	17	38.6%		27	61.4%		0.317
	MMC	11	34.4%		21	65.6%		
	BCG	19	51.4%		18	48.6%		

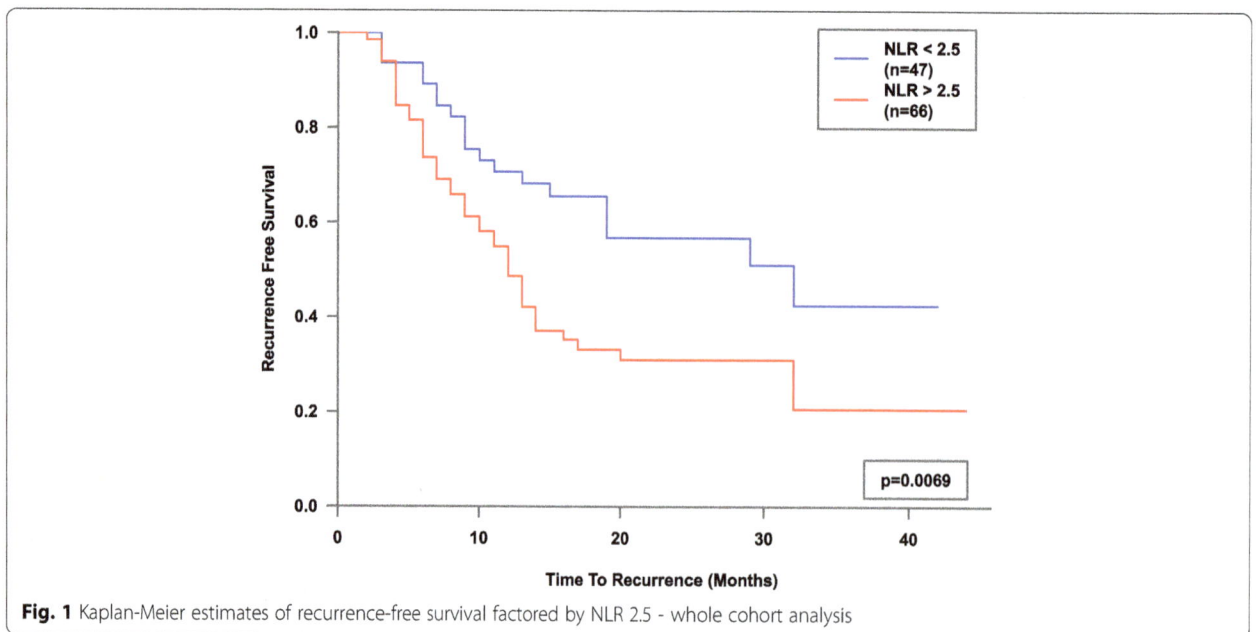

Fig. 1 Kaplan-Meier estimates of recurrence-free survival factored by NLR 2.5 - whole cohort analysis

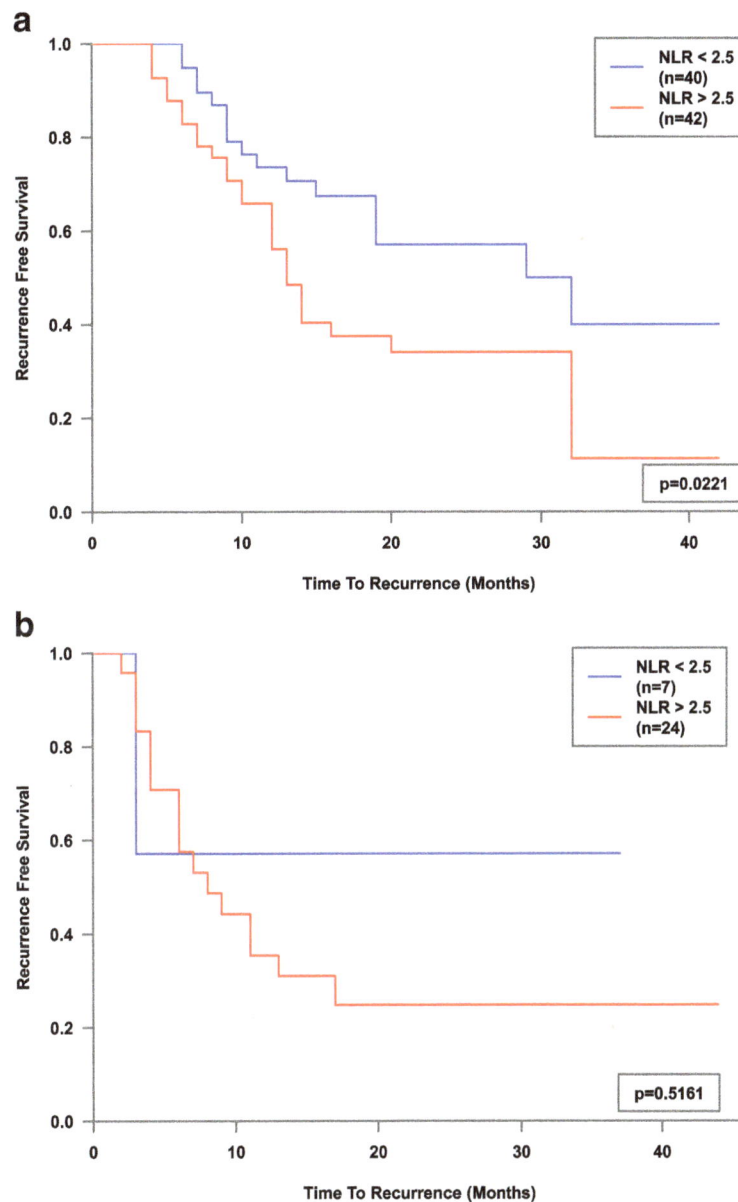

Fig. 2 Kaplan-Meier estimates of recurrence-free survival factored by NLR 2.5 for non-muscle invasive stages Ta (**a**) and T1 (**b**)

that the probability of recurrence is increased at least 2-fold for a person with NLR > 2.5 compared with NLR < 2.5 in this whole cohort analysis. After stratification by Treatment Type, NLR2.5 was only found significant for the 'BCG' subgroup ($p = 0.023$) with Hazard Ratio of 3.792 (CI 1.2–11.9) and not for the 'No Treatment' and 'MMC' subgroups ($p = 0.123$ and $p = 0.96$ respectively). (Table 3).

An identical Cox analysis was then done for the EORTC Score, which resulted in a significance only for the 'No Treatment' subgroup ($p = 0.024$) with Hazard ratio of 1.278 (CI 1.03–1.58), and interestingly not for the whole cohort ($p = 0.132$) or the other subgroups. (Table 4).

When NLR2.5 and the EORTC Score are analyzed together as a multivariate Cox model, the results per subgroups are retained: the EORTC Score is only significant for the 'No Treatment' subgroup ($p = 0.039$) and NLR2.5 is only significant for the BCG subgroup ($p = 0.025$). Although in contrast to the Univariate models, EORTC is very close to significance ($p = 0.058$, HR 1.11, CI 0.996–1.241) when taken together with NLR2.5 ($p = 0.012$, HR 2.098, CI 1.174–3.75). (Table 5).

Discussion

The main advantage of this study is its prospective nature, which to our knowledge, is one of the firsts to deal with

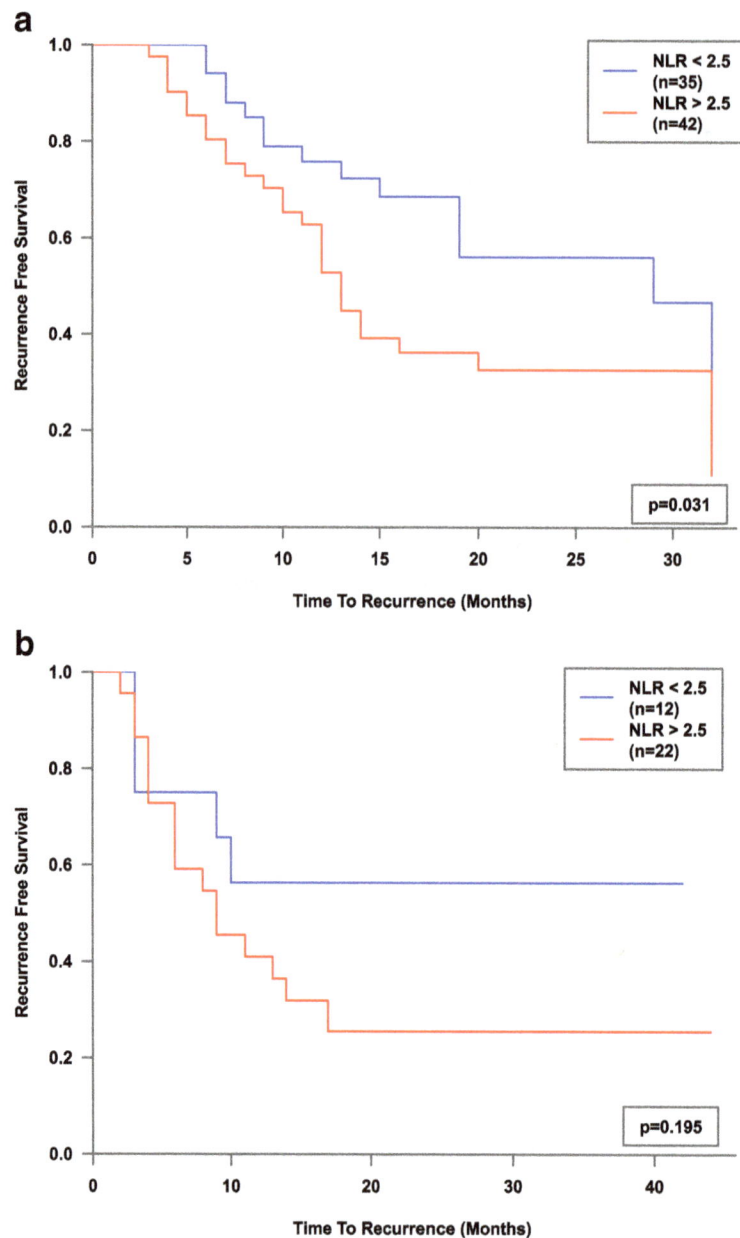

Fig. 3 Kaplan-Meier estimates of recurrence-free survival factored by NLR 2.5 for low (**a**) and high (**b**) pathological grades

NLR as a predictor for NMIBC. Upon diagnosis, NMIBC is initially treated with complete TUR-BT, after which an adjuvant therapy is considered. Based on clinical and pathological factors, patients can be assigned to risk groups, such as the EORTC Score for the assessment of disease recurrence and progression [5]. However, these predictive tools are far from optimal for the individual patient – what is the progression probability cutoff that justifies cystectomy? How aggressive an intra-vesical treatment should be with a 35% risk of recurrence per year? To be able to answer these kinds of questions in a more evidence-based manner, new and novel predictors are a necessity.

In the current study, we prospectively assessed the predictive value of NLR versus and in conjunction to the EORTC score in a group of NMIBC patients. The first main finding for the whole cohort include a statistically significant association between high NLR (> 2.5) and increased probability of recurrence – a finding that manifests in shorter time to recurrence.

In addition, high NLR was consistently associated with worse outcomes in all the sub-groups, although significance was demonstrated only for the Ta Stage, G1 Grade and the BCG treatment group. We believe that given a larger cohort per sub-group, a statistical significance is

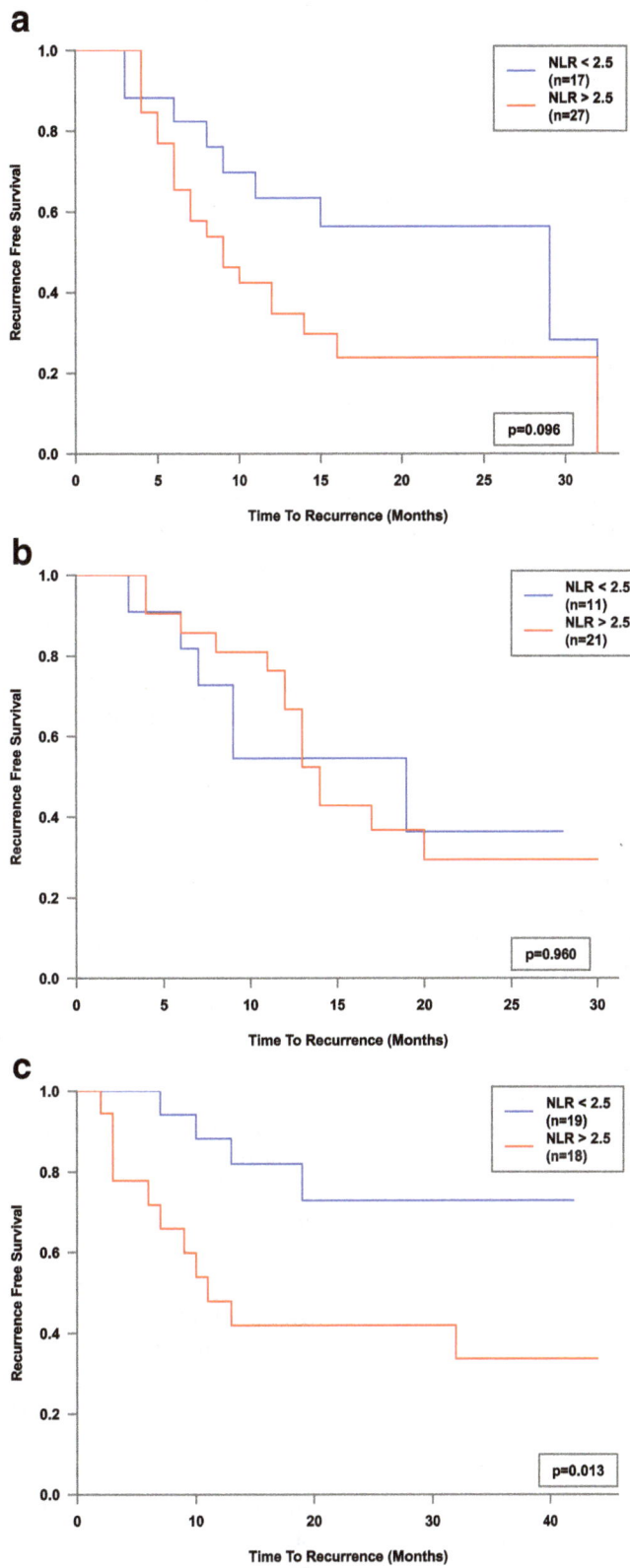

Fig. 4 Kaplan-Meier estimates of recurrence-free survival factored by NLR 2.5 for 'No Intravesical Treatment' (**a**), 'MMC' (**b**) and 'BCG' (**c**) and subgroups

Table 3 Univariate Cox Regression for recurrence using the NLR 2.5 cutoff, stratified by treatment subgroups

Group	P-Value	Hazard Ratio	95.0% CI for HR Lower	Upper
Whole Cohort	0.010	2.029	1.185	3.472
No Treatment	0.123	1.866	0.845	4.123
MMC	0.960	1.025	0.392	2.677
BCG	0.023	3.793	1.203	11.956

probable. Nevertheless, the trend is clear – patients with higher NLR presented with worse recurrence-free survival in each stratification. NLR ratio was more significant in patients who received BCG compare to those who received MMC. We may assume that as an immune modulator BCG has better effect in patients with lower NLR. As this is a new finding arising from a prospective study our aim is to keep on analyzing this subgroup in our next prospective study.

The second main finding is the apparent synergistic effect between NLR (> 2.5) and the EORTC score, as the significance of the score increased substantially when calculated alongside the NLR2.5 variable. The EORTC score was used as a measure of reference, as it has been already established for thousands of patients. However, the EORTC score was never designed to be used when BCG intra-vesical treatment is chosen, as was clearly stated in reference [5]. This limitation of the EORTC score matches our results, as this score is undoubtedly significant for the group that received no treatment, but insignificant for whole cohort which includes the BCG treated patients. Luckily, the NLR > 2.5 is specifically significant for the BCG subgroup, in a manner that complements the EORTC score and improves the overall prediction for the whole-cohort.

While the pathophysiology is not yet clear, it has been suggested that the relative neutrophilia increases the number of inflammatory markers that include pro-angiogenic factors (VEGF), growth factors (CXCL8), proteases and anti-apoptotic markers (NF-kB) – all of which support tumor growth and progression. In addition, the lymphocytopenia is suggested to hurt cell-mediated immune response and thus worsening prognosis [16].

Table 4 Univariate Cox Regression for recurrence using the EORTC score, stratified by treatment subgroups

Group	P-Value	Hazard Ratio	95.0% CI for HR Lower	Upper
Whole Cohort	0.132	1.085	0.976	1.207
No Treatment	0.024	1.278	1.033	1.580
MMC	0.266	1.128	0.913	1.393
BCG	0.934	1.008	0.841	1.207

Table 5 Multivariate Cox Regression for recurrence using both the EORTC score and NLR 2.5 Cutoff, stratified by treatment subgroups

Group	Variable	P-Value	Hazard Ratio	95.0% CI for HR Lower	Upper
Whole Cohort	NLR2.5	0.012	2.098	1.174	3.750
	EORTC	0.058	1.112	0.996	1.241
No Treatment	NLR2.5	0.273	1.673	0.666	4.201
	EORTC	0.039	1.267	1.012	1.587
MMC	NLR2.5	0.640	1.285	0.449	3.682
	EORTC	0.233	1.138	0.920	1.408
BCG	NLR2.5	0.025	3.962	1.193	13.159
	EORTC	0.396	1.086	0.898	1.312

Pretreatment NLR is readily available, and higher values have been shown to correlate with higher stage tumors and adverse treatment outcomes in a wide variety of cancers including malignancies of the gastrointestinal and genitourinary tracts, including urothelial carcinoma of the bladder [6, 7, 12, 13].

Focusing on bladder cancer, several previous studies have evaluated the predictive value of NLR, most of which were conducted on patients undergoing radical cystectomy [9, 17–19]. Based on these studies, NLR may be used in the pre-operative setting to predict tumor invasiveness, or in the post-operative setting, together with pathologic tumor characteristics, to predict outcome. Can et al. found a correlation between muscle invasive disease in TURBT specimens and preoperative NLR > 2.57, patient age, female gender and platelet count, and suggested using NLR > 2.57 in a risk formula which may assist in deciding which patients may benefit from early cystectomy [17]. Similarly, Krane et al. found that patients with a NLR > 2.5 had a significantly higher likelihood of extravesical disease at radical cystectomy, suggesting that they may benefit from neoadjuvant chemotherapy [10]. Finally, Viers et al. found an association between higher pre-operative NLR and significantly increased risk of extravesical tumor extension and lymph node involvement, in a large group of bladder cancer patients undergoing radical cystectomy [9].

Curiously, most of the studies investigating the role of NLR in patients with NMIBC specifically have been retrospective – including our own two previously published articles [12, 13]. To date, only two prospective studies on the matter have been published, after this study's initiation. Favilla et al. further established the predictive value of NLR on recurrence, but did not elaborate regarding the relationship between NLR and the EORTC score [20]. Sebahattin et al. argued that correction for age might alter the results, so a logistic regression analysis (backwards, conditional) of the NLR2.5 and Age as a covariate, was performed. This regression resulted in only NLR2.5 as a significant variable ($p = 0.005$) with Odds ratio of 3.045 (CI 1.392–6.661), meaning that there is an average of at least 3-fold higher probability of recurrence for a person with NLR > 2.5 compared with NLR < 2.5. Age was removed from the model because of insignificance ($p = 0.988$) [21].

Limitations

A prominent limitation dealing with the NLR marker is the volatility of the Neutrophil and Lymphocyte counts. While we did actively exclude patients with hematologic malignances and with active infections, it is possible that some chronic medications or antibiotics affect the NLR value. An argument can be made that this approach might skew results, but as mentioned in the 'Materials' section – we strived to examine the effect of NLR on as much patients as possible, with the intention to generalize, and not marginalize, the NLR usability. We believe that the inclusive cohort in this study (i.e. including a small number of possible antibiotic users) can be regarded more like hurdle rather than a helpful measure, and thus the results are more meaningful. Evidence to this claim can be found on our previous publication, which dealt with a much more 'distilled' cohort [13].

Another limitation of the study is the small cohort per different subgroups. This has resulted in a discrepancy between the literature and our data regarding the known incidence rates of concomitant CIS. A possible explanation can either be attributed to chance, or the notion that many patients with concomitant CIS are discovered already in T2 stage, and thus were not included in this study.

We believe that given a larger cohort per sub-groups such as treatment type or pathological stage, a statistical significance is probable. A larger prospective study may be required to further solidify the place of NLR in predicting disease recurrence in patients with NMIBC and to incorporate it in the current risk calculation tools.

Conclusions

NLR > 2.5 was found to be a significant predictor of disease recurrence and demonstrated high hazard ratio and worse recurrence-free survival in patients with NMIBC, especially in those treated with BCG. Additionally, our data demonstrated statistical evidence that NLR > 2.5 might have an improving effect on the EORTC score's prediction when calculated together. Thus, we propose to consider the incorporation of NLR > 2.5 in the next revisions of the EORTC score.

Abbreviations

AUA: American Urological Association; BCG: Bacillus Calmette–Guérin; CBC: Complete blood count; EORTC: European Organization for Research and Treatment of Cancer; MMC: Mitomycin C; NLR: Neutrophil-to-lymphocyte ratio; NMIBC: Non-muscle invasive bladder cancer; TUR-BT: Trans-urethral resection of bladder tumor

Authors' contributions

IG project development, data collection, data analysis, manuscript writing. ZB project development, data collection, manuscript writing. ON project development. JR project development, data analysis, manuscript editing. SH project development, data collection, manuscript writing. All authors read and approved the final manuscript.

Author details

[1]Department of Urology, Bnai Zion Medical Center, Faculty of Medicine, Technion - Israel Institute of Technology, Golomb 47, 31048 Haifa, Israel. [2]Department of Mathematics, Technion - Israel Institute of Technology, Haifa, Israel.

References

1. Ferlay J, Soerjomataram I, Dikshit R, Eser S, Mathers C, Rebelo M, et al. Cancer incidence and mortality worldwide: sources, methods and major patterns in GLOBOCAN 2012. Int J Cancer. 2015;136(5):E359–86.
2. Babjuk M, Burger M, Zigeuner R, Shariat SF, van Rhijn BWG, Compérat E, et al. EAU guidelines on non–muscle-invasive Urothelial carcinoma of the bladder: update 2013. Eur Urol. 2013;64(4):639–53.
3. Brausi M, Witjes JA, Lamm D, Persad R, Palou J, Colombel M, et al. A Review of Current Guidelines and Best Practice Recommendations for the Management of Nonmuscle Invasive Bladder Cancer by the International Bladder Cancer Group. J Urol. 2011:2158–67. Available from: http://linkinghub.elsevier.com/retrieve/pii/S002253471104506X.
4. Hidas G, Pode D, Shapiro A, Katz R, Appelbaum L, Pizov G, et al. The natural history of secondary muscle-invasive bladder cancer. BMC Urol. 2013;13:23.
5. Sylvester RJ, van der Meijden APM, Oosterlinck W, Witjes JA, Bouffioux C, Denis L, et al. Predicting recurrence and progression in individual patients with stage ta T1 bladder Cancer using EORTC risk tables: a combined analysis of 2596 patients from seven EORTC trials. Eur Urol. 2006;49(3):466–77 Available from: http://linkinghub.elsevier.com/retrieve/pii/S0302283805008523.
6. Chua W, Charles KA, Baracos VE, Clarke SJ. Neutrophil/lymphocyte ratio predicts chemotherapy outcomes in patients with advanced colorectal cancer. Br J Cancer. 2011;104(8):1288–95.
7. Lee BS, Lee SH, Son JH, Jang DK, Chung KH, Lee YS, et al. Neutrophil–lymphocyte ratio predicts survival in patients with advanced cholangiocarcinoma on chemotherapy. Cancer Immunol Immunother. 2016;65(2):141–50.
8. Viers BR, Houston Thompson R, Boorjian SA, Lohse CM, Leibovich BC, Tollefson MK. Preoperative neutrophil-lymphocyte ratio predicts death among patients with localized clear cell renal carcinoma undergoing nephrectomy. Urol Oncol Semin Orig Investig. 2014;32(8):1277–84.
9. Viers BR, Boorjian SA, Frank I, Tarrell RF, Thapa P, Karnes RJ, et al. Pretreatment neutrophil-to-lymphocyte ratio is associated with advanced pathologic tumor stage and increased Cancer-specific mortality among patients with Urothelial carcinoma of the bladder undergoing radical cystectomy. Eur Urol. 2014;66(6):1157–64.
10. Krane LS, Richards KA, Kader AK, Davis R, Balaji KC, Hemal AK. Preoperative neutrophil/lymphocyte ratio predicts overall survival and Extravesical disease in patients undergoing radical cystectomy. J Endourol. 2013;27(8):1046–50 Available from: http://online.liebertpub.com/doi/abs/10.1089/end.2012.0606.
11. Gondo T, Nakashima J, Ohno Y, Choichiro O, Horiguchi Y, Namiki K, et al. Prognostic value of Neutrophil-to-lymphocyte ratio and establishment of novel preoperative risk stratification model in bladder cancer patients treated with radical cystectomy. Urology. 2012:1085–91. Available from: https://www.ncbi.nlm.nih.gov/pubmed/22446338.
12. Mano R, Baniel J, Shoshany O, Margel D, Bar-On T, Nativ O, et al. Neutrophil-to-lymphocyte ratio predicts progression and recurrence of non-muscle-invasive bladder cancer. Urol Oncol. 2015;33(2):67.e1–7.
13. Rubinstein J, Bar-On T, Bahouth Z, Mano R, Shoshany O, Baniel J, et al. A mathematical model for predicting tumor recurrence within 24 months following surgery in patients with T1 high-grade bladder cancer treated with BCG immunotherapy. Bladder. 2015;2(2):e18.

14. Montironi R, Lopez-Beltran A. The 2004 WHO classification of bladder tumors: a summary and commentary. Int J Surg Pathol. 2005;13(2):143–53 Available from: http://www.ncbi.nlm.nih.gov/pubmed/15864376.

15. Chang SS, Boorjian SA, Chou R, Clark PE, Daneshmand S, Konety BR, et al. Diagnosis and treatment of non-muscle invasive bladder cancer: AUA/SUO guideline. J Urol. 2016;196(4):1021–9.

16. Paramanathan A, Saxena A. A systematic review and meta-analysis on the impact of pre-operative neutrophil lymphocyte ratio on long term outcomes after curative intent resection of solid tumours. Surg Oncol. 2014: 31–9 Available from: http://www.elsevier.com/locate/suronc%5Cnhttp://ovidsp.ovid.com/ovidweb.cgi?T=JS&PAGE=reference&D=emed12&NEWS=N&AN=2014201553.

17. Can C, Baseskioglu B, Yılmaz M, Colak E, Ozen A, Yenilmez A. Pretreatment parameters obtained from peripheral blood sample predicts invasiveness of bladder carcinoma. Urol Int. 2012;89(4):468–72.

18. Potretzke A, Hillman L, Wong K, Shi F, Brower R, Mai S, et al. NLR is predictive of upstaging at the time of radical cystectomy for patients with urothelial carcinoma of the bladder. Urol Oncol Semin Orig Investig. 2014; 32(5):631–6.

19. Zhang G-M, Zhu Y, Luo L, Wan F-N, Zhu Y-P, Sun L-J, et al. Preoperative lymphocyte-monocyte and platelet-lymphocyte ratios as predictors of overall survival in patients with bladder cancer undergoing radical cystectomy. Tumor Biol. 2015;36(11):8537–43.

20. Favilla V, Castelli T, Urzì D, Reale G, Privitera S, Salici A, et al. Neutrophil to lymphocyte ratio, a biomarker in non-muscle invasive bladder cancer: a single-institutional longitudinal study. Int Braz J Urol. 2016;42(4):685–93.

21. Albayrak S, Zengin K, Tanik S, Atar M, Unal SH, Imamoglu MA, et al. Can the neutrophil-to-lymphocyte ratio be used to predict recurrence and progression of non-muscle-invasive bladder cancer? Kaohsiung J Med Sci. 2016;32(6):327–33. Available from:. https://doi.org/10.1016/j.kjms.2016.05.001.

22

Relapsed papillary urothelial neoplasm of low malignant potential (PUNLMP) of the young age

Palma Maurizi[1], Michele Antonio Capozza[1], Silvia Triarico[1]* (ID), Maria Luisa Perrotta[2], Vito Briganti[2] and Antonio Ruggiero[1]

Abstract

Background: Papillary Urothelial Neoplasm of Low Malignant Potential (PUNLMP) are exceptionally rare in the first decade of life (mostly if multifocal) and there is a lack of standardized recommendations for the pediatric age.

Case presentation: We describe the case of a 9-year-old boy with a diagnosis of PUNLMP, who underwent to cystoscopic lesion removal and later to endoscopic lesion removal and intra-bladder Mitomycin-c (MMC) instillations for relapsed disease. Follow-up investigations at five years showed disease negativity.

Conclusions: Intra-bladder MMC instillation may allow obtaining the complete remission with bladder-sparing for paediatric patients with a high-risk relapsed PUNLMP.

Keywords: Papillary urothelial bladder neoplasm, Low grade of malignancy, Relapsed disease, Intrabbladder chemotherapy

Background

Urothelial bladder neoplasms are extremely rare in the first decades of life, with an incidence of 0.1–0.4% and less than 35 cases described in children below ten years of age [1–3].

The most typical form of young age is the Papillary Urothelial Neoplasm of Low Malignant Potential (PUNLMP), which is biologically indolent and low tumour grading and staging. Survival at five years of age is reported at about 95% [4].

Multifocal forms are sporadic and there are currently no cases described in the literature in children under ten years. Although these tumours are mostly superficial and low grading, it is difficult to clearly define the aetiology, the invasive potential, the optimal treatment and expected survival [5].

Case presentation

We describe the case of an otherwise healthy 9-y-old boy with a bladder neoplasm, whose clinical history started a year before years with macroscopic haematuria.

The cystoscopy showed the presence at the right ureteral meatus of papillomatous structure (of about 2 cm of diameters), which was entirely removed through transurethral resection (TUR). The histology revealed "urothelial papillary neoplasia with a low degree of malignancy, without infiltration of the sub-epithelial connective tissue", according to the 2004 WHO/ISUP (World Health Organization/International Society of Urological Pathology) classification.

Then, the patient underwent a six-monthly follow-up, with regular clinical and radiologic screening.

However, the ultrasonography of bladder performed one year later revealed a dendriform intravesical tumour of the lateral walls and of the bladder bottom. The cystoscopy confirmed the presence of a multifocal relapse of the disease (Figs. 1a and b). The lesions appeared superficial and not infiltrating, sited at the

* Correspondence: silviatriarico@libero.it
[1]Pediatric Oncology Unit, Foundation "A. Gemelli" Hospital IRCCS - Catholic University of Sacred Hearth, Largo A. Gemelli 8, 00168 Rome, Italy
Full list of author information is available at the end of the article

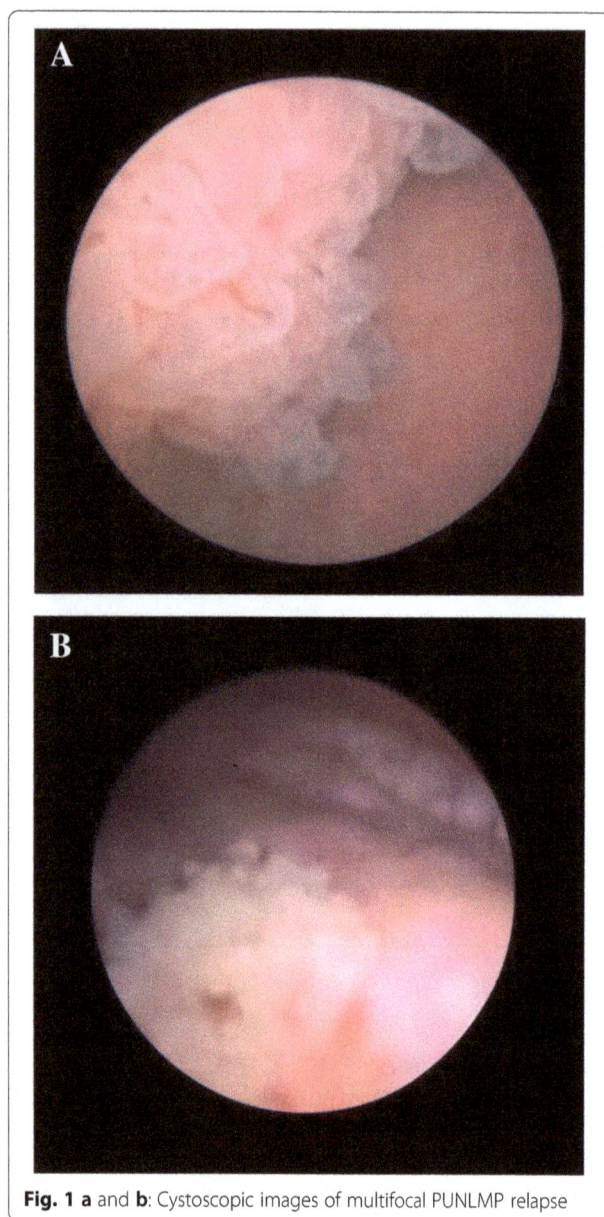

Fig. 1 a and **b**: Cystoscopic images of multifocal PUNLMP relapse

lateral walls and the bladder bottom, with a maximum diameter of 3.5 cm. The histological analysis confirmed the prior diagnosis of PUNLMP.

The computerized tomography with urographic scans (uro-CT) excluded any infiltration of the bladder detrusor muscle and the presence of metastatic disease.

Owing to the clinical history, the histology and the stage of the disease, intra-bladder chemotherapy was adopted. The treatment consisted of a first induction phase comprising mono-weekly intra-bladder instillations of Mitomycin-c (MMC) at a dose of 20 mg for a total of 8 weeks. The cystoscopy performed at the end of the induction phase showed the complete regression of the lesions.

Therefore, maintenance therapy was performed with monthly instillations of MMC at the dose of 20 mg for a

total of 6 months. The treatment was well tolerated, without significant complications.

After a month, we performed a close follow-up with renal function, renal and urinary ultrasound, urodynamic evaluation, which was found normal.

Two months later, chemical and cytological urinary tests and cystoscopy were achieved and the random biopsies of the primarily affected areas resulted regular. A TUR was performed during the cystoscopy performed at one year.

Afterward, the child was examined with chemical and cytological urinary tests every three months, besides the renal and urinary ultrasound, the urodynamic evaluation and the cystoscopy were performed every six months in the next two years.

Currently, at five years from the end of the chemotherapy, clinical and instrumental follow-up checks detect the absence of the disease and normal urinary function.

Discussion and conclusions PUNLMP is a histopathological entity introduced firstly in the 1998 WHO/ISUP classification.

These neoplasms have a high propensity to local recurrence mostly in the adult population (with a risk of relapse between 40 and 70%), with lower recurrence risk (about 13%) in the young population [6].

The treatment varies widely according to the group of risk. The European Organization for Researches and Treatment of Cancer (EORTC) classifies adult patients based on six different prognostic factors: number of lesions and size of the tumour, previous relapse rate, invasiveness of the lamina propria, concomitant presence of carcinoma in situ and histological grading [7]. Another important prognostic factor is the result of the cystoscopy performed at three months after the TUR [3].

Despite the smallness of the cases, the articles published in the last twenty years suggest overlooking intra-bladder chemotherapy after TUR for the paediatric population with PUNLMP. Although this approach, after one year our patient presented a multifocal recurrence with low-grade and superficial lesions, not infiltrating the lamina propria. Because of the features of the recurrence, the patient belonged to the high-risk group and for the multifocality of the lesions, he would have been subjected to radical cystectomy. Although the lack of standardized recommendations for the treatment of multifocal relapsed PUNLMP of the young age, intra-bladder chemotherapy was suggested for saving organ function [8].

The therapeutic options currently available for adult patients include immunotherapy with the Calmette-Guerin bacillus (BCG) and intra-bladder chemotherapy with MMC, Doxorubicin and Epirubicin [9, 10]. Considering the patient's age and systemic toxicity related to BCG therapy, we decided to perform treatment with endoscopic intra-bladder MMC instillations. The therapy was well tolerated, with complete remission of the disease at the end of the induction phase.

Then, we made a close follow-up, because of PUNLMP of young age, even if less rarely than in adults, may present an aggressive behavior in terms of recurrence and invasiveness [6, 11, 12].

Concerning the follow-up, although the absence of shared recommendations, the key-examination remains the ultrasound of the urinary tract, which may reduce the frequency of execution of cystoscopy among the paediatric patients [13]. Conversely, cystoscopy remains imperative and should be associated with urinary cytology in the cases of recurrent neoplasms [1, 3, 14].

Intra-bladder MMC instillation seems a safe and effective therapeutic option for paediatric patients with a high-risk relapsed PUNLMP, allowing to achieve the complete remission of disease and the bladder sparing.

Given the paucity of cases and the lack of treatment and follow-up guidelines, it would be necessary to prospectively validate treatment recommendations and share follow-up programs for pediatric patients with PUNLMP.

Abbreviations
BCG: Calmette-Guerin Bacillus; EORTC: European Organization for Researches and Treatment of Cancer; MMC: Mitomycin-c; PUNLMP: Papillary Urothelial Neoplasm of Low Malignant Potential; TUR: Transurethral resection; Uro-TC: Computerized tomography with urographic scans; WHO/ISUP: World Health Organization / International Society of Urological Pathology

Acknowledgements
Not applicable.

Authors' contributions
PM and MLP made substantial contribution to conception and design, moreover they collected the patient data. VB, AR reviewed the literature and performed the discussion, ST and MAC made analysis and interpretation of data, furthermore they were the major contributors in writing the manuscript. All authors read and approved the final manuscript. Each author participated adequately in the work to take public responsibility for appropriate portions of the content and agreed to be accountable for all aspects of the work.

Author details
[1]Pediatric Oncology Unit, Foundation "A. Gemelli" Hospital IRCCS - Catholic University of Sacred Hearth, Largo A. Gemelli 8, 00168 Rome, Italy. [2]Pediatric Surgery Unit, San Camillo Forlanini Hospital, Rome, Italy.

References
1. Berrettini A, Castagnetti M, Salerno A, Nappo SG, Manzoni G, Rigamonti W, Caione P. Bladder urothelial neoplasms in pediatric age: Experience at three tertiary centers. J Pediatr Urol. 2015;11:26.e1e26.e5.
2. Stanton ML, Xiao L, Czerniak BA, Guo CC. Urothelial tumors of the urinary bladder in young patients: a clinicopathologic study of 59 cases. Arch Pathol Lab Med. 2013;137(10):1337–41.
3. Paner GP, Zehnder P, Amin AM, Husain AN, Desai MM. Urothelial neoplasms of the urinary bladder occurring in young adult and pediatric patients: a comprehensive review of literature with implications for patient management. Adv Anat Pathol. 2011;18:79–89. https://doi.org/10.1097/PAP.0b013e318204c0cf.
4. Alanee S, Shukla AR. Bladder malignancies in children aged <18 years: results from the surveillance, epidemiology and end results database. BJU Int. 2009;106:557e60.
5. McGuire EJ, Weiss RM, Baskin AM. Neoplasms of transitional cell origin in first twenty years of life. Urology. 1973;1:57e9.
6. Fine SW, Humphrey PA, Dehner LP, Amin MB, Epstein J. Urothelial neoplasms in patients 20 years or younger: a clinicopathological analysis using the world health organization 2004 bladder consensus classification. J Urol. 2005;174:1976e80.
7. Sylvester RJ, van der Meijden AP, Oosterlinck W, et al. Predicting recurrence and progression in individual patients with stage ta T1 bladder cancer using EORTC risk tables: a combined analysis of 2596 patients from seven EORTC trials. Eur Urol. 2006;49:466–5.
8. Di Carlo D, Ferrari A, Perruccio K, D'Angelo P, Fagnani AM, Cecchetto G, Bisogno G. Management and follow-up of urothelial neoplasms of the bladder in children: a report from the TREP project. Pediatr Blood Cancer. 2005;62:1000–3.
9. Resnick MJ, Bassett JC, Clark PE. Management of superficial and muscle-invasive urothelial cancers of the bladder. Curr Opin Oncol. 2013;25:281–8.
10. Sternberg C. Linee guida Carcinoma della Vescica, AIOM. 2017. http://media.aiom.it/userfiles/files/doc/LG/2017_LGAIOM_Urotelio.pdf.
11. Migaldi M, Rossi G, Maiorana A, et al. Superficial papillary urothelial carcinomas in young and elderly patients: a comparative study. BJU Int. 2004;94:311e65.
12. Yossepowitch O, Dalbagni G. Transitional cell carcinoma of the bladder in young adults: presentation, natural history and outcome. J Urol. 2002;168:61e6.
13. Hoenig DM, McRae S, Chen SC, Diamond DA, Rabinowitz R, Caldamone AA. Transitional cell carcinoma of the bladder in the pediatric patient. J Urol. 1996;156:203–5.
14. Lerena J, Krauel L, Garcia-Aparicio L, Vallasciani S, Suñol M, Rodó J. Transitional cell carcinoma of the bladder in children and adolescents: six case series and review of the literature. J Pediatr Urol. 2010;6:481–5.

23

The long-term efficacy of one-shot neoadjuvant intra-arterial chemotherapy combined with radical cystectomy versus radical cystectomy alone for bladder cancer: a propensity-score matching study

Wasilijiang Wahafu[1], Sai Liu[1], Wenbin Xu[3], Mengtong Wang[1], Qingbao He[1], Liming Song[1], Mingshuai Wang[1], Feiya Yang[1,2], Lin Hua[3], Yinong Niu[1*] and Nianzeng Xing[1,2*]

Abstract

Background: Bladder cancer is a complex disease associated with high morbidity and mortality. Management of bladder cancer before radical cystectomy continues to be controversial. We compared the long-term efficacy of one-shot neoadjuvant intra-arterial chemotherapy (IAC) versus no IAC (NIAC) before radical cystectomy (RC) for bladder cancer.

Methods: We performed a retrospective review of patients who underwent either one-shot IAC or NIAC before RC between October 2006 and November 2015. A propensity-score matching (1:3) was performed based on key characters. The Kaplan-Meier method was utilized to estimate survival probabilities, and the log-rank test was used to compare survival outcomes between different groups. A multivariable Cox proportional hazard model was used to estimate survival outcomes.

Results: Twenty-six patients were treated using IAC before RC, and 123 NIAC patients also underwent RC. After matching, there was no significant difference between groups in baseline characteristics, perioperative variables, complication outcomes or tumor characteristics. Compared with clinical tumor stages, pathological tumor stages demonstrated a significant decrease ($P = 0.002$) in the IAC group. There was no significant difference in overall survival (OS, $p = 0.354$) or cancer-specific survival (CSS, $p = 0.439$) between the groups. Among all patients, BMI significantly affected OS ($p = 0.004$), and positive lymph nodes (PLN) significantly affected both OS ($p < 0.001$) and CSS ($p = 0.010$).

Conclusions: One-shot neoadjuvant IAC before RC shows safety and tolerability and provides a significant advantage in pathological downstaging but not in OS or CSS. Further study of neoadjuvant combination therapeutic strategies with RC is needed.

Keywords: Bladder cancer, Neoadjuvant chemotherapy, Intra-arterial infusion, Cystectomy, Treatment outcome

* Correspondence: 18601020160@163.com; nianzengxing@yeah.net
[1]Institute of Urology, Capital Medical University, Department of Urology,
Capital Medical University Beijing Chao-Yang Hospital, Beijing 100020, China
Full list of author information is available at the end of the article

Background

Bladder cancer is a complex disease associated with high morbidity and mortality rates. Approximately 75% of newly diagnosed patients present with non-muscle-invasive bladder cancer (MIBC), which is characterized by a high recurrence rate and 5-yr survival of ~ 90% [1]. Once the disease becomes MIBC, the 5-year overall survival is a dismal outcome at 47% compared with the 81% survival rate of patients with non-muscle-invasive disease [2]. Approximately 50% of MIBC patients will develop metastasis and have a 5-yr survival of only ~ 5% [3, 4]. Despite radical cystectomy (RC) with bilateral pelvic lymph node dissection (PLND) as the gold standard treatment, RC only permits a 5-yr survival in approximately 50% of patients [3, 5–8]. In fact, there was no significant improvement in bladder cancer outcomes over the last three decades.

Although several high-quality clinical trials have demonstrated improved survival and pathologic downstaging with the use of chemotherapy prior to RC, adoption of neoadjuvant chemotherapy for MIBC has been slow. Several hypotheses, such as the significant toxicities and delayed surgery, especially the inability to identify which patients could derive the most benefit from neoadjuvant chemotherapy, were slow during the adoption of neoadjuvant treatment. Additionally, 25 to 33% of patients are unable to receive adjuvant chemotherapy after RC due to postoperative problems, such as perioperation complications or deterioration of renal function [9, 10]. Therefore, we hypothesized that one-shot neoadjuvant intra-arterial chemotherapy (IAC) would have less toxicity and better disease control than RC alone. Moreover, this strategy would allow patients to complete therapy quickly and move on to the next form of therapy.

Therefore, we compared the long-term efficacy of one-shot neoadjuvant IAC versus no IAC (NIAC) before RC for bladder cancer in this study.

Methods

To evaluate the long efficacy of one-shot neoadjuvant IAC versus NIAC before RC for bladder cancer, we retrospectively reviewed all patients treated with RC/PLND between October 2006 and November 2015 for urothelial carcinoma of the bladder without distant metastasis in the Department of Urology, Beijing Chao-Yang Hospital. This study was approved by the Institutional Review Board of Beijing Chao-Yang Hospital. To prevent selection bias of the learning curve, we chosen patients who operations were performed by the same laparoscopic surgeon (Xing).

Patient eligibility and selection

The diagnosis of bladder cancer was made using imaging findings (ultrasonography, computed tomography, magnetic resonance imaging), chest radiography with or without cystoscopic biopsy, and routine laboratory analysis. The TNM classification was staged according to the American Joint Committee on Cancer staging system (7th 2010). Clinical staging was based on the physical examination, imaging findings, and biopsies of bladder tumors before the start of therapy. All patients had pathologic documentation of urothelial carcinoma, which was defined as local disease (pT2-4 N0/+M0) or non-muscle-invasive bladder cancer (NMIBC), but the patients were at high risk for tumors [T1G3 with concurrent carcinoma in situ (CIS) at diagnosis, multiple and/or large T1G3, recurrent T1G3]. The pathological results were reviewed by the two genitourinary pathologists after matching the two groups. Patient with pelvic lymph node metastasis diagnosed by imaging studies were eligible. Patients who underwent neoadjuvant intravesicle chemotherapy but not adjuvant chemotherapy were ineligible. Patients who had nonurothelial carcinoma ($n = 11$), preoperative pelvic irradiation ($n = 5$), missing clinical information (n = 11) or who were lost during follow-up ($n = 17$) were excluded, leaving 149 patients available for analysis.

IAC treatment protocol

Gemcitabine (700–1000 mg/m^2) and cisplatin (35–70 mg/m^2) were infused into the femoral artery to the internal iliac artery using the Seldinger technique. The approach of 15 patients was from the bilateral internal iliac artery, while the unilateral internal iliac artery was used in 11 patients, and the approach was based on tumor location as determined by imaging tests, cystoscopy and digital subtraction angiography. Complete blood counts and biochemical studies were performed every 2 weeks. Patients were evaluated for treatment responses using imaging tests and were assigned to receive RC/PLND 4 weeks after IAC to allow adequate recovery.

Statistical analysis

Baseline comparison between the intra-arterial and no intra-arterial groups

Key baseline characteristics [gender, age, Body mass index (BMI), hypertension, diabetes, age-adjusted Charlson comorbidity index (CCI), American Society of Anesthesiologists (ASA) score, Eastern Cooperative Oncology Group performance status (ECOG PS), smoking history, time between tumor confirmation and RC, preoperative irradiations, and follow-up duration)]were compared between the IAC and NIAC groups.

Continuous characters were compared by independent sample t-tests when the data were normally distributed and by Wilcoxon rank sum test when the data were nonnormally distributed. The Pearson chi-square test or Fisher's exact test was performed to calculate p values for categorical factors. The Wilcoxon rank sum test was performed to compare ordinal values.

Propensity-score matching

We performed matched group analysis to control for differences between groups due to selection bias and confounding factors. Propensity-score matching was performed based on key characters, including gender, age, BMI, hypertension, diabetes, age-adjusted CCI, ASA score, ECOG PS, smoking history, time between tumor confirmation and RC, preoperative irradiations and follow-up duration. Propensity scores were estimated using a logistic regression model. A 1:3 matching with no replacement was applied using the nonrandom package in R (http://www.r-project.org). A t-test or Wilcoxon rank sum test, or Pearson's chi-square test or Fisher's exact test, was applied to compare differences in covariates after matching to demonstrate that matching enhanced the balance between groups.

Oncological outcomes in the matched group

We compared oncological outcomes in a matched cohort using a t-test, a Wilcoxon rank sum test, Pearson's chi-square tests and Fisher's exact test. The Kaplan-Meier method was utilized to estimate survival probabilities, and the log-rank test was used to compare survival outcomes between different groups. A multivariable Cox proportional hazard model was used to estimate survival outcomes.

All statistical analyses, except for propensity-score matching, were performed with IBM SPSS version 19.0 (IBM corp., Armonk, NY). Statistical significance was considered at two-sided $p < 0.05$. All statistical plots were drawn in GraphPad prism version 6.0 (GraphPad Software Inc., La Jolla, CA 92037 USA).

Results

A total of 26 patients underwent one-shot neoadjuvant IAC, and 123 patients were treated using RC/PLND alone. The baseline characteristics of patients enrolled are listed in Table 1. All key variables except follow-up duration (88 mo vs 26 mo, $p = 0.002$) were not different at baseline between the two groups. To reduce the differences between groups due to selection bias, we performed a matched analysis based on follow-up duration Additional file 2 Figure S1.

The matching algorithm was 1:3, which was the optimal weight for each key variable. The patients were followed up for a median period of 88 months in the IAC group and for 56 months in the NIAC group ($p = 0.161$). There were no significant differences between the groups in patient demographics and clinical characteristics. Table 1 lists the baseline characteristics for the matched cohorts.

There was no significant difference in perioperative variables between the IAC and NIAC groups (Table 2). In the type of urinary diversion, more than 50% of patients received orthotopic neobaldders in both groups. IAC treatment did not affect renal function in terms of serum creatinine ($P = 0.702$) or blood urea nitrogen ($P = 0.119$) levels. The proportion of those who remained in

Table 1 Baseline characteristics of the patients in the IAC and NIAC before and after matched groups (1:3)

	Intra-arterial	Before matched groups		After matched groups (1:3)	
		No intra-arterial	p value	No intra-arterial	p value
Patients (n)	26	123		78	
Gender			1.000		1.000
Female, n (%)	4(15.4%)	19(15.4%)		10(12.8%)	
Male, n (%)	22(84.6%)	104(84.6%)		68(87.2%)	
Age, yr, median (IQR)	60.0(55.0–71.0)	63.0(56.0–72.0)	0.328	62.5(56.0–69.3)	0.799
Body mass index (kg/m2)	25.2 ± 3.12	24.1 ± 3.8	0.184	24.3 ± 3.1	0.202
Hypertension, n (%)	12(46.2%)	38(30.9%)	0.134	27(34.6%)	0.293
Diabetes, n (%)	4(15.4%)	16(13.0%)	0.995	8(10.3%)	0.723
Age-adjusted CCI	4.0(3.0–7.0)	4.0(3.0–5.0)	0.625	4.0(3.0–6.0)	0.909
ASA score	2.0(1.8–2.0)	2.0(2.0–2.0)	0.221	2.0(2.0–2.0)	0.188
ECOG PS	1.0(0.0–1.0)	1.0(0.0–1.0)	0.490	1.0(1.0–1.0)	0.394
Smoking history, n (%)	15(57.7%)	58(47.2%)	0.329	40(51.3%)	0.571
Time between confirmed tumor and RC, mo, median (IQR)	3.0(1.0–6.8)	5.0(1.0–18.0)	0.133	5.0(1.0–18.0)	0.173
TURBT before RC	7(25.9%)	57(46.3%)	0.048	32(41.0%)	0.100
Preoperative irradiation, n (%)	0(0.0%)	5(4.1%)	0.587	3(3.8%)	0.571
Follow-up length, mo, median (IQR)	88.0(37.0–109.0)	26.0(14.0–65.0)	0.002	56.0(30.8–91.3)	0.161

IAC, intra-arterial chemotherapy; NIAC, no-intra-arterial chemotherapy; IQR = interquartile range; RC = radical cystectomy; ASA = American Society of Anesthesiologists; CCI = Charlson comorbidity index; ECOG PS = Eastern Cooperative Oncology Group performance status

Table 2 Perioperative variables of the matched groups

	Intra-arterial	No Intra-arterial	p value
Patients (n)	26	78	
Type of urinary diversion, n (%)			0.840
Cutaneous ureterostomy	2(7.7%)	5(6.4%)	
Ileal conduit	9(34.6%)	32(41.0%)	
Orthotopic neobladder	15(57.7%)	41(52.6%)	
Operating time, min, mean (IQR)	369.0(300.0–420.0)	382.9(306.0–420.0)	0.574
Estimated blood loss, ml, mean (IQR)	411.5(187.5–525.0)	348.1(200.0–400.0)	0.456
Removed Jackson-Pratt drain, day, mean (IQR)	12.6(9.0–14.3)	14.7(8.0–19.0)	0.591
Passing flatus, day, mean (IQR)	4.9(3.0–6.0)	4.0(3.0–5.0)	0.189
Adjuvant chemotherapy, n (%)	4(15.4%)	12(15.4%)	1.000
Pre-op laboratory studies			
HGB (g/L), median (IQR)	134.0(122.3–142.3)	132.5(119.8–146.3)	0.943
HCT (%), median (IQR)	38.6(36.9–41.5)	39.8(36.1–42.4)	0.615
WBC, median (IQR)	6.4(5.0–7.6)	6.5(5.3–7.8)	0.286
Platelets, median (IQR)	218.5(193.0–262.5)	216.5(187.3–258.5)	0.768
BUN(mmol/L), median (IQR)	5.7(4.7–7.0)	6.1(4.6–8.0)	0.119
Creatinine(μmol/L), median (IQR)	84.2(70.3–113.5)	82.2(70.1–99.9)	0.702
Albumin (g/L), median (IQR)	35.1(32.8–39.0)	36.0(33.0–39.9)	0.931
Overall complications, n (%), Clavien grade	24(92.3%)	75(96.2%)	0.791
Perioperative complications (< 30 d), n (%),			0.930
0	2(7.7%)	3(3.8%)	
1	0(0.0%)	2(2.6%)	
2	21(80.8%)	66(84.6%)	
3	3(11.5%)	5(6.4%)	
4	0(0.0%)	0(0.0%)	
Short-term complications (< 90 d), n (%)			0.516
0	24(92.3%)	68(87.2%)	
1	0(0.0%)	4(5.1%)	
2	1(3.8%)	3(3.8%)	
3	1(3.8%)	3(3.8%)	
4	0(0.0%)	0(0.0%)	
Long-term complications (>90 d), n (%)			0.616
0	24(92.3%)	74(94.9%)	
1	0(0.0%)	0(0.0%)	
2	0(0.0%)	0(0.0%)	
3	1(3.8%)	3(3.8%)	
4	1(3.8%)	1(1.3%)	
Surgery intensive care unit stay, n (%)	0(0.0%)	8(10.3%)	0.196

IQR = interquartile range; HGB = hemoglobin; HCT = hematocrit; WBC = white blood cell; BUN = blood urea nitrogen

the intensive care unit after surgery was lower in the IA group than in the NIAC group (0% vs 10.3%; $p = 0.196$). The total complication rate was not significantly different between the two groups (92.3% vs 96.2%; $p = 0.791$). However, Clavien grade 2 complications (>80%) were more common in the perioperative period (< 30 d).

Tumor characteristics are listed in Table 3. The pathology results of all patients showed urothelial cell carcinoma of the urinary bladder. Positive surgical margins were reported in the NIAC group (3.8%). Compared with clinical TNM stages, pathological TNM staging demonstrated similar in the NIAC group after matching

Table 3 Tumor characteristics of the matched groups

	Intra-arterial	No intra-arterial	p value
Patients (n)	26	78	
Pathologic stage outcome, n (%)			0.414
pT1	9(34.6%)	26(33.3%)	
pT2a	6(23.1%)	11(14.1%)	
pT2b	1(3.8%)	14(17.9%)	
pT3a	6(23.1%)	11(14.1%)	
pT3b	3(11.5%)	3(3.8%)	
pT4a	1(3.8%)	13(16.7%)	
Histology grade, n (%)			0.566
Low grade	6(23.1%)	14(17.9%)	
High grade	20(76.9%)	64(82.1%)	
Pathology, n (%)			0.399
Urothelial cancer	21(80.8%)	71(91.0%)	
Urothelial cancer with squamous differentiation	3(11.5%)	4(5.1%)	
Urothelial cancer with glandular differentiation	2(7.7%)	3(3.8%)	
Nodes removed, median (IQR)	17.0(11.8–21.3)	14.0(8.0–19.0)	0.304
PLN, median (range)	0.0(6.0)	0.0(27.0)	0.904
Lymph-node-positive patients, n (%)	7(26.9%)	18(23.1%)	0.691
Positive surgical margins, n (%)	0(0.0%)	3(3.8%)	0.571
Associated CIS, no. (%)	4(15.4%)	12(15.4%)	1.000

IQR = interquartile range; CIS = carcinoma in situ; PLN = positive lymph nodes

($P = 0.519$, Additional file 1 Table S1 and Additional file 2 Figure S2); however, a significant decrease showed in the IAC group ($P = 0.002$): 7 (26.9%) patients had no stage change, 17 (65.4%) patients exhibited a stage decrease, and 2 (7.7%) patients exhibited a stage increase (Additional file 1 Table S2 and Additional file 2 Figure S3). There was one patient with severe gross hematuria that was diagnosed as NMIBC by CT. Conservative measures and attempts to achieve hemostasis by cystoscopy were unsuccessful at controlling bleeding. The patient therefore underwent endovascular treatment with intra-arterial chemotherapy and

superselective embolization of the vesical arteries 2 weeks before RC/PLND.

Of the 26 patients in the IAC group, two (7.7%) died because of cancer, and one (3.8%) died due to another reason. Among the 78 patients in the NIAC group, eleven (14.1%) suffered cancer-specific mortality, and five (6.4%) died due to another reason. There was no significant difference in the rates along the curve for overall mortality ($p = 0.354$) or cancer-specific mortality ($p = 0.439$) between the IAC and NIAC groups (Fig. 1).

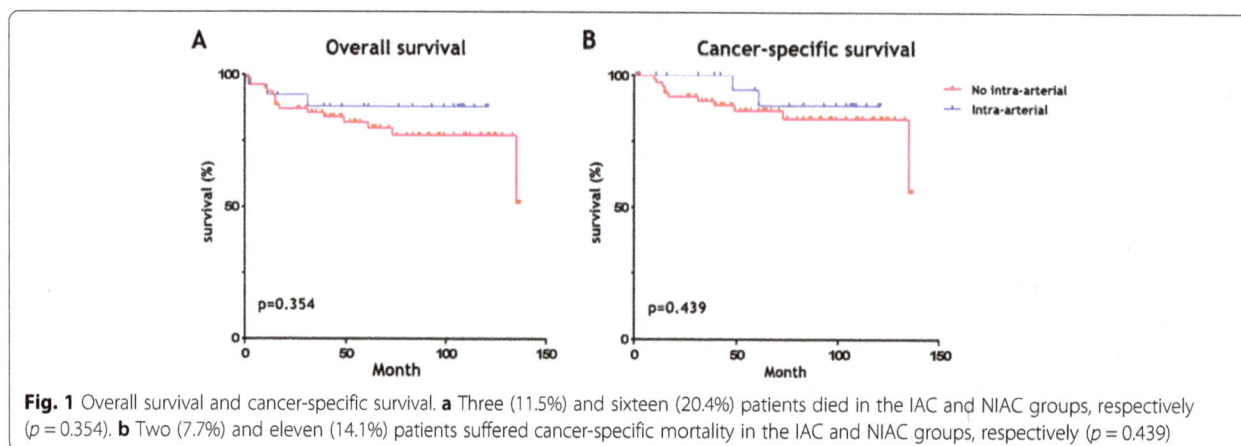

Fig. 1 Overall survival and cancer-specific survival. **a** Three (11.5%) and sixteen (20.4%) patients died in the IAC and NIAC groups, respectively ($p = 0.354$). **b** Two (7.7%) and eleven (14.1%) patients suffered cancer-specific mortality in the IAC and NIAC groups, respectively ($p = 0.439$)

Multivariable Cox proportional hazards regression analysis (Table 4) showed that several variables have an impact on overall survival. In all samples, BMI ($p = 0.005$), diabetes ($p = 0.002$), ASA score (p = 0.005), PLN (p<0.001) and perioperative complications ($p = 0.020$) were influencing factors.

When these potential factors were used to calculate the Kaplan-Meier survival curve, some were associated with OS and CSS (Fig. 2). BMI less than 25 kg/m² was associated with OS ($p = 0.004$) but not CSS ($p = 0.050$), and PLN was associated with OS (p<0.001)and CSS ($p = 0.010$). The survival time and cumulative survival rate (1-, 5- and 10-year rates) are depicted in Table 5.

Discussion

Our present results show that there was a downstaging advantage with one-shot neoadjuvant IAC before RC for MIBC (p = 0.002), but it did not significantly improve OS ($p = 0.354$) or CSS ($p = 0.439$) compared to those treated without IAC. We performed Cox regression to assess risk factors association with survival in all samples and found that BMI (less than a 25 kg/m²) significantly affected OS (p = 0.004), and PLN significantly affected both OS (p<0.001 = and CSS (p = 0.010). Besides, we are curious about the potential risk factors affecting survival outcomes in the IAC and NIAC group and their difference in the two groups. So, despite the small sample size of IAC and NIAC group, we used Cox regression to explore the risks in the both groups exploratorily. The exploratory analysis found that diabetes ($P = 0.029$, RR = 14.649) was an influencing factor in IAC group, whereas BMI ($P = 0.015$, RR = 0.802), PLN ($P < 0.001$, RR = 7.474) and smoking history ($P = 0.043$, RR = 3.388) were influencing factors in NIAC group (Additional file 1 Table S3). Furthermore, when these potential factors were used to calculate the Kaplan-Meier survival curve, some were associated with OS and CSS in IAC groups and NIAC groups (Additional file 1 Table S4-S7 and Additional file 2 Figure S4). In brief, one-shot neoadjuvant resulted in significant downstaging; for RC, only BMI and PLN correlate with survival in our long-term data.

RC usually occurs 4 to 6 weeks after MIBC diagnosis in our center, and this time offers an opportunity to preoperatively perform neoadjuvant therapy. Although standard neoadjuvant cisplatin-based combination chemotherapy followed by RC is supported by level 1 evidence for resectable (cT2-T4aN0M0) MIBC, the inability to identify which patients may derive most benefit from neoadjuvant chemotherapy was slow during the adoption of neoadjuvant treatment. Nevertheless, approximately 50% of patients with urothelial carcinoma are considered ineligible to receive cisplatin based on renal dysfunction and impaired performance status, and a subset of patients also refuse to receive neoadjuvant chemotherapy [11]. Notably, adherence to adjuvant and neoadjuvant chemotherapy regimens was observed in a similarly low proportion of patients (approximately 21% each) in the USA, and the majority of patients with resectable bladder cancer received no chemotherapy at all [12]. Therefore, the treatment algorithm for MIBC tumors in a short window before RC is still evolving.

Neoadjuvant IAC is not a new concept. In the 1980s–1990s, multiple efforts were made to improve oncological outcomes by adding various IAC treatment modalities plus RC to treatment regimens for MIBC. A summary of the published neoadjuvant IAC papers, including key information on chemotherapy regimens, is provided in Table 6 (Additional file 2 Figure S5) [13–21]. Although most of the literature is early in its use, the drugs also have differences, but all show varying degrees of pathological downstaging or even complete response (CR; pT0). Pathological downstaging or pathological CR to neoadjuvant chemotherapy is a well-recognized biomarker of improved OS [22]. Because it was such a short period of therapy, we felt that achieving pathological CR would be quite challenging in our study. Although OS and CSS for the study cohort remained disappointing, one-shot neoadjuvant IAC showed an encouraging pathological downstaging rate of greater than 60% ($P = 0.002$). Meanwhile, the safety and tolerability profile for IAC was quite favorable. In particular, no chemotherapy-related adverse events have been reported in the IAC group, which did not delay planned surgery. Moreover, no differences in perioperative, short-term or long-term complications were recorded compared with patients undergoing RC only. Similarly, intraoperative performance (operating time, estimated blood loss, blood transfusion, number of nodes removed and surgical margins) was not compromised by neoadjuvant IAC. Therefore, our treatment produced major pathologic responses, indicating that the side effects of chemotherapy can be reliably avoided when using one-shot IAC.

Bladder cancer is a heterogeneous disease, which means that only single treatment is not enough. Current research is actively exploring novel combinations and ideal sequencing with various treatment modalities, especially immunotherapy combined with chemotherapy, radiotherapy or targeted therapies. Although bladder

Table 4 Multivariable Cox proportional hazards model to estimate survival outcomes

Variables	Total	
	p value	RR(95%CI)
BMI	0.005	0.767(0.638–0.922)
Diabetes	0.002	8.716(2.263–33.563)
ASA score	0.005	4.846(1.600–14.682)
Positive lymph nodes	<0.001	11.886(3.912–36.119)
Perioperative complication	0.020	4.416(1.259–15.488)

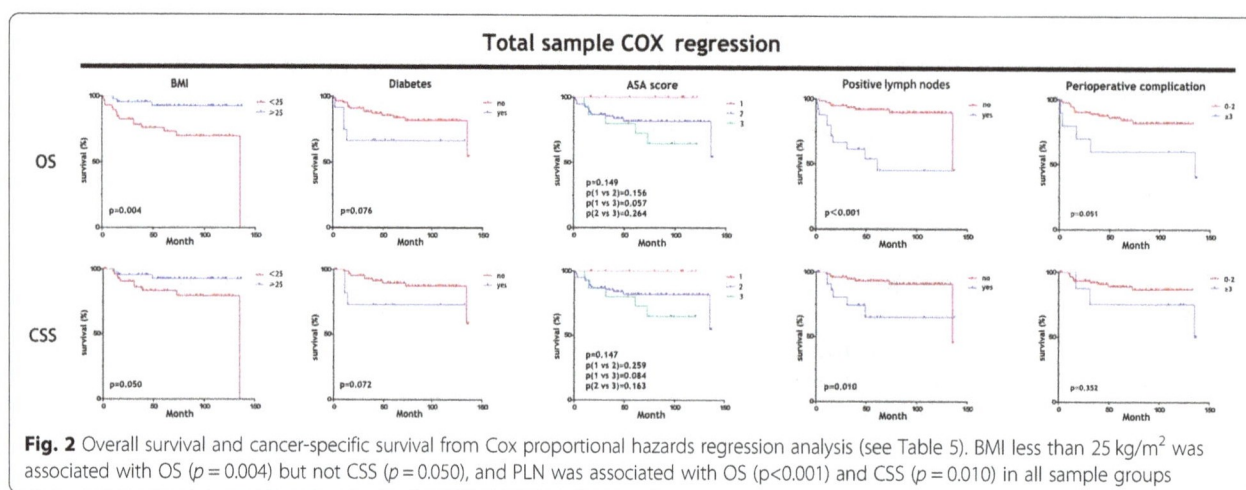

Fig. 2 Overall survival and cancer-specific survival from Cox proportional hazards regression analysis (see Table 5). BMI less than 25 kg/m^2 was associated with OS ($p = 0.004$) but not CSS ($p = 0.050$), and PLN was associated with OS ($p<0.001$) and CSS ($p = 0.010$) in all sample groups

cancer carries the third highest mutation rate of all studied cancers, suggesting the possibility of increased immunogenicity via the development of neoantigens, it is clear from existing data that the majority of patients will not respond to monotherapy [23–25]. Interestingly, chemotherapeutic agents have direct cytotoxic effects on tumor cells that release tumor antigens but also have positive effects on immune effector T cells [26]. Therefore, in theory, one-shot IAC can play a synergistic role as a single immunotherapy. Moreover, chemotherapy may substantially prolong the total duration of neoadjuvant immunotherapy [27]. However, patient selection must be optimized. In addition to having good renal function, it is also necessary to pay attention to the patient's nutritional status and immune system, which may be hampered by an aged-related reduction in functional decline. With an average age of 73 years at diagnosis, perioperative immunonutrition has a significant impact on surgery and the efficacy of immunotherapy [28]. According to our findings, BMI, diabetes and ASA score were associated with survival and may be the modifiable predictors in older and sicker patient populations.

Additionally, the optimization of toxicity and tolerability of combination therapies through appropriate dosing and sequencing should be determined using well-designed clinical trials.

The strengths of our study are the selection of only one surgeon's cases for minimizing the influence of different levels of maturity and the use of propensity-score matching to reduce the inherent biases. As a result, patients who were matched only on the basis of key variables were selected. However, an important limitation is our drawing conclusions from small sample and highly selected patients with retrospective, nonrandomized data, which might introduce possible selection biases that we did not control for. Another limitation of the present study was that there was no consistent record of recurrence-free survival (RFS) in the long-term follow-up period. Although the final pathology showed no difference between the cohorts, the proportion of positive surgical margins was higher in NIAC cohort. It is possible that NIAC cohort had lower stage disease to begin with which would affect the RFS of patients. However, it should be noted that OS is the gold standard and the

Table 5 Description of survival of groupings in the entire set of patients (see Fig. 2)

	Mean ST (mo)	Medium ST (mo)	1-year CSR (95%CI)	5-year CSR (95%CI)	0-year CSR (95%CI)
OS of BMI grouping					
<25	102.35	135.00	0.897(0.784–0.952)	0.733(0.587–0.835)	0.699(0.541–0.811)
≥25	129.00	–	0.956(0.0–1.0)	0.927(0.0–1.0)	0.927 (0.0–1.0)
OS of PLN grouping					
No	124.81	135.00	0.975(0.903–0.994)	0.920(0.830–0.963)	0.897(0.793–0.951)
Yes	75.65	61.00	0.800(0.000–1.000)	0.540(0.002–0.943)	0.450(0.006–0.884)
CSS of PLN grouping					
No	126.37	135.00	0.987(0.913–0.998)	0.932(0.843–0.971)	0.909(0.804–0.959)
Yes	98.10	–	0.861(0.000–1.000)	0.649(0.000–0.985)	0.649(0.000–0.985)

ST: survival time; CSR: cumulative survival rate; OS: overall survival; CSS: cancer-specific surival; BMI: body mass index; PLN: positive lymph nodes

Table 6 Summary of the published papers on neoadjuvant intra-arterial chemotherapy followed by radical cystectomy

Study	Year	Country	Type of study	Sample size (RC/total)	Chemotherapy regimen	No. of cycles	Interval to RC, (wks.)	Downstaging, (%), only RC	OS (only RC)
Kanoh et al. [13]	1983	Japan	Retrospective	7/13	ADM	2/wk. (≥3 wks)	6.7	5 (71.4)	2 died (14.6)
Kamidono et al. [14]	1984	Japan	Retrospective	11/11	ADM, MMC	1	4.2	7 (63.6)	3 died (17.5)
Maatman et al. [15]	1986	Italia	Prospective	16/25	CDDP, ADM	1–4	4	4 (25)	1 died (15.7)
Kanoh et al. [16]	1987	Japan	Retrospective	15/32	ADM ± CDDP	10–23 (17)	–	–	1 died, 5-year OS 87.5%
Kakizaki et al. [17]	1987	Japan	Retrospective	29/29	MMC, CPM, thio-TEPA, 5-FU, ADM, CDDP	1	2	–	–
Jacobs et al. [18]	1989	USA	Retrospective	16/30	CDDP	1	4	15 (93.8)	3 N+ average 13 mo 8 N0 average 28 ± 8 mo
Galetti et al. [19]	1989	USA	Phase II	4/8(only IA)	CDDP	1	–	3 (75)	37mo (6–56)
Arima et al. [20]	1997	Japan	Retrospective	80/120	ADM + CDDP	1–4	–	75 (62.5)	–
Miyata et al. [21]	2015	Japan	Retrospective	17/50	CDDP, ADM, EPI	2 ± 0.2	4–8	–	–
Recent study	2019	China	Retrospective	26/26	GC	1	4	17 (65.4)	3 died (2 from cancer: 11 and 31mo)

RC, radical cystectomy; OS, overall survival; ADM, adriamycin or doxorubicin; MMC, mitomycin C; CDDP, cisplatin; EPI, epirubicin; GC, gemcitabine + cisplatin; –, not available

most dependable end point in clinical cancer research to support treatment algorithms. Furthermore, CSS may be a surrogate endpoint for RFS. Nevertheless, we were not able to detect statistically significant differences between the groups in OS or CSS. At the same time, more than half of our patients were from all over the country, and some proportion of patients did not have clear data on disease recurrence. Therefore, RFS is not as important. Finally, we should know that there was not a specific marker to judge the safety, tolerability, or clinical benefit of the treatments in the subgroups of patients. Answers to some of these questions will become clearer as these studies begin to mature with clinical readouts.

Conclusions

This long-term follow-up, retrospective study of one-shot neoadjuvant IAC in patients who underwent RC from 2006 to 2015 shows significant advantages in pathological downstaging but not in OS or CSS. Moreover, this study demonstrates the safety and tolerability of this treatment and provides a basis for combination therapy. Future efforts to improve survival in patients with bladder cancer is warranted and further study of the ideal neoadjuvant therapeutic strategies followed by RC is needed.

Supplementary information

Additional file 1: Table S1. Pathological staging before and after surgery in the NIAC group after matching (see Fig. S2), **Table S2.**

Pathological staging before and after surgery in the IAC group (see Fig. S3), **Table S3.** Multivariable Cox proportional hazard model to estimate survival outcomes in IAC and NIAC groups, **Table S4.** Description of OS of diabetes groupings in the IAC group (see Fig. S4A), **Table S5.** Description of OS of BMI groupings in the NIAC group (see Fig. S4B), **Table S6.** Description of OS of PLN groupings in the NIAC group (see Fig. S4B), **Table S7.** Description of CSS of PLN groupings in the NIAC group (see Fig. S4B)

Additional file 2: Figure S1. Propensity-score matching analysis based on follow-up duration (Box plot), (A), Distribution of different groups of patients by follow-up time before the match (B), Distribution of different groups of patients by follow-up time after 1:3 matching, **Figure S2.** Tumor staging changes in the NIAC group after matching (see Table S1), **Figure S3.** Tumor staging changes in the IAC group (see Table S2), **Figure S4.** Overall survival and cancer-specific survival from Cox proportional hazards regression analysis (see Table S3-S6), (A), Diabetes is associated with only OS (p = 0.004) in the IAC group. (B). BMI was only associated with OS (p = 0.014), and PLN was associated with both OS (p< 0.001 = and CSS (p = 0.017) in the NIAC group, **Figure S5.** Flow diagram of the article selection process

Abbreviations
ADM: adriamycin or doxorubicin; ASA: American Society of Anesthesiologists; BMI: body mass index; BUN: blood urea nitrogen; CCI: Charlson Comorbidity Index; CDDP: cisplatin; CIS: carcinoma in situ; CSS: cancer-specific survival; ECOG PS: Eastern Cooperative Oncology Group performance status; EPI: epirubicin; HCT: hematocrit; HGB: hemoglobin; IAC: intra-arterial chemotherapy; IQR: interquartile range; MMC: mitomycin C; NIAC: no-intra-arterial chemotherapy; OS: overall survival; PLN: positive lymph nodes; PLND: pelvic lymph node dissection; RC: radical; WBC: white blood cell; GC: gemcitabine + cisplatin.; ST: survival time; CSR: cumulative survival rate

Acknowledgements
We wish to thank all our colleagues in the Department of Urology, Beijing Chao-Yang Hospital, without you, we could not have completed the work.

Authors' contribution
Author contributions: L.S., M.W. and F.Y. had full access to all of the data in the study and take responsibility for the integrity of the data and the

accuracy of the data analysis. Acquisition of data: S.L., M.W. and Q.H. Study concept and design: Y.N. and N.X. Manuscript writing: W.W. and W.X. Statistical analysis: W.X. and L.H. Revision of the manuscript for intellectual content: Y.N. and N.X. Correspondence: Y.N. and N.X. All authors read and approved the final manuscript.

Author details
[1]Institute of Urology, Capital Medical University, Department of Urology, Capital Medical University Beijing Chao-Yang Hospital, Beijing 100020, China. [2]Department of Urology, National Cancer Center/National Clinical Research Center for Cancer/Cancer Hospital, Chinese Academy of Medical Sciences and Peking Union Medical College, Beijing 100021, China. [3]School of Biomedical Engineering, Capital Medical University, Beijing 100069, China.

References
1. Babjuk M, Bohle A, Burger M, Capoun O, Cohen D, Comperat EM, et al. EAU guidelines on non-muscle-invasive Urothelial carcinoma of the bladder: update 2016. Eur Urol. 2017;71(3):447–61.
2. Miller KD, Siegel RL, Lin CC, Mariotto AB, Kramer JL, Rowland JH, et al. Cancer treatment and survivorship statistics, 2016. CA Cancer J Clin. 2016; 66(4):271–89.
3. Stein JP, Lieskovsky G, Cote R, Groshen S, Feng AC, Boyd S, et al. Radical cystectomy in the treatment of invasive bladder cancer: long-term results in 1,054 patients. J Clin Oncol. 2001;19(3):666–75.
4. von der Maase H, Sengelov L, Roberts JT, Ricci S, Dogliotti L, Oliver T, et al. Long-term survival results of a randomized trial comparing gemcitabine plus cisplatin, with methotrexate, vinblastine, doxorubicin, plus cisplatin in patients with bladder cancer. J Clin Oncol. 2005;23(21):4602–8.
5. Stein JP, Skinner DG. Radical cystectomy for invasive bladder cancer: long-term results of a standard procedure. World J Urol. 2006;24(3):296–304.
6. Dalbagni G, Genega E, Hashibe M, Zhang ZF, Russo P, Herr H, et al. Cystectomy for bladder cancer: a contemporary series. J Urol. 2001;165(4): 1111–6.
7. Bassi P, Ferrante GD, Piazza N, Spinadin R, Carando R, Pappagallo G, et al. Prognostic factors of outcome after radical cystectomy for bladder cancer: a retrospective study of a homogeneous patient cohort. J Urol. 1999;161(5): 1494–7.
8. Ghoneim MA. el-Mekresh MM, el-Baz MA, el-attar IA, Ashamallah a. radical cystectomy for carcinoma of the bladder: critical evaluation of the results in 1,026 cases. J Urol. 1997;158(2):393–9.
9. Donat SM, Shabsigh A, Savage C, Cronin AM, Bochner BH, Dalbagni G, et al. Potential impact of postoperative early complications on the timing of adjuvant chemotherapy in patients undergoing radical cystectomy: a high-volume tertiary cancer center experience. Eur Urol. 2009;55(1):177–85.
10. Thompson RH, Boorjian SA, Kim SP, Cheville JC, Thapa P, Tarrel R, et al. Eligibility for neoadjuvant/adjuvant cisplatin-based chemotherapy among radical cystectomy patients. BJU Int. 2014;113(5b):E17–21.
11. Galsky MD, Hahn NM, Rosenberg J, Sonpavde G, Hutson T, Oh WK, et al. Treatment of patients with metastatic urothelial cancer "unfit" for Cisplatin-based chemotherapy. J Clin Oncol. 2011;29(17):2432–8.
12. Reardon ZD, Patel SG, Zaid HB, Stimson CJ, Resnick MJ, Keegan KA, et al. Trends in the use of perioperative chemotherapy for localized and locally advanced muscle-invasive bladder cancer: a sign of changing tides. Eur Urol. 2015;67(1):165–70.
13. Kanoh S, Umeyama T, Nemoto S, Ishikawa S, Nemoto R, Rinsho K, et al. Long-term intra-arterial infusion chemotherapy with adriamycin for advanced bladder cancer. Cancer Chemother Pharmacol. 1983;11(Suppl): S51–8.
14. Kamidono S, Fujii A, Hamami G, Nakano Y, Umezu K, Oda Y, et al. New preoperative chemotherapy for bladder cancer using combination hemodialysis and direct hemoperfusion: preliminary report. J Urol. 1984; 131(1):36–40.
15. Maatman TJ, Montie JE, Bukowski RM, Risius B, Geisinger M. Intra-arterial chemotherapy as an adjuvant to surgery in transitional cell carcinoma of the bladder. J Urol. 1986;135(2):256–60.
16. Kanoh S, Noguchi R, Ohtani M, Ishikawa S, Nemoto R, Koiso K, et al. Intra-arterial chemotherapy for bladder cancer. Cancer Chemother Pharmacol. 1987;20(Suppl:S6–9).
17. Kakizaki H, Suzuki H, Kubota Y, Numasawa K, Suzuki K. Preoperative one-shot intra-arterial infusion chemotherapy for bladder cancer. Cancer Chemother Pharmacol. 1987;20(Suppl:S15–9).
18. Jacobs SC, Menashe DS, Mewissen MW, Lipchik EO. Intraarterial cisplatin infusion in the management of transitional cell carcinoma of the bladder. Cancer. 1989;64(2):388–91.
19. Galetti TP, Pontes JE, Montie J, Medendorp SV, Bukowski R. Neoadjuvant intra-arterial chemotherapy in the treatment of advanced transitional cell carcinoma of the bladder: results and followup. J Urol. 1989;142(5):1211–4 discussion 4-5.
20. Arima K, Tochigi H, Sugimura Y, Kawamura J. Balloon-occluded arterial infusion as a useful neoadjuvant chemotherapy for bladder cancer. Br J Urol. 1997;80(3):417–20.
21. Miyata Y, Nomata K, Ohba K, Matsuo T, Hayashi N, Sakamoto I, et al. Efficacy and safety of systemic chemotherapy and intra-arterial chemotherapy with/without radiotherapy for bladder preservation or as neo-adjuvant therapy in patients with muscle-invasive bladder cancer: a single-Centre study of 163 patients. Eur J Surg Oncol. 2015;41(3):361–7.
22. Chism DD, Woods ME, Milowsky MI. Neoadjuvant paradigm for accelerated drug development: an ideal model in bladder cancer. Oncologist. 2013; 18(8):933–40.
23. Cancer Genome Atlas Research N. Comprehensive molecular characterization of urothelial bladder carcinoma. Nature. 2014;507(7492): 315–22.
24. Lawrence MS, Stojanov P, Polak P, Kryukov GV, Cibulskis K, Sivachenko A, et al. Mutational heterogeneity in cancer and the search for new cancer-associated genes. Nature. 2013;499(7457):214–8.
25. Siefker-Radtke AO, Apolo AB, Bivalacqua TJ, Spiess PE, Black PC. Immunotherapy with checkpoint blockade in the treatment of Urothelial carcinoma. J Urol. 2018;199(5):1129–42.
26. Krantz D, Hartana CA, Winerdal ME, Johansson M, Alamdari F, Jakubczyk T, et al. Neoadjuvant chemotherapy reinforces antitumour T cell response in Urothelial urinary bladder Cancer. Eur Urol. 2018;74(6):688–92.
27. Necchi A, Anichini A, Raggi D, Briganti A, Massa S, Luciano R, et al. Pembrolizumab as Neoadjuvant Therapy Before Radical Cystectomy in Patients With Muscle-Invasive Urothelial Bladder Carcinoma (PURE-01): An Open-Label, Single-Arm, Phase II Study. J Clin Oncol. 2018:JCO1801148.
28. Tobert CM, Hamilton-Reeves JM, Norian LA, Hung C, Brooks NA, Holzbeierlein JM, et al. Emerging impact of malnutrition on surgical patients: literature review and potential implications for cystectomy in bladder Cancer. J Urol. 2017;198(3):511–9.

24

Continuous saline bladder irrigation for two hours following transurethral resection of bladder tumors in patients with non-muscle invasive bladder cancer does not prevent recurrence or progression compared with intravesical Mitomycin-C

Andrew T. Lenis[1,2,3] ![ORCID], Kian Asanad[1], Maher Blaibel[4], Nicholas M. Donin[1,2,3] and Karim Chamie[1,2,3*]

Abstract

Background: Intravesical Mitomycin-C (MMC) following transurethral resection of bladder tumor (TURBT), while efficacious, is associated with side effects and poor utilization. Continuous saline bladder irrigation (CSBI) has been examined as an alternative. In this study we sought to compare the rates of recurrence and/or progression in patients with NMIBC who were treated with either MMC or CSBI after TURBT.

Methods: We retrospectively reviewed records of patients with NMIBC at our institution in 2012–2015. Perioperative use of MMC (40 mg in 20 mL), CSBI (two hours), or neither were recorded. Primary outcome was time to recurrence or progression. Descriptive statistics, chi-squared analysis, Kaplan-Meier survival analysis, and Cox multivariable regression analyses were performed.

Results: 205 patients met inclusion criteria. Forty-five (22.0%) patients received CSBI, 71 (34.6%) received MMC, and 89 (43.4%) received no perioperative therapy. On survival analysis, MMC was associated with improved DFS compared with CSBI ($p = 0.001$) and no treatment ($p = 0.0009$). On multivariable analysis, high risk disease was associated with increased risk of recurrence or progression (HR 2.77, 95% CI: 1.28–6.01), whereas adjuvant therapy (HR 0.35, 95% CI: 0.20–0.59) and MMC (HR 0.43, 95% CI: 0.25–0.75) were associated with decreased risk.

Conclusions: Postoperative MMC was associated with improved DFS compared with CSBI and no treatment. The DFS benefit seen with CSBI in other studies may be limited to patients receiving prolonged irrigation. New intravesical agents being evaluated may consider saline as a control given our data demonstrating that short-term CSBI is not superior to TURBT alone.

Keywords: Bladder cancer, Therapeutic irrigation, Mitomycin-C, Recurrence, Outcome assessment

* Correspondence: kchamie@mednet.ucla.edu
[1]David Geffen School of Medicine at the University of California Los Angeles, 300 Stein Plaza, Suite 348, Los Angeles, California 90095, USA
[2]Department of Urology, Health Services Research Group, David Geffen School of Medicine at UCLA, Los Angeles, California, USA
Full list of author information is available at the end of the article

Background

Non-muscle invasive bladder cancer (NMIBC) accounts for approximately 70% of new cases of urothelial carcinoma of the bladder. [1] NMIBC has been considered a chronic disease due to its high risk of future complications, including recurrence, which necessitates frequent monitoring and surveillance. The lifelong risk of recurrence and repeated interventions contributes to poor physician and patient compliance with published guidelines, and it significantly burdens the healthcare system from a financial standpoint. [2, 3] Therefore, strategies to prevent recurrence and future complications are paramount to reducing long-term morbidity and mortality.

The standard adjuvant therapy following transurethral resection of bladder tumor (TURBT) for NMIBC is intravesical instillation of Mitomycin-C (MMC), which has been shown to decrease rates of recurrence by approximately 11%, although this is variable depending on the number of and time from prior recurrences. [4, 5] The posited mechanism of action is to prevent free-floating tumor cells in the urine following TURBT from re-implanting onto the bladder wall. Although rare, MMC can potentially cause several significant side effects, including severe lower urinary tract symptoms, persistent chronic bladder pain, and even bladder necrosis in case reports. [6] Furthermore, MMC is contraindicated when there is a concern for bladder perforation and when there is significant post-operative gross hematuria. Considering these limitations, there is an urgent need for alternative strategies to prevent the re-implantation of tumor cells following TURBT, to reduce recurrence and minimize the morbidity of the disease. A 2012 Cochrane review of intravesical gemcitabine yielded conflicting results. [7] Apaziquone is a novel intravesical alkylating agent that has demonstrated safety and tolerability in patients as a post-TURBT instillation and is being evaluated in Phase 3 clinical trials (NCT02563561). [8] Alternatively, several groups have utilized sterile water and saline irrigation over 18–24 h as a strategy to lyse floating tumors cells and prevent the re-implantation of cells into the bladder wall. [9, 10] In our current study, we sought to evaluate continuous bladder irrigation with isotonic (0.9% NaCl) normal saline (CBSI) for two hours following TURBT as a strategy to reduce recurrence or progression in patients with NMIBC.

Methods

Patient cohort

Patients undergoing endoscopic resection of bladder tumors at our institution between March 2012 and July 2015 were identified from the medical record by Current Procedure Terminology (CPT)-4 codes for transurethral biopsy and resection (52204, 52214, 52224, 52234, 52235, 52240). Pathologic and clinical reports were reviewed, and patients with NMIBC were selected for inclusion in the cohort. We excluded all patients with variant histology, including small cell, squamous cell, adenocarcinoma, lymphepithelioid, sarcomatoid, and micropapillary disease. We also excluded patients with a diagnosis of upper tract urothelial carcinoma within one year, unresectable volume of tumor, known metastatic disease, less than three months of follow-up, or patients who underwent cystectomy within three months of diagnosis. Patients were categorized based on a modified AUA Risk Stratification for NMIBC. [11] Low risk was defined as a solitary LG lesion < 2 cm. Intermediate risk was defined as any LG T1, solitary LG Ta > 2 cm, multiple LG Ta, solitary HG Ta < 2 cm, or a history of LG NMIBC. High risk was defined as any CIS, HG T1, HG Ta > 2 cm, multiple HG Ta, or any history of HG Ta lesions or BCG recurrence. Modification of the AUA risk groups was made in order to conform to the size criteria used in the current procedural terminology codes for TURBT. Follow-up was calculated based on the time of the last cystoscopy. All study conduct was approved by the Institutional Review Board at our institution.

Independent variables

All patients received adjuvant CSBI, adjuvant MMC, or no adjuvant treatment at the discretion of the operating surgeon. Typically, patients for whom there was a concern for bladder perforation were not given CSBI or MMC. MMC was given as an instillation of 40 mg in 20 mL of saline. Following a dwell time of 60–90 min, the MMC was drained from the bladder and the catheter was left in place if deemed necessary by the surgeon. CSBI was performed by placement of a three-way Foley catheter at the conclusion of the case and was left running for approximately two hours post-operatively. The rate was kept at maximum flow without titration for this time. Patients did not require an overnight stay specifically for CSBI.

Dependent variables

Our dependent variable of interest was time to recurrence or progression. Recurrence was defined as the presence of pathologically confirmed urothelial carcinoma on biopsy or repeat resection. Patients who were found to have a lesion visible on cystoscopy that warranted intervention in the office (e.g. fulguration) were also classified as having disease recurrence. Cytology results obtained at the time of office fulguration were recorded. Progression was defined as any increase in grade or stage of disease.

Statistical analysis

Comparisons between categorical variables were tested using Chi-squared analysis and Fisher's exact test when appropriate. The two-sample Student's t-test was used to test for differences between continuous variables. Differences in disease-free survival (DFS) were analyzed using the Kaplan-Meier method. Cox proportional hazards models were used to estimate hazards ratios for covariates of interest. All statistical analyses were performed with Stata statistical software version 14 (StataCorp, College Station, TX).

Results

A total of 205 patients underwent TURBT for NMIBC during the study period and met all inclusion criteria. Mean age was 71.9 (SD = 11.4) years and 81.5% were male. Low grade (LG) and high grade (HG) were the primary grades in 105 (51.2%) and 100 (48.8%) patients, respectively. Stage was Ta without CIS, Ta with CIS, T1 without CIS, T1 with CIS, and CIS alone in 126 (61.5%), 12 (5.9%), 36 (17.6%), 13 (6.3%), and 18 (8.8%) patients, respectively. Tumor size was < 0.5 cm, 0.5–2 cm, 2–5 cm, and > 5 cm in 20 (9.8%), 90 (43.9%), 45 (21.9%), and 50 (24.4%) patients, respectively. Multiple tumors were present in 105 (51.2%) patients and 75 (36.6%) had a history of NMIBC. A modified AUA risk stratification as discussed in the methods resulted in 23 (11.2%) low risk patients, 80 (39%) intermediate risk patients, and 102 (49.8%) high risk patients. As immediate perioperative therapy, a total of 45 (22.0%) patients had CSBI, 71 (34.6%) had MMC, and 89 (43.4%) had no perioperative therapy. Only 36 (19.8%) of patients with intermediate or high risk disease underwent a restaging TURBT. Eighty-six (42.0%) patients received adjuvant intravesical therapy, most commonly with bacillus Calmette-Guérin (BCG n = 76), BCG + interferon (n = 6), Gemcitabine (n = 2), or MMC (n = 2). Table 1 and Table 2 summarize the cohort characteristics stratified by perioperative treatment and recurrence and progression, respectively.

Median follow-up time for the entire cohort was 16 [Interquartile range (IQR): 8–28] months. A total of 74 (36.1%) patients recurred at a median of 9.5 [IQR: 4–14] months and 16 (7.8%) progressed at a median of 16 [IQR: 6–31.5] months. The median DFS was 25 months for those who received no perioperative treatment, 55 months for those receiving MMC, and 16 months for those receiving CSBI. The Kaplan-Meier survival curve is presented in Fig. 1 and demonstrates a significant DFS advantage of MMC compared with either CSBI or no perioperative treatment (log rank test: $p < 0.01$). Kaplan-Meier curves for patients with a combination of low and intermediate risk NMIBC (log rank test: p = 0.02) and high risk NMIBC (log rank test: $p = 0.04$), and are presented in Figs. 2 and 3, respectively.

Lastly, we created a multivariable model incorporating age, AUA risk stratification, use of additional adjuvant therapy, and type of perioperative therapy (None, MMC, or CSBI). On Cox multivariable modeling, high risk was associated with increased risk of recurrence or progression (HR 2.77, 95% CI: 1.28–6.01), whereas adjuvant therapy (HR 0.35, 95% CI: 0.20–0.59) and MMC (HR 0.43, 95% CI: 0.25–0.75) were associated with decreased risk of recurrence or progression (Table 3).

Discussion

The burden of NMIBC includes high financial costs to the healthcare system, significant risk of recurrence that necessitates life-long invasive surveillance, and uncertainty of possible progression that would prompt future radical operative intervention, especially in the highest-risk patients. Strategies to reduce the risk of recurrence and progression, including intravesical chemotherapy and immunotherapy, have been shown to be effective. [4, 12] However, none of these are without risk of potential significant side effects. In our current study we sought to utilize postoperative CSBI in a fashion similar to MMC, as an immediate, one-time postoperative treatment following surgery. This strategy avoids the toxicity of intravesical chemotherapy, as well as the inconvenience of an overnight hospital stay for prolonged CSBI.

In our cohort, however, post-operative CSBI for two hours was not equivalent to a single dose of perioperative MMC. Given the small numbers of patients in the low risk subgroup, we combined patients from low risk and intermediate risk groups for analysis. In the low and intermediate risk patients, there was a significant improvement in DFS with MMC compared with CSBI. In fact, CSBI performed no better than no perioperative treatment. In the high risk subgroup, a similar trend was observed. In our study the absolute risk reduction of postoperative MMC compared with no treatment at one year was 12.3%, which is similar to what is reported in the literature (11.7%). [4, 13] This benefit of MMC holds true even in our Cox multivariable model.

With respect to the efficacy of CSBI, our data stands in contrast to results published by others, albeit with some important differences in study design. Onishi et al. performed a non-randomized study comparing 18–22 h of post-operative CSBI to a full year of induction and maintenance MMC in patients with European Organization for Research and Treatment of Cancer (EORTC) intermediate risk NMIBC and showed no difference in several outcomes, including recurrence-free rates, time to first recurrence, and frequency of recurrences. [10] In this manuscript, the authors alluded to a planned prospective study that was recently published. [14] In their follow-up study, 227 patients with primary EORTC low- to intermediate-risk (all LG) NMIBC were randomized 1:1 to receive CSBI for 18 h or a single dose of 30 mg of MMC in 30 mL of saline. After a median follow-up of 37 months, 29% of patients experienced a recurrence. Recurrence-free rates at 1, 3, and 5 years were similar between the CSBI

Table 1 Cohort characteristics stratified by perioperative treatment

Variable	No treatment	MMC	CSBI	p-value
Total no. of patients	89	71	45	–
Age, mean (SD)	73.2 (11.2)	68.2 (12.3)	75.3 (8.9)	< 0.002+
Gender, n (%)				0.54
Male	75 (84.3)	55 (77.5)	37 (83.2)	
Female	14 (15.7)	16 (22.5)	8 (17.8)	
Grade, n (%)				0.9
High	45 (50.6)	34 (47.9)	21 (46.7)	
Low	44 (49.4)	37 (52.1)	24 (53.3)	
Stage, n (%)				0.03*
Ta without CIS	55 (61.8)	41 (57.8)	30 (66.7)	
Ta with CIS	3 (3.4)	4 (5.6)	5 (11.1)	
T1 without CIS	13 (14.6)	18 (25.4)	5 (11.1)	
T1 with CIS	4 (4.5)	6 (8.5)	3 (6.7)	
CIS only	14 (15.7)	2 (2.8)	2 (4.4)	
Tumor size, n (%)				0.12*
< 0.5 cm	11 (12.36)	3 (4.2)	6 (13.3)	
0.5–2.0 cm	33 (37.1)	41 (57.8)	16 (35.6)	
2.0–5.0 cm	22 (24.7)	13 (18.3)	10 (22.2)	
> 5.0 cm	23 (25.8)	14 (19.7)	13 (28.9)	
Multiple tumors, n (%)	47 (52.8)	36 (50.7)	22 (48.9)	0.91
Recurrent disease, n (%)	40 (45.0)	23 (32.4)	12 (26.7)	0.08
AUA Risk Stratification				0.72
Low risk	10 (11.2)	6 (8.5)	7 (15.6)	
Intermediate risk	34 (38.2)	31 (43.7)	15 (33.3)	
High risk	45 (50.6)	34 (47.9)	23 (51.1)	
Restaging resection, n (%)	8 (9.0)	18 (25.4)	10 (22.2)	0.02
Adjuvant therapy, n (%)	35 (39.3)	35 (49.3)	16 (35.6)	0.28
Follow-up in months, median [IQR]	14 [6–28]	23 [11–32]	13 [9–19]	< 0.01§

MMC Mitomycin-C, *CSBI* continuous saline bladder irrigation, *SD* standard deviation, *CIS* carcinoma in situ. +One-way ANOVA. *Fisher's exact test. §non-parametric equality of medians test

and MMC groups on Kaplan-Meier analysis. Subgroup analysis showed no difference when stratified between the low- and intermediate-risk tumors. Adverse events were also compared and the MMC group was found to have significantly higher rates of gross hematuria, irritative bladder symptoms, and dysuria (including retention). While the equivalence of CSBI and MMC demonstrated by Onishi et al. could be explained in part by patient selection (all LG patients), we did not replicate this result even in the low and intermediate risk subgroups of our cohort. One important difference in our protocols is the dose of MMC, which was the standard 40 mg in our study and 30 mg in the study by Onishi et al. The most striking difference between our studies, however, is in the duration of CSBI. We intentionally restricted CSBI to two hours to limit the need for overnight hospital stays. While similarly

efficacious to one instillation of MMC, CSBI used by Onishi et al. was titrated over 18 h, and it was not reported how many of these patients required an overnight stay. While the authors debate the cost advantages of saline compared with MMC, we question whether this may be offset by even a small fraction of patients requiring overnight admissions for CSBI. Nevertheless, this data demonstrates that in addition to a standard dose of 40 mg of MMC, duration may be an important component of the efficacy of CSBI in preventing tumor cell re-implantation.

Our results also appear to conflict with the results of a recent meta-analysis utilizing individual patient data from randomized trials comparing immediate intravesical instillation of various chemotherapy agents to TURBT alone or instillation of control solution (saline

Table 2 Cohort characteristics stratified by Recurrence or Progression

Variable	Recurrence or Progression	No Recurrence or Progression	p-value
Total no. of patients	90	115	–
Age, mean (SD)	73.6 (10.8)	70.6 (11.8)	0.07+
Gender, n (%)			0.81
Male	74 (82.2)	93 (80.9)	
Female	16 (17.8)	22 (19.1)	
Grade, n (%)			0.38
High	47 (52.2)	53 (46.1)	
Low	43 (47.8)	62 (53.9)	
Stage, n (%)			0.09*
Ta without CIS	55 (61.1)	71 (61.7)	
Ta with CIS	3 (3.3)	9 (7.8)	
T1 without CIS	14 (15.6)	22 (19.1)	
T1 with CIS	5 (5.6)	8 (7.0)	
CIS	13 (14.4)	5 (4.4)	
Tumor size, n (%)			0.09
< 0.5 cm	14 (15.6)	6 (5.2)	
0.5–2.0 cm	37 (41.1)	53 (46.1)	
2.0–5.0 cm	17 (18.9)	28 (24.4)	
> 5.0 cm	22 (24.4)	28 (24.3)	
Multiplicity of tumor, n (%)	56 (62.2)	49 (42.6)	< 0.01
Recurrent disease, n (%)	42 (46.7)	33 (28.7)	< 0.01
AUA Risk Stratification			0.07
Low risk	9 (10.0)	14 (12.2)	
Intermediate risk	28 (31.1)	52 (45.2)	
High risk	53 (58.9)	49 (42.6)	
Restaging resection, n (%)	12 (13.3)	24 (20.9)	0.16
Adjuvant therapy, n (%)	32 (35.6)	54 (47.0)	0.10
Perioperative treatment, n (%)			0.004
None	47 (52.2)	42 (36.5)	
MMC	20 (22.2)	51 (44.4)	
CSBI	23 (25.6)	22 (19.1)	

MMC Mitomycin-C, *CSBI* continuous saline bladder irrigation, *SD* standard deviation, *CIS* carcinoma in situ. +One-way ANOVA. *Fisher's exact test

or water). [5] Upon closer examination, however, we are unable to compare the protocols included as published in the meta-analysis or in the original manuscripts to our brief post-operative irrigation protocol. Of the 13 included studies, the use of post-operative irrigation was only documented as consistently used in four of these studies. Irrigation protocols were not detailed in the meta-analysis and review of the original data could not identify specific protocols. Furthermore, at least one study utilized distilled water for irrigation, which has the theoretical advantage of an osmotic cytotoxic effect but the disadvantages of being hypotonic. Therefore, despite a 21% relative reduction in recurrences found in this

meta-analysis with use of post-operative irrigation alone, we can only cautiously compare this result with our data without more detailed information about the irrigation protocols used.

The concept of utilizing irrigation for eradication of residual tumor cells following surgery for cancer is not a new concept, nor is it limited to urology or even endoscopic surgery. Surgeons have traditionally irrigated surgical sites to mechanically wash away debris, dilution of bacterial loads, and as a method of tumor cell lysis, depending on the tonicity of the fluid. A survey in England found that 74% of general surgeons perform intraoperative peritoneal lavage during cancer operations (36%

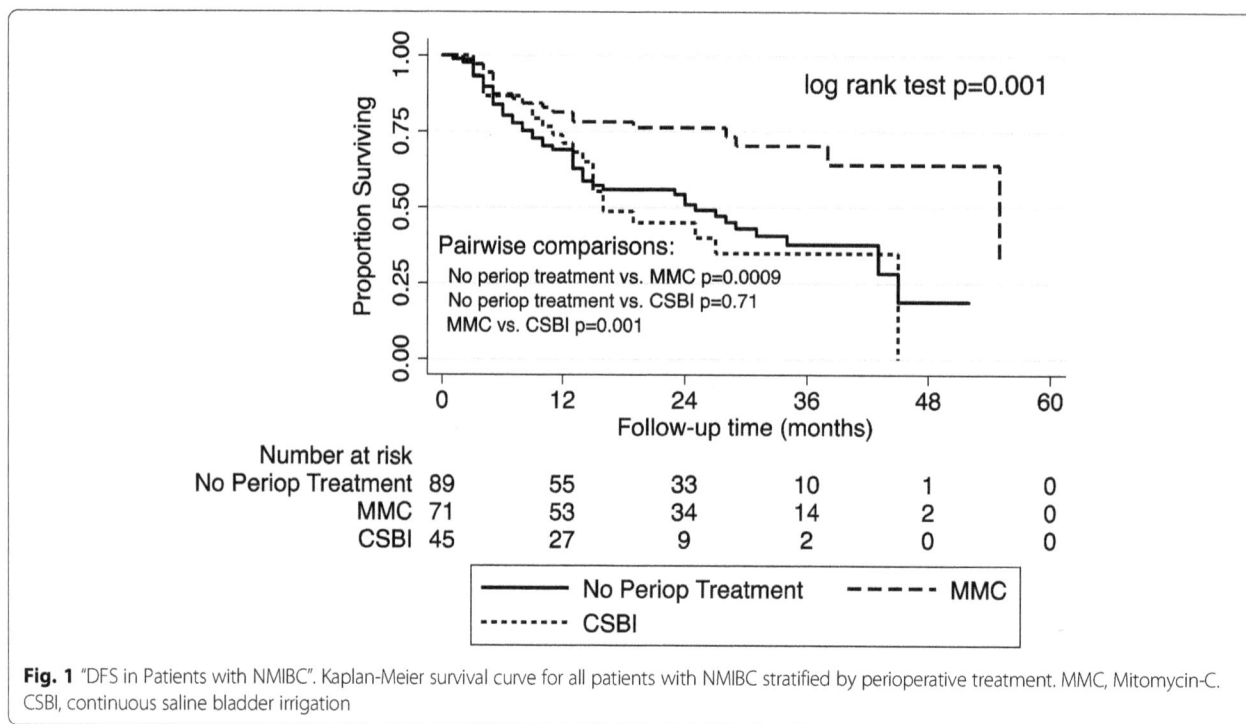

Fig. 1 "DFS in Patients with NMIBC". Kaplan-Meier survival curve for all patients with NMIBC stratified by perioperative treatment. MMC, Mitomycin-C. CSBI, continuous saline bladder irrigation

with water, 21% with saline, and 17% with betadine). [15] However, efficacy data on irrigation type is conflicting. Sweitzer et al. designed an experiment in mice to evaluate whether distilled water or sterile saline irrigation could reduce the burden of orthotopically implanted melanoma tumor cells. [16] Unfortunately, they found that neither the mechanical process of irrigation nor the hypotonicity of water reduced the tumor burden. In contrast, Fumito et al. demonstrated the superiority of water irrigation to saline irrigation following laparotomy in a mouse model of colorectal cancer tumor spillage. [17] In head and neck cancer models, both the type of irrigation and type of cancer cell line contributed to efficacy. [18, 19] These and other conflicting data suggest that multiple

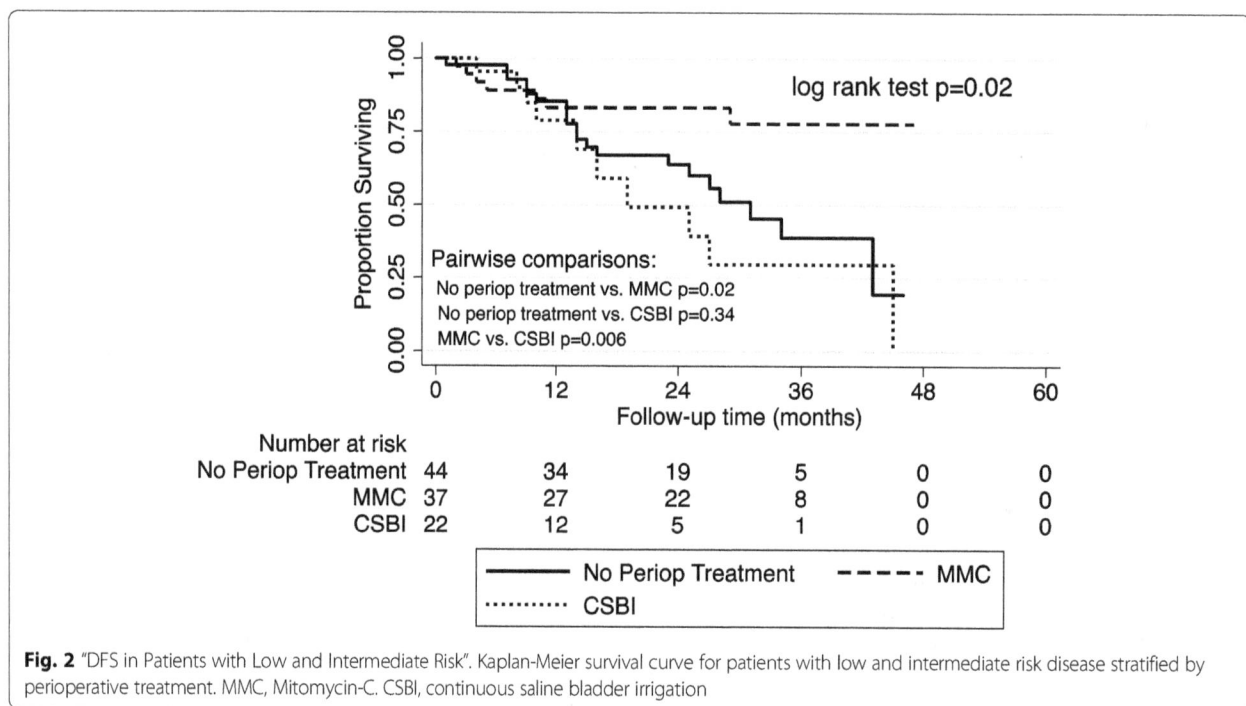

Fig. 2 "DFS in Patients with Low and Intermediate Risk". Kaplan-Meier survival curve for patients with low and intermediate risk disease stratified by perioperative treatment. MMC, Mitomycin-C. CSBI, continuous saline bladder irrigation

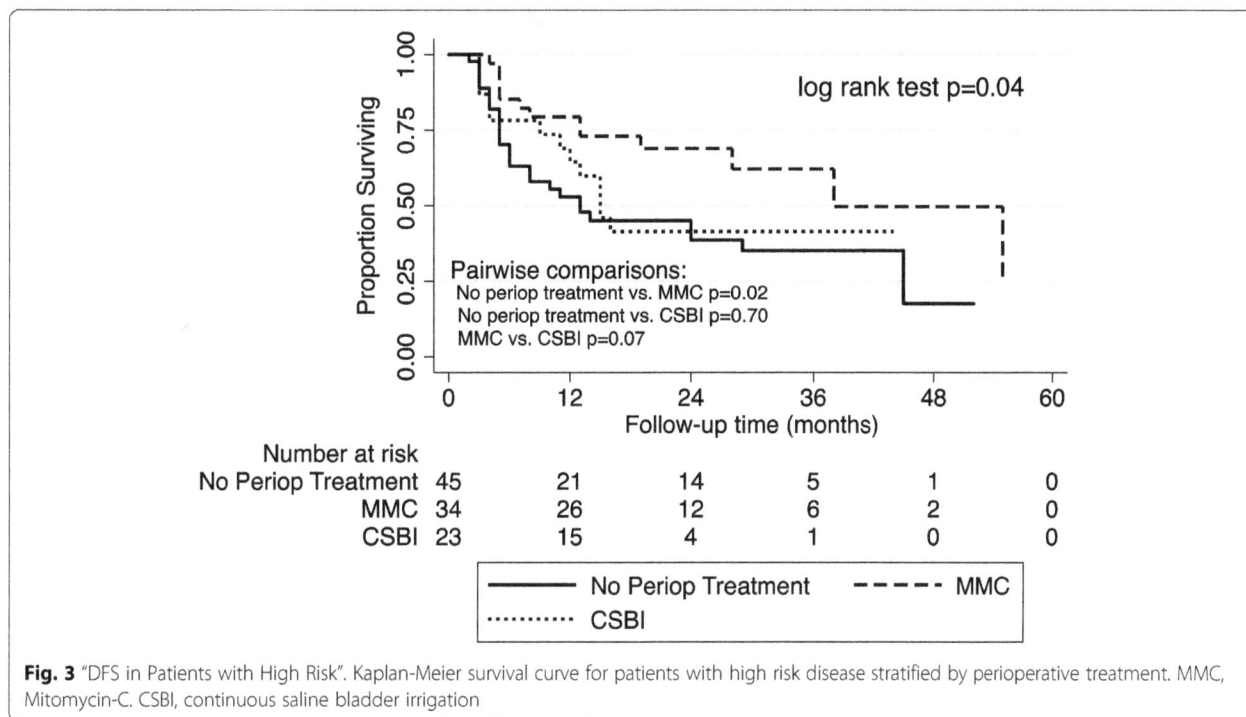

Fig. 3 "DFS in Patients with High Risk". Kaplan-Meier survival curve for patients with high risk disease stratified by perioperative treatment. MMC, Mitomycin-C. CSBI, continuous saline bladder irrigation

factors play a role with respect to the eradication of residual tumor burden, potentially related to the microenvironment and tumor cell-specific factors, such as cell adhesion properties and degree of de-differentiation.

The literature does strongly support irrigation following intra-luminal surgery in other surgical fields. For example, Zhou et al. performed a meta-analysis of studies evaluating intra-luminal washout following anterior resection for rectal cancer and concluded that washout leads to reduced rates of local recurrence. [20] In the urologic literature, Moskovitz et al. first postulated in 1987 that intravesical irrigation with distilled water during and after TURBT would lead to fewer recurrences. [21] While several small studies have demonstrated conflicting results regarding the use of water irrigation compared with no perioperative treatment, no studies have compared CSBI to MMC until the aforementioned studies by Onishi et al. [10, 14, 22, 23] Our study is the first to compare a shorter, perioperative duration of CSBI to both MMC and no perioperative treatment, and to evaluate this strategy in a heterogeneous patient population with low, intermediate, and high risk disease.

Table 3 Cox multivariable model for Recurrence or Progression

Variable	Hazard Ratio	95% Confidence Interval	p-value
Age (per year of age)	1.00	0.98–1.02	0.92
AUA Risk Stratification			
Low Risk	Reference	Reference	
Intermediate Risk	0.84	0.39–1.80	0.66
High Risk	2.77	1.28–6.01	0.01
Adjuvant therapy			
No	Reference	Reference	
Yes	0.35	0.20–0.59	< 0.001
Perioperative treatment			
No perioperative treatment	Reference	Reference	
MMC	0.43	0.25–0.75	0.003
CSBI	0.96	0.58–1.60	0.89

LG low grade, *HG* high grade, *CIS* carcinoma in situ, *MMC* Mitomycin-C, *CSBI* continuous saline bladder irrigation

Our results, however, should be considered within the context of several limitations. Although this was a hypothesis-based study driven by pre-clinical and clinical data, it was not a randomized controlled study, and was limited to the data available in medical records. Furthermore, the study is underpowered and longer term follow-up is required to fully realize the potential differences between treatment groups. It is possible that a larger cohort with longer term follow up could confirm the null hypothesis, suggesting that no difference exists between treatment groups. However, at our institution we are mainly utilizing intravesical gemcitabine based on recently published data that suggests efficacy at a fraction of the cost and with reduced side effects compared with MMC. [24] Consequently, in combination with the current data that suggests inefficacy of 2 h of CSBI, we are unlikely to treat more patients with adjuvant CSBI. Primarily one surgeon (KC) performed CSBI during the study period while most other surgeons in the department utilized either MMC or no additional perioperative therapy. Therefore, referral patterns may have contributed to patient heterogeneity between groups. Despite some baseline differences between treatment groups described in our results, the data remains consistent when controlling for factors such as tumor grade, stage, and recurrence disease, among others, in a multivariable model. A consistent surveillance cystoscopy protocol was not used for all patients and could have helped standardize follow-up and limit detection bias. Finally, we utilized a clinical definition of recurrence that included any suspicious lesion during office cystoscopy that warranted an intervention (usually fulguration), which may have artificially increased our recurrence rates.

Nevertheless, our study comparing perioperative CSBI, perioperative MMC, and no perioperative treatment answers important questions regarding CSBI as prophylaxis following endoscopic resection for NMIBC. While CSBI for two hours postoperatively should not replace current guideline-recommended perioperative MMC, it does appear that longer duration of CSBI may increase its efficacy. [10, 14] Research is needed to determine whether the duration can be reduced to limit the number of additional hospital stays and whether other, novel perioperative instillations may reduce recurrences and limit side effects.

Conclusions

Our data demonstrates that perioperative CSBI for two hours following TURBT is not equivalent to postoperative MMC in terms of rates of recurrence or progression. CSBI for two hours appears to be equivalent to no perioperative treatment, regardless of tumor grade. It is possible that CSBI may be required for a longer duration to reduce tumor cell re-implantation and, in turn, decrease rates of recurrence or progression.

Acknowledgements

This work was supported by the National Institutes of Health Loan Repayment Program (L30 CA154326 (Principal Investigator: KC)), the STOP Cancer Foundation (Principal Investigator: KC), the H & H Lee Surgical Resident Research Award (Recipient: ATL), and the Short Term Training Program (STTP) at the David Geffen School of Medicine at UCLA (Recipient: KA).

Authors' contributions

ATL was primarily involved in protocol/project development, data collection/management, data analysis, manuscript writing/editing. KA was involved in data collection/management and manuscript writing. MB was involved in data collection/management and manuscript writing. NMD was involved in protocol/project development, data collection/management, data analysis, manuscript writing/editing. KC supervised and was responsible for all study oversight. All authors read and approved the final manuscript.

Author details

[1]David Geffen School of Medicine at the University of California Los Angeles, 300 Stein Plaza, Suite 348, Los Angeles, California 90095, USA. [2]Department of Urology, Health Services Research Group, David Geffen School of Medicine at UCLA, Los Angeles, California, USA. [3]Jonsson Comprehensive Cancer Center, David Geffen School of Medicine at UCLA, Los Angeles, California, USA. [4]Riverside School of Medicine, University of California, Riverside, California, USA.

References

1. Clark PE, Agarwal N, Biagioli MC, Eisenberger MA, Greenberg RE, Herr HW, et al. Bladder cancer J Natl Compr Canc Netw. 2013:446–75.
2. James AC, Gore JL. The costs of non-muscle invasive bladder cancer. Urol. Clin. North Am. 2013:40:261–9 Available from: http://www.ncbi.nlm.nih.gov/pubmed/23540783.
3. Chamie K, Saigal CS, Lai J, Hanley JM, Setodji CM, Konety BR, et al. Compliance with guidelines for patients with bladder cancer: variation in the delivery of care. Cancer. 2011;117:5392–401 Available from: http://www.pubmedcentral.nih.gov/articlerender.fcgi?artid=3206145&tool=pmcentrez&rendertype=abstract.
4. Sylvester RJ, Oosterlinck W, van der Meijden APM. A single immediate postoperative instillation of chemotherapy decreases the risk of recurrence in patients with stage ta T1 bladder cancer: a meta-analysis of published results of randomized clinical trials. J Urol. 2004;171:2186–90 quiz2435.
5. Sylvester RJ, Oosterlinck W, Holmäng S, Sydes MR, Birtle A, Gudjonsson S, et al. Systematic review and individual patient data meta-analysis of randomized trials comparing a single immediate instillation of chemotherapy after transurethral resection with transurethral resection alone in patients with stage pTa-pT1 urothelial carcinoma of the bladder: which patients benefit from the instillation? Eur Urol. 2016;69:231–44.
6. Doherty AP, Trendell-Smith N, Stirling R, Rogers H, Bellringer J. Perivesical fat necrosis after adjuvant intravesical chemotherapy. BJU Int. 1999;83:420–3.
7. Jones G, Cleves A, Wilt TJ, Mason M, Kynaston HG, Shelley M. Intravesical gemcitabine for non-muscle invasive bladder cancer. Cochrane Database Syst Rev John Wiley & Sons, Ltd. 2012;1:CD009294.
8. Hendricksen K, Cornel EB, de Reijke TM, Arentsen HC, Chawla S, Witjes JA. Phase 2 study of adjuvant intravesical instillations of apaziquone for high risk nonmuscle invasive bladder cancer. J Urol. 2012;187:1195–1199.
9. Taoka R, Williams SB, Ho PL, Kamat AM. In-vitro cytocidal effect of water on bladder cancer cells: the potential role for intraperitoneal lavage during radical cystectomy. CUAJ. 2015;9:E109–13.
10. Onishi T, Sasaki T, Hoshina A, Yabana T. Continuous saline bladder irrigation after transurethral resection is a prophylactic treatment choice for non-muscle invasive bladder tumor. Anticancer Res. 2011;31:1471–4.
11. Chang SS, Boorjian SA, Chou R, Clark PE, Daneshmand S, Konety BR, et al. Diagnosis and treatment of non-muscle invasive bladder Cancer: AUA/SUO guideline. J Urol. 2016;196:1021–9.
12. Sylvester RJ, van der Meijden APM, Lamm DL. Intravesical bacillus Calmette-Guerin reduces the risk of progression in patients with superficial bladder cancer: a meta-analysis of the published results of randomized clinical trials. J Urol. 2002;168:1964–70 Available from: http://www.ncbi.nlm.nih.gov/pubmed/12394686.

13. Abern MR, Owusu RA, Anderson MR, Rampersaud EN, Inman BA. Perioperative intravesical chemotherapy in non-muscle-invasive bladder cancer: a systematic review and meta-analysis. J Natl Compr Cancer Netw. 2013;11:477–84.

14. Onishi T, Sugino Y, Shibahara T, Masui S, Yabana T, Sasaki T Randomized controlled study of the efficacy and safety of continuous saline bladder irrigation after transurethral resection for the treatment of n... - PubMed - NCBI. BJU international. 2016.

15. Whiteside OJH, Tytherleigh MG, Thrush S, Farouk R, Galland RB. Intra-operative peritoneal lavage--who does it and why? Ann R Coll Surg Engl. 2005;87:255–8.

16. Sweitzer KL, Nathanson SD, Nelson LT, Zachary C. Irrigation does not dislodge or destroy tumor cells adherent to the tumor bed. J Surg Oncol. 1993;53:184–90.

17. Ito F, Camoriano M, Seshadri M, Evans SS, Kane JM, Skitzki JJ. Water: a simple solution for tumor spillage. Ann Surg Oncol Springer-Verlag. 2011;18:2357–63.

18. Lodhia KA, Dale OT, Winter SC. Irrigation solutions in head and neck cancer surgery: a preclinical efficacy study. Ann Otol Rhinol Laryngol SAGE Publications. 2015;124:68–71.

19. Hah JH, Roh DH, Jung YH, Kim KH, Sung M-W. Selection of irrigation fluid to eradicate free cancer cells during head and neck cancer surgery. Head neck. Wiley subscription services, Inc. A Wiley Company. 2012;34:546–50.

20. Zhou C, Ren Y, Li J, Li X, He J, Liu P. Systematic review and meta-analysis of rectal washout on risk of local recurrence for cancer. - PubMed - NCBI. J Surg Res. 2014;189:7–16.

21. Moskovitz B, Levin DR. Intravesical irrigation with distilled water during and immediately after transurethral resection and later for superficial bladder cancer. Eur Urol. 1987;13:7–9.

22. Sakai Y, Fujii Y, Hyochi N, Masuda H, Kawakami S, Kobayashi T, et al. A large amount of distilled water ineffective for prevention of bladder cancer cell implantation at the time of transurethral resection. Hinyokika Kiyo. 2006;52:173–5.

23. Amos S, Gofrit ON. Prevention of bladder tumor recurrence. Evolving trends in urology. In: Sashi S Kommu, editor. 1st ed. Rijeka, Croatia: InTech; 2012. pp. 69–76. https://doi.org/10.5772/38495.

24. Messing EM, Tangen CM, Lerner SP, Sahasrabudhe DM, Koppie TM, Wood DP, et al. Effect of Intravesical instillation of gemcitabine vs saline immediately following resection of suspected low-grade non-muscle-invasive bladder Cancer on tumor recurrence: SWOG S0337 randomized clinical trial. JAMA. 2018;319:1880–8.

25

Effects of biofeedback-based sleep improvement program on urinary symptoms and sleep patterns of elderly Korean women with overactive bladder syndrome

Jooyeon Park[1], Choal Hee Park[2], Sang-Eun Jun[1], Eun-Ju Lee[1], Seung Wan Kang[3] and Nahyun Kim[1]* (iD)

Abstract

Background: The prevalence of overactive bladder syndrome (OAB) increases with age. Sleep disturbances in elderly individuals with OAB is a common problem. The purpose of this study was to examine the effects of a biofeedback-based sleep improvement (BBSI) program on urinary symptoms and sleep patterns in elderly Korean women with OAB.

Methods: A non-equivalent control group pre–/post-test design was used. Elderly women with OAB were assigned to an intervention group ($n = 20$) or a control group ($n = 18$). The BBSI program was implemented in the intervention group for 12 weeks, while two educational sessions of general sleep hygiene and lifestyle modification were provided to the control group. Using SPSS 23.0, the data were analyzed by descriptive analysis using the chi-square test, Fisher's exact test, Mann-Whitney test, and Wilcoxon test.

Results: After the 12-week BBSI program, significant improvements were found in the intervention group's the square root of the mean squared differences of successive R-R intervals ($p = 0.025$), low frequency/high frequency ratio ($p = 0.006$), and epinephrine ($p = 0.039$). We also observed a significant difference in urinary symptoms, sleep efficiency, wake after sleep onset, number of awakenings, and number of awakenings within 3 h after sleep onset ($p < 0.001$, $p = 0.004$, $p = 0.001$, $p = 0.001$, and $p = 0.048$, respectively). However, no significant changes were found in these variables in the control group.

Conclusions: The BBSI program effectively improved urinary symptoms and sleep patterns of elderly Korean women with OAB. Further longitudinal research is required to investigate the sustainability and effects of the BBSI program.

Keywords: Overactive bladder syndrome, Sleep, Autonomic nervous system

* Correspondence: drkim@kmu.ac.kr
[1]College of Nursing, Keimyung University, Daegu, Republic of Korea
Full list of author information is available at the end of the article

Background

Sleep disorders in elderly individuals with overactive bladder syndrome (OAB) are a common problem. The prevalence of OAB in elderly individuals in the United States and Europe is 16.9 and 11.8%, respectively [1, 2]. OAB is characterized by major lower urinary tract dysfunction that causes urinary frequency, nocturia, and urinary urgency irrespective of urge incontinence [3]. Its prevalence increases with age [2] and lower physical activity [4] and is higher in females than in males [1]. Nocturia is the most uncomfortable lower urinary tract symptom in elderly individuals; it directly causes sleep disturbances and increases the risk of falls and fractures [5]. Frequent awakening due to symptoms of OAB disturbs the quality of sleep, resulting in severe fatigue in daytime activities [6].

The cause of OAB has not been identified yet; however, one or more physiological changes are thought to play a role in its development [7]. OAB without the presence of a neurological disease has been attributed to autonomic nervous system (ANS) abnormalities based on the role of the ANS in regulating bladder function [8]. The parasympathetic nervous system induces bladder contractions, while the sympathetic nervous system regulates the contractions of the bladder neck and urethral smooth muscle and relaxation of the bladder body [9]. Therefore, ANS imbalances can result in abnormal bladder activity [8].

Although elderly individuals can suffer from sleep disorders secondary to OAB, aging itself causes ANS changes, leading to increased and decreased activities of the sympathetic and parasympathetic nervous systems, respectively, thereby lowering the sleep quality [10]. Excessive sympathetic nervous system activity leads to frequent awakening and interferes with deep sleep, suggesting that sleep interventions in elderly women should be directed towards maintaining balance in the ANS [11, 12].

However, active efforts to solve such problems are lacking because most patients tend to perceive this issue as a natural phenomenon due to aging. Few studies have examined the management of symptoms in the elderly at the physiological level and few interventions are available to address sleep disorders. Sleep disorders are often considered characteristic of elderly patients. Additionally, there are limited drug therapies that can be used to improve sleep problems in elderly people with OAB. Anti-muscarinic drugs are the most commonly used ones in the treatment of OAB; however, long-term adherence to the management is very low due to the side effects, such as constipation and dry mouth [13, 14]. Particularly, elderly patients may be on multiple drugs for various comorbidities; therefore, care must be taken in prescribing these drugs. For this reason, several studies have suggested that multicomponent treatment should be considered as the first-line therapy for OAB in elderly people [15, 16].

In this study, we aimed to use mechanism-based interventions to improve sleep in elderly people with OAB and focused on using mechanisms to balance the ANS. A therapeutic approach towards balancing the ANS is essential to be an effective sleep intervention in elderly patients with OAB. The use of biofeedback from the sympathetic and parasympathetic nervous systems to balance the ANS appears to be an important approach in alleviating the symptoms of OAB. Additionally, biofeedback has been reported to be not only an effective intervention in patients with physical and psychological disorders secondary to ANS imbalances but also a suitable sleep intervention as well [17].

In the literature, changes in autonomic functions might be the underlying cause of OAB and lowered sleep quality. OAB also could be one of the major factors that interfere with deep sleep in the elderly. Therefore, we hypothesized that stabilizing the autonomic functions might reduce the symptoms of OAB and improve sleep.

Methods

Study design

This experimental study used a multi-site nonequivalent control group pre- and post-test design.

Participants and procedures

This study was conducted between March and September 2018. Our study population was selected from the elderly women registered in two senior welfare centers in Korea. The inclusion criteria were the following: (1) age ≥ 65 years; (2) Overactive Bladder Symptom Score (OABSS) ≥ 3, and urgency score ≥ 2 [18]; (3) Pittsburgh Sleep Quality Index (PSQI) score ≥ 5 [19]; (4) Mini-Mental State Examination (MMSE) ≥ 24 [20]; and (5) no history of participation in other programs to improve sleep over the previous 6 months. Participants were excluded if they were consuming sleeping pills or OAB medications, had a history of urinary tract infection at the time of the survey, were diagnosed with neurological or psychiatric disorders or autonomic neuropathy, or were diagnosed with other diseases affecting autonomic function.

To recruit the participants, we visited each senior welfare center and obtained permission to explain the study to prospective elderly participants. We then explained the study's purpose and procedures and invited interested elderly patients to participate. We also used posters to invite elderly women to participate. After consulting the chief of each center, using a coin toss, one center was assigned to provide the experimental group and the other the control group. The intervention was initiated a week after the categorization. The flowchart of patient selection is depicted in Fig. 1. Of the 55 enrolled women, 9 women refused to participate in the study; therefore, 23 were included in the biofeedback-based sleep improvement (BBSI) program, while another 23 patients were only managed in terms of sleep hygiene and lifestyle modifications. Overall, eight patients were lost to follow-up and dropping out; the remaining 38 were followed up for 12 weeks (20 in the BBSI group vs. 18 in the control group).

For the pre-test, the participants arrived at the study location and rested for more than 30 min. Three research assistants administered the questionnaire and measured heart rate variability (HRV). For HRV measurements, the participants were suggested to relax and instructed to breathe comfortably without speaking. After the 12-week intervention, a follow-up evaluation was conducted with the same contents as those in the pre-test. The research

assistants examined the same items as in the pre-test to minimize measurement errors.

Sample size estimation

The sample size of this study was determined using the G power version 3.1.9 program. The sample size was calculated based on a two-sided test with significance level of 0.05, power of 0.80, and effect size of (d) 0.99 [21] in the study of sleep disorders. As a result, there were a total of 36 participants, 18 of whom were required in each group to evaluate differences between the two groups. Its actual power was 0.82. In the present study, 23 in the experimental group and 23 in the control group were chosen as candidates for participation in the program based on a dropout rate of 20%.

Intervention

The intervention program was developed to improve sleep in elderly women with OAB. We designed the

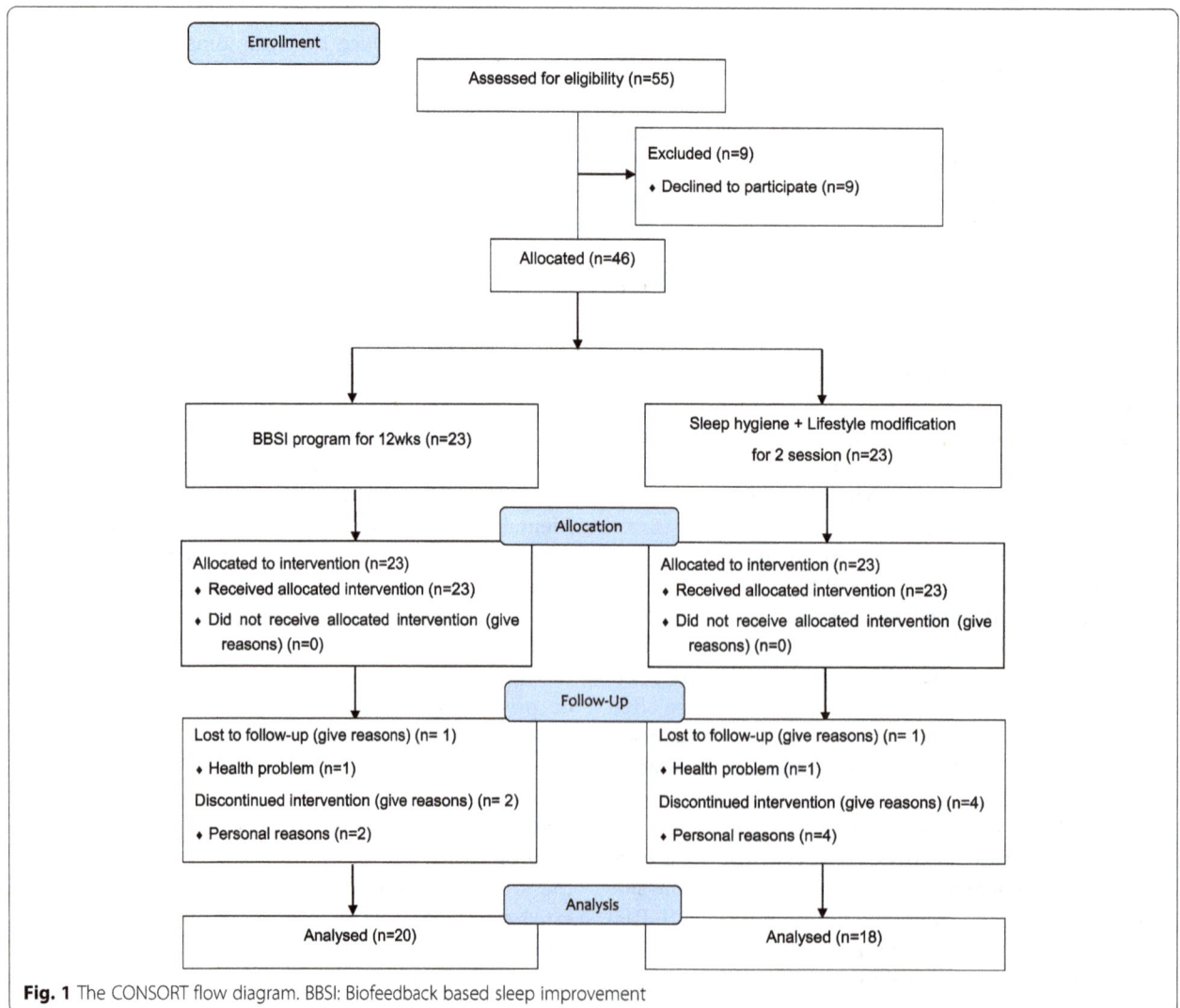

Fig. 1 The CONSORT flow diagram. BBSI: Biofeedback based sleep improvement

program with an emphasis on ANS balance, including individual intervention, group education, and telephone coaching. We prepared an intervention plan by reviewing the literature based on Overactive Bladder Syndrome Treatment Guidelines [22] and Sleep Hygiene Education provided by the Korean Society of Sleep Medicine [23]. The components of the program consisted of direct and indirect elements that have been previously reported to be effective for autonomic balance. Biofeedback was used for the direct approach for ANS balance [24], and lifestyle modifications, physical activity, and depression management—which were reported to be effective for ANS balance—were used as indirect approaches [25–27]. Additionally, behavioral therapy is very important in sleep disorders with OAB. Therefore, the participants were educated regarding sleep hygiene in consideration of OAB characteristics and pelvic floor muscle (PFM) contraction exercises were included in the program [28, 29]. The main outlines of the BBSI program were as follows: (1) individual intervention: HRV biofeedback training—a key component of ANS balance; (2) group training: behavioral therapy to reduce OAB symptoms and improve sleep, including lifestyle modifications, sleep hygiene, pelvic muscle contractions, physical activity, and depression management; and (3) telephone coaching: emotional support and individual goal setting. An additional file shows this in more detail [see Additional file 1].

The individual interventions consisted of weekly biofeedback training for 20 min for 12 weeks. For biofeedback training, a computerized biofeedback system (Procomp, Thought Technology, Montreal, QC, Canada) was used. By analyzing the changes in the visual heart rhythm and respiration, HRV biofeedback balances the ANS by controlling the respiratory rate. The intervention provider was an experienced urology nurse who was well-trained to provide biofeedback. Biofeedback confirmed the participant's baseline status in pre-testing and maintained an ideal state (close to 1.5) of low frequency (LF) to high frequency (HF) ratio (LF/HF) during training [30].

Group education was conducted for 40 min once a week for 12 weeks. It consisted of sleep hygiene education, lifestyle modifications, PFM contraction exercises, physical activity, and depression management. The lifestyle modification program included body mass index control, caffeine restriction, and alcohol restriction. A pedometer was provided to increase each participant's amount of physical activity. After each round of group training, individual counseling was provided to encourage each participant to achieve their goals.

Telephone coaching was conducted to encourage goal achievement and provide emotional support. We encouraged the use of biofeedback-based respiration techniques every day and set individual and daily goals to promote physical activity. We then confirmed that they

practiced the same. Emotional support was provided after identifying the participants' environmental and psychological statuses. Also, for positive reinforcement, the program provided participants with a workbook at the beginning of the program and rewarded participants who achieved the goal well during the mid-term check.

The control group received 40 min of training on sleep hygiene and lifestyle modifications in the 4th and 8th sessions of intervention, respectively. In order to maintain consistency in the contents of the two groups, education was conducted by the same educators in both groups. Additionally, before the program began, the researchers agreed on the materials to be provided to both groups and conducted the training in accordance with the agreed content. Sleep hygiene education consisted of the same 11 sleep hygiene items as those of the intervention group. Regarding lifestyle modifications, the control group was instructed to restrict caffeine and water intake, perform PFM exercises, and increase physical activity.

Outcome measures
Measures of HRV
HRV was used to assess the sympathetic and parasympathetic activities since it enables qualitative, quantitative, and noninvasive analysis of global autonomic function [17, 31]. To assess ANS activity, HRV was measured with a heart rate monitoring device (Polar V800, Polar Electro Oy, Kempele, Finland). All R-R intervals collected through the wireless chest strap of the heart rate monitor were recorded with a 1000-Hz wireless heart rate monitor suitable for HRV analyses. After the measurement, the raw data were extracted by the Pro-trainer Polar 5 (version 5.40.171, Polar Electro) program and transferred to Kubios (version 2.0, 2008, Biosignal Analysis and Medical Imaging Group, Finland). We evaluated HRV with the converted values in Kubios.

The results of HRV demonstrate the values in time and frequency domains for ANS activity. The parameters of the time domain analysis were the standard deviation of Normal to Normal R-R intervals (SDNN) and the square root of the mean squared differences of successive R-R intervals (RMSSD). SDNN estimates the overall HRV, while RMSSD represents parasympathetic activity. The parameters of the frequency domain analysis were total power (TP), LF, HF, and LF/HF ratio. TP reflects the control capacity of the ANS, LF (0.04–0.15 Hz) represents sympathetic activity, and HF (0.15–0.4 Hz) represents the parasympathetic activity. The LF/HF ratio represents the interaction and balance between the two systems [32].

With the participants breathing normally, we calculated SDNN, RMSSD, TP, LF, HR, and LF/HF ratio. The participants were instructed not to smoke or drink alcohol or caffeinated beverages after 10 pm on the night before data collection. Each participant was seated on a comfortable chair and the HRV monitor was placed on the left wrist. Participants were asked not to talk and breathe at a normal rate during the 5-min measurement.

Plasma catecholamine level

Epinephrine (epi) and norepinephrine were assayed using blood samples. Each participant was instructed to lie quietly for 30 min before the blood sampling. Venous blood (5 mL) was obtained in a heparin anticoagulation vacuum tube. Catecholamine levels were measured by high-performance liquid chromatography (Acclaim, Bio-Rad, United States of America).

OAB symptoms

OAB symptom severity was measured using 8 of the 33 items of the Overactive Bladder Questionnaire (OAB-q) developed by Cyone et al. [33]. The 8-item questionnaire consisted of 4 sub-areas: frequency, urgency, nocturia, and urge incontinence. Each item consists of a 6-point Likert scale ranging from "not affected at all" (1 point) to "strongly affected" (6 points). The symptom severity scale was calculated by the converted scores given by Coyne et al. [33] using a range of 0–100. The higher the score, the greater the severity of OAB symptoms. Cronbach's α was 0.86 [33] vs. Cronbach's α of 0.79 in our study.

Sleep patterns

We measured sleep efficiency (SE), wake after sleep onset (WASO), number of awakenings, and number of awakenings within 3 h of sleep onset using actigraphy (W-GT3X-BT, Actigraph, Inc., Pensacola FL, United States of America) to assess sleep. The actigraphy device can be worn on the waist or wrist using an elastic belt. In elderly individuals, wearing an actigraphy device on the wrist reportedly reduces the sensitivity of low-intensity activities when using walking aids [34, 35]; therefore, we chose to place it on the waist. The data collected by the actigraphy device was analyzed by Actilife 6 software to obtain SE, WASO, number of awakenings, and number of awakenings within 3 h of sleep onset. In this study, sleep was scored using medium threshold settings and default parameters for sleep scoring based on 1-min epochs. Since the measurement period of the actigraphy is at least 3 consecutive days [36], the participants wore the actigraphy device during sleep for 3 days. We also asked the participants to accurately collect information regarding bedtime and rise time for each night while they were wearing the actigraphy device.

Data analysis

The data were analyzed using SPSS for Windows version 20.0 (SPSS Inc., Armonk, NY, United States of America). We used the Chi-square test, Fisher's exact test, and Mann–Whitney test to test the homogeneity of the general characteristics of the experimental and control groups. The efficacy of the BBSI program was analyzed using the Wilcoxon test. Cronbach's test was used to confirm reliability. P values < 0.05 were considered to be statistically significant.

Results

Twenty elderly women with OAB treated with the BBSI program (BBSI group) and 18 with OAB without the BBSI program (control group) were included in the present study. The patients' basic characteristics, clinical and laboratory parameters of ANS activity, OAB symptoms, and sleep patterns are summarized in Table 1. The mean age in the BBSI group and control group was 80.05 ± 4.21 and 81.06 ± 4.32 years, respectively. There were no intergroup differences in the educational level, marital status, monthly income, parity, caffeine intake, water intake, BMI, or OAB duration. Regarding the parameters of HRV, catecholamines, OAB symptoms, and sleep patterns did not differ between the groups.

The effects of the 12-week BBSI program on the HRV parameters and plasma catecholamine levels are summarized in Table 2. Significant decreases were observed in RMSSD (37.02 ± 35.56 vs. 51.93 ± 49.61, $p = 0.025$), LF/HF ratio (2.59 ± 2.23 vs. 1.03 ± 0.27, $p = 0.006$), and epinephrine levels (42.31 ± 13.58 vs. 34.69 ± 12.83, $p = 0.039$) in the BBSI group after the intervention, whereas SDNN, TP, LF, and HF did not differ after the intervention. All the parameters related to HRV and plasma catecholamine levels in the control group did not change in the control group after the 12-week period.

The effects of the 12-week BBSI intervention on OAB symptoms measured by OAQ-q are summarized in Table 3. At baseline, no significant difference was found in the frequency, urgency, nocturia, or urgency incontinence between the patients and controls (Table 1). After the 12-week intervention, the BBSI group demonstrated a significant improvement in the urgency score (8.5 ± 1.5 vs. 7.5 ± 0.82, $p = 0.004$), nocturia (9.35 ± 2.08 vs. 6.85 ± 1.42, $p < 0.001$), and total score (48.81 ± 10.59 vs. 33.96 ± 7.31, $p < 0.001$).

Table 4 shows that, regarding sleep patterns, in the BBSI group, we observed a significant difference in SE, WASO, number of awakenings, and number of awakenings within three hours after sleep onset ($p = 0.004$, $p = 0.001$, $p = 0.001$, and $p = 0.048$, respectively).

Discussion

In this study, we aimed to develop, apply, and analyze the efficacy of a BBSI program in elderly women with

Table 1 Homogeneity test for general characteristics and baseline of variables (N = 38)

Variables		BBSI (n = 20)	Control (n = 18)	p
		Mean ± SD or n (%)		
Age (yr)		80.05 ± 4.21	81.06 ± 4.32	.472
Education level	<Elementary school	17 (80.0)	15 (83.4)	.383
	≥ Middle school	3 (15.0)	3 (16.6)	
Spouse	Yes	3 (15.0)	3 (16.7)	.616†
	No	17 (85.0)	15 (83.3)	
Monthly income	< 100	20 (100.0)	17 (95.0)	.474†
(10,000 won)	≥ 100	0 (0.0)	1 (5.0)	
Parity (number)		3.80 ± 1.58	3.17 ± 1.92	.272
Caffeine intake (cup/day)	< 4	10 (50.0)	11 (61.1)	.492
	≥ 4	10 (50.0)	7 (38.9)	
Water intake (cc/day)	< 1000	12 (60.0)	15 (83.3)	.113†
	≥ 1000	8 (40.0)	3 (16.7)	
Regular exercise (/week)	< 3	17 (85.0)	15 (83.3)	.263†
	≥ 3	3 (15.0)	3 (16.7)	
BMI (kg/m²)		23.95 ± 3.96	24.13 ± 2.94	.882
OAB duration (yr)		2.35 ± 2.38	1.58 ± 1.29	.225§
HRV				
SDNN (ms)		29.79 ± 29.13	25.54 ± 19.48	.826§
RMSSD (ms)		37.02 ± 35.56	28.97 ± 23.93	.682§
TP (ms²)		2893.95 ± 6692.99	1303.61 ± 3158.63	.748§
LF (ms²)		1429.35 ± 3794.62	735.39 ± 1657.95	.815§
HF (ms²)		856.20 ± 1579.64	638.89 ± 1562.95	501§
LF/HF ratio		2.59 ± 2.23	2.81 ± 2.13	.520§
Catecholamines				
E (pg/mL)		42.31 ± 13.58	50.56 ± 18.73	.126§
NE (pg/mL)		472.84 ± 198.28	511.77 ± 195.55	.520§
OAB symptom severity		42.81 ± 10.59	38.54 ± 11.83	.248§
Sleep				
SE (%)		86.89 ± 4.93	87.77 ± 5.39	.619§
WASO (min)		69.20 ± 27.57	56.27 ± 22.94	.128§
Number of awakenings		10.85 ± 4.16	10.14 ± 4.80	.609§
Number of awakenings in 3 h after sleep onset		4.48 ± 1.74	4.09 ± 1.81	.702§

†Fisher's exact test; § Mann-Whitney test; *BBSI* Biofeedback-based sleep improvement program, *OAB* Overactive bladder syndrome, *SDNN* Standard deviation of all normal to normal R-R intervals, *RMSSD* Root mean square differences of successive R-R intervals, *TP* Total power, *LF* Low frequency, *HF* High frequency, *Epi* Epinephrine, *NE* Norepinephrine, *SE* Sleep efficiency, *WASO* Wake after sleep onset

OAB who were assumed to have an overall ANS imbalance due to excessive sympathetic activity. The program included biofeedback training using HRV, lifestyle modifications, physical activity, depression management, sleep hygiene, and PFM exercises. After the 12-week program, RMSSD—a key indicator of HRV—had increased significantly, while the LF/HF ratio and epinephrine secretion decreased significantly. Furthermore, OAB symptoms had alleviated. These results improved sleep by decreasing WASO, number of awakenings during sleep, number of awakenings within 3 h of sleep onset, and increasing sleep efficiency (SE).

Notable results of this study were that post-intervention RMSSD in the experimental group increased significantly, whereas the post-intervention LF/HF ratio decreased significantly. No differences were observed in these indicators in the control group after completion of the study. Biofeedback using HRV effectively treated the psychological issues, such as depression, panic, and insomnia through ANS balance [17]. The

Table 2 Effects of the BBSI program on the levels of heart rate variability parameters and catecholamines ($N = 38$)

Variables	BBSI ($n = 20$)			Control ($n = 18$)		
	Pre	Post		Pre	Post	
	Mean ± SD	Mean ± SD	p	Mean ± SD	Mean ± SD	p^*
SDNN (ms)	29.79 ± 29.13	47.47 ± 37.51	.113	25.54 ± 19.48	21.63 ± 11.50	.420
RMSSD (ms)	37.02 ± 35.56	51.93 ± 49.61	.025	28.97 ± 23.93	29.39 ± 22.45	.758
TP (ms^2)	2893.95 ± 6692.99	2036.60 ± 4422.05	.550	1303.61 ± 3158.63	2302.22 ± 5030.27	.983
LF (ms^2)	1429.35 ± 3794.62	804.85 ± 2132.54	.455	735.39 ± 1657.95	1074.83 ± 2463.03	.433
HF (ms^2)	856.20 ± 1579.64	1147.25 ± 2163.45	.709	638.89 ± 1562.95	844.33 ± 1893.83	.647
LF/HF ratio	2.59 ± 2.23	1.03 ± 0.27	.006	2.81 ± 2.13	2.42 ± 1.30	.446
Epi (pg/mL)	42.31 ± 13.58	34.69 ± 12.83	.039	50.56 ± 18.73	59.20 ± 23.59	.076
NE (pg/mL)	472.84 ± 198.28	434.91 ± 180.38	.218	511.77 ± 195.55	457.87 ± 210.90	.129

BBSI Biofeedback-based sleep improvement program, *OAB* Overactive bladder syndrome; *p*: difference from pre-test to post-test in BBSI groups *p**: difference from pre-test to post-test in control groups, *SDNN* Standard deviation of normal to normal R-R intervals, *RMSSD* Root mean square differences of successive R-R intervals, *TP* Total power, *LF* Low frequency, *HF* High frequency, *E* Epinephrine, *NE* Norepinephrine

ANS also demonstrated other benefits, such as decreased pulse, increased body temperature, and improved blood circulation [37].

According to previous studies in females with OAB, the LF/HF ratio is significantly increased when the bladder is full [38, 39]. Hsiao et al. emphasized that the sympathetic nervous system is relatively overactive in OAB because the LF/HF ratio is higher in women with OAB than that in healthy adults, even when the bladder is empty [40]. Similarly, Choi et al. [41] reported that HF—a frequency domain indicator of RMSSD and parasympathetic nerve activity—was decreased in women with OAB compared to healthy adults. RMSSD increased and LF/HF ratio decreased after the intervention in this study—a finding that was consistent with ANS changes that may help alleviate OAB symptoms. Furthermore, Hubeaux et al. suggested that ANS dysfunction due to sympathetic predominance may be implied in the generation of abnormal bladder sensations, such as urgency [38, 39]. In contrast, increased parasympathetic nerve activity has been reported as a cause of OAB [7, 42] or nocturia [43]. There are differences in the participants and data collection methods in these studies; therefore, direct comparison is difficult. However, our biofeedback protocol was designed to activate the parasympathetic nerves while keeping the LF/HF ratio at an appropriate value during biofeedback training, which may have been an important factor in alleviating OAB symptoms. Considering the results of previous studies, the results of this study confirm the possibility of ANS imbalance due to sympathetic dominance as the cause of OAB. ANS changes associated with senescence involve increase and decrease in the activities of the sympathetic and parasympathetic nervous systems, respectively [10, 44]. Such changes lead to sleep disturbances, including frequent awakening and reduced rapid eye movement (REM) sleep [44]. In one study, RMSSD was reported to be lower in elderly individuals than that in younger individuals, and this finding was more common in females [45]. Therefore, increased RMSSD may induce deep sleep and stabilize sleep structure. Further, serum epinephrine was significantly reduced after 12 weeks in the BBSI group. The LF/HF ratio is well-known to better reflect sympathetic nervous system balance than any other single indicator [30], whereas the circulating epinephrine level is directly related to sympathetic activity. Therefore, serum epinephrine level is a powerful tool for evaluating the program efficacy.

Table 3 Effects of BBSI program on the severity of OAB symptoms, as measured by OAB-q ($N = 38$)

Variables	BBSI ($n = 20$)			Control ($n = 18$)		
	Pre	Post		Pre	Post	
	Mean ± SD	Mean ± SD	p	Mean ± SD	Mean ± SD	p^*
Frequency	2.00 ± 0.79	1.95 ± 0.51	.782	2.22 ± 0.73	1.94 ± 0.54	.132
Urgency	8.50 ± 1.50	7.50 ± 0.82	.004	7.50 ± 1.00	7.39 ± 1.58	.756
Nocturia	9.35 ± 2.08	6.85 ± 1.42	<.001	8.44 ± 2.06	8.39 ± 1.29	.979
Urgency incontinence	6.70 ± 2.11	6.00 ± 1.84	.100	6.33 ± 3.12	5.33 ± 2.33	.055
Total	42.81 ± 10.59	33.96 ± 7.31	<.001	38.54 ± 11.83	35.53 ± 9.44	.214

BBSI Biofeedback-based sleep improvement program, *OAB* Overactive bladder syndrome, *OAB-q* Overactive bladder questionnaire; *p*: difference from pre-test to post-test in BBSI groups; *p**: difference from pre-test to post-test in control groups

Table 4 Effects of the BBSI program on the patterns of sleep parameters (N = 38)

Variables	BBSI (n = 20)			Control (n = 18)		
	Pre	Post		Pre	Post	
	Mean ± SD	Mean ± SD	p	Mean ± SD	Mean ± SD	p*
SE (%)	86.89 ± 4.93	90.54 ± 4.36	.004	87.77 ± 5.39	86.71 ± 6.07	.717
WASO (min)	69.20 ± 27.57	37.28 ± 21.16	.001	56.27 ± 22.94	59.48 ± 22.87	.281
Number of awakenings	10.85 ± 4.16	7.12 ± 2.89	.001	10.14 ± 4.80	10.94 ± 4.21	.236
Number of awakenings in 3 h after sleep onset	4.48 ± 1.74	3.44 ± 1.74	.048	4.09 ± 1.81	4.65 ± 2.29	.256

BBSI Biofeedback-based sleep improvement program, *OAB* Overactive bladder syndrome; *p*: difference from pre-test to post-test in BBSI groups; *p**: difference from pre-test to post-test in control groups; *SE* Sleep efficiency, *WASO* Wake after sleep onset

Urinary symptom severity was significantly decreased in the experimental group, while no differences were noted in the control group. Symptoms of OAB are directly affected by changes in sleep structure due to aging, such as decreased REM and slow wave sleep [5]. Active interventions for these direct factors play an important role in improving sleep in elderly individuals [46]. The primary intervention for alleviating urinary symptoms is behavioral therapy, especially in elderly patients. This treatment is safer and has fewer side effects than drug therapy or surgery [47, 48] and has better subjective assessment of symptoms than drug therapy [49].

Few previous studies have focused on ANS as a mediator in the relief of OAB symptoms. Cho et al. [50] attempted to alleviate OAB symptoms by inducing ANS changes using Tai-chi. No change in ANS activity was observed but urinary symptoms were alleviated without improvement in nocturia [50]. However, in the present study, nocturia and urgency were improved—but not frequency and urgency incontinence. We believe that this difference in the outcome was due to the focus of the intervention. In OAB patients—especially those with urgency incontinence—it is important to acquire skills to respond to urgency situations, such as PFM contraction and relaxation techniques [48]. However, the intervention program of this study was composed mainly of factors that reduce nocturia by emphasizing the practice of sleep hygiene—including water and caffeine restriction—urination before bedtime, and performing appropriate exercise to reduce awakening. These results indicate that urinary symptoms are related to several factors and that a customized intervention for each symptom is necessary for symptomatic relief [47].

In this study, SE increased, while wakefulness after sleep onset, number of awakenings during sleep, and number of awakenings within 3 h after sleep onset decreased, and overall sleep improved in the experimental group after the program. In elderly women with OAB, SE reduced and WASO increased significantly due to decreased urinary symptoms and exacerbated changes that occur during the normal aging process [5, 51]. Furthermore, since sympathetic nervous activity may affect

REM sleep and induce nocturia [52], these results suggest that increasing RMSSD and decreasing the LF/HF ratio improves sleep in elderly women with OAB. Particularly, lower sleep quality due to nocturia is a problem due to which patients with OAB are the most inconvenienced [53]. Decreased wakefulness after sleep onset is associated with reduced nocturnal enuresis. Additionally, the frequency of awakening due to urination in the initial stages of sleep is a key parameter for clinically assessing the quality of sleep and life [54]. The frequency of awakening during sleep is known to increase with age and this frequency is important in terms of sleep quality in elderly individuals with OAB because it can be difficult to return to sleep after awakening [55]. The elderly demonstrate slow sleep—which is deep sleep for 3 h after sleep onset—during which arousal has the greatest effect on daytime drowsiness and disruption of daily activities [56]. The decrease in awakening frequency seems to positively affect sleep quality by increasing sleep continuity.

This study introduced a method to effectively treat sleep disorders using a program that addresses the physiological issues to alter ANS imbalances. A strong point of the program is that it addresses the issue integrally by approaching sleep disruption in view of the characteristics of OAB. Additionally, as an early study of sleep problems in patients with OAB, considerable results were obtained that confirm that ANS stabilization is effective in improving OAB and sleep. Based on the results of this study, it also may be possible to apply ANS stabilization to OAB patients more easily in daily life, such as relaxation and meditation therapy [57].

Despite the strengths, the study has some limitations. First, the study has the potential for bias due to the use of a non-randomized controlled trial design and no blinding between the researchers and participants. Second, HRV measurements—reflecting ANS—were evaluated during daytime stability and do not reflect changes in sleep and bladder activity at other times of the day. Third, the findings should be generalized with caution as there is the possibility of interference from external variables and the fact that only two senior welfare centers in Korea were included. Finally, it is difficult for the participants to apply the BBSI program's protocol to their daily life on their own. Further studies with larger samples with randomized control trial designs and direct ANS activity measurements are needed to evaluate the precise relationships between ANS activity, bladder activity, and sleep patterns. Additionally, simplifying the elements of the program and making it easier to apply in everyday life will help the participants manage the disorders on their own.

Conclusions

This study tested a BBSI program in elderly women with OAB in a coordinated manner and demonstrated that the program could improve ANS balance, alleviate urinary symptoms, and improve sleep. The results of this intervention study demonstrate that it is meaningful to consider physiological factors in sleep interventions. Therefore, the program is expected to positively affect the quality of sleep and life in elderly women with OAB.

Supplementary information

> **Additional file 1.** Biofeedback-based sleep improvement program

Abbreviations
ANS: Autonomic nervous system; BBSI: Biofeedback-Based Sleep Improvement; Epi: Epinephrine; HF: High frequency; HRV: Heart rate variability; LF: Low frequency; MMSE: Mini-Mental State Examination; NE: Norepinephrine; OAB: Overactive bladder syndrome; OABSS: Overactive bladder symptom scores; PFM: Pelvic floor muscle; PSQI: Pittsburgh Sleep Quality Index; RMSSD: Square root of the mean squared differences of successive N-N intervals; SDNN: Standard deviation of the N-N interval; SE: Sleep efficiency; TP: Total power; WASO: Wake after sleep onset

Acknowledgements
Not applicable.

Authors' contributions
Conceived and designed the present study: JP, NK. Acquired the data: JP, CHP, NK. Analyzed and interpreted the data: JP, CHP, SE, EL, SWK. Drafted the manuscript: JP, NK. Provided significant input regarding the content of the manuscript: SWK, SE, EL. All authors read and approved the final manuscript for publication.

Author details
[1]College of Nursing, Keimyung University, Daegu, Republic of Korea.
[2]Department of Urology, Keimyung University School of Medicine, Daegu, Republic of Korea. [3]College of Nursing, Seoul National University, Seoul, Republic of Korea.

References
1. Irwin DE, Milsom I, Hunskaar S, Reilly K, Kopp Z, Herschorn S, et al. Population-based survey of urinary incontinence, overactive bladder, and other lower urinary tract symptoms in five countries: results of the EPIC study. Eur Urol. 2006;50:1306–14 discussion 14-5.
2. Stewart W, Van Rooyen J, Cundiff G, Abrams P, Herzog A, Corey R, et al. Prevalence and burden of overactive bladder in the United States. World J Urol. 2003;20:327–36.
3. Haylen BT, de Ridder D, Freeman RM, Swift SE, Berghmans B, Lee J, et al. An international Urogynecological association (IUGA)/international continence society (ICS) joint report on the terminology for female pelvic floor dysfunction. Int Urogynecol J. 2010;21:5 26.
4. Rohrmann S, Crespo CJ, Weber JR, Smit E, Giovannucci E, Platz EA. Association of cigarette smoking, alcohol consumption and physical activity with lower urinary tract symptoms in older American men: findings from the third National Health and Nutrition Examination Survey. BJU Int. 2005; 96:77–82.
5. Weiss JP, Blaivas JG. Nocturnal polyuria versus overactive bladder in nocturia. Urology. 2002;60:28–32.
6. Ge TJ, Vetter J, Lai HH. Sleep disturbance and fatigue are associated with more severe urinary incontinence and overactive bladder symptoms. Urology. 2017;109:67–73.
7. Aydogmus Y, Uzun S, Gundogan FC, Ulas UH, Ebiloglu T, Goktas MT. Is overactive bladder a nervous or bladder disorder? Autonomic imaging in patients with overactive bladder via dynamic pupillometry. World J Urol. 2017;35:467–72.
8. Gillespie J. The autonomous bladder: a view of the origin of bladder overactivity and sensory urge. BJU Int. 2004;93(4):478–83.
9. Steers WD. Pathophysiology of overactive bladder and urge urinary incontinence. Rev Urol. 2002;4:S7.
10. Nagendra R, Maruthai N, Kutty B. Meditation and its regulatory role on sleep. Front Neurol. 2012;3:54.
11. Viola AU, Tobaldini E, Chellappa SL, Casali KR, Porta A, Montano N. Short-term complexity of cardiac autonomic control during sleep: REM as a potential risk factor for cardiovascular system in aging. PLoS One. 2011;6:e19002.
12. Crasset V, Mezzetti S, Antoine M, Linkowski P, Degaute JP, Van De Borne P. Effects of aging and cardiac denervation on heart rate variability during sleep. Circulation. 2001;103:84–8.
13. Usmani SA, Reckenberg K, Johnson O, Stranges PM, Teshome BF, Kebodeaux CD, et al. Relative risk of adverse events and treatment discontinuations between older and non-older adults treated with antimuscarinics for overactive bladder: a systematic review and meta-analysis. Drugs Aging. 2019;36:639–45.
14. Vouri SM, Kebodeaux CD, Stranges PM, Teshome BF. Adverse events and treatment discontinuations of antimuscarinics for the treatment of overactive bladder in older adults: a systematic review and meta-analysis. Arch Gerontol Geriatr. 2017;69:77.
15. Vaughan CP, Bilwise DL. Sleep and nocturia in oder adults. Sleep Med Clin. 2018;13:107–11.
16. Shiri R, Hakama M, Häkkinen J. Uvinen a, Huhtala H, Tammela TL, et al. the effects of lifestyle factors on the incidence of nocturia. J Urol. 2008;180: 2059–62.
17. Jester DJ, Rozek EK, McKelley RA. Heart rate variability biofeedback: implications for cognitive and psychiatric effects in older adults. Aging Ment Health. 2018;30:1–7.
18. Jeong SJ, Homma Y, Oh S-J. Korean version of the overactive bladder symptom score questionnaire: translation and linguistic validation. Int Neurourol J. 2011;15:135.
19. Buysse DJ, Germain A, Moul DE, Franzen PL, Brar LK, Fletcher ME, et al. Efficacy of brief behavioral treatment for chronic insomnia in older adults. Arch Intern Med. 2011;171:887–95.
20. Kang Y, Na DL, Hahn S. A validity study on the Korean mini-mental state examination (K-MMSE) in dementia patients. J Korean Neurol Assoc. 1997;15: 300–8.
21. Chung BY, Park HS. Effects of non-pharmacological interventions for adults with insomnia in Korea: a meta-analysis. KAIS. 2017;18(1):95–106.
22. Korean Continence Society. Overactive bladder syndrome treatment guidelines. 3rd ed. Seoul: Aplus; 2018.
23. Korean Society of Sleep Medicine. Sleep Hygiene Education. 2008. http://www.sleepmed.or.kr/content/info/hygiene.html. Accessed 28 Apr. 2008.
24. Lehrer PM. Heart rate variability biofeedback and other psychophysiological procedures as important elements in psychotherapy. Int J Psychophysiol. 2018;131:89–95.
25. Melo R, Santos MD, Silva E, Quitério RJ, Moreno MA, Reis MS, et al. Effects of age and physical activity on the autonomic control of heart rate in healthy men. Braz J Med Biol Res. 2005;38:1331–8.
26. Radtke T, Khattab K, Brugger N, Eser P, Saner H, Wilhelm M. High-volume sports club participation and autonomic nervous system activity in children. Eur J Clin Investig. 2013;43:821–8.
27. Van der Kooy KG, Van Hout HP, Van Marwijk HW, et al. Differences in heart rate variability between depressed and non-depressed elderly. Int J Geriatr Psychiatry. 2006;21:147–50.

28. Patel D, Steinberg J, Patel P. Insomnia in the elderly: a review. J Clin Sleep Med. 2018;14(6):1017–24.

29. Wooldridge LS. Overactive bladder. J Am Acad Nurse Pract. 2016;3:251–68.

30. Xhyheri B, Manfrini O, Mazzolini M, Pizzi C, Bugiardini R. Heart rate variability today. Prog Cardiovasc Dis. 2012;55:321–31.

31. Choi JB, Lee JG, Kim YS. Characteristics of autonomic nervous system activity in men with lower urinary tract symptoms (LUTS): analysis of heart rate variability in men with LUTS. Urology. 2010;75:138–42.

32. Bilchick KC, Berger RD. Heart rate variability. J Cardiovasc Electrophysiol. 2006;17:691–4.

33. Coyne K, Revicki D, Hunt T, Corey R, Stewart W, Bentkover J, et al. Psychometric validation of an overactive bladder symptom and health-related quality of life questionnaire: the OAB-q. Qual Life Res. 2002;11:563–74.

34. Ancoli-Israel S, Martin JL, Blackwell T, Buenaver L, Liu L, Meltzer LJ, et al. The SBSM guide to actigraphy monitoring: clinical and research applications. Behav Sleep Med. 2015;13:S4–38.

35. Schrack JA, Cooper R, Koster A, Shiroma EJ, Murabito JM, Rejeski WJ, et al. Assessing daily physical activity in older adults: unraveling the complexity of monitors, measures, and methods. J Gerontol Series A. 2016;71:1039–48.

36. Smith MT, McCrae CS, Cheung J, Martin JL, Harrod CG, Heald JL, et al. Use of actigraphy for the evaluation of sleep disorders and circadian rhythm sleep-wake disorders: an American Academy of sleep medicine clinical practice guideline. J Clin Sleep Med. 2018;14:1231–7.

37. Lehrer P, Vaschillo E. The future of heart rate variability biofeedback. Biofeedback. 2008;36:11–4.

38. Hubeaux K, Deffieux X, Ismael SS, Raibaut P, Amarenco G. Autonomic nervous system activity during bladder filling assessed by heart rate variability analysis in women with idiopathic overactive bladder syndrome or stress urinary incontinence. J Urol. 2007;178:2483–7.

39. Hubeaux K, Deffieux X, Raibaut P, Le Breton F, Jousse M, Amarenco G. Evidence for autonomic nervous system dysfunction in females with idiopathic overactive bladder syndrome. Neurourol Urodyn. 2011;30:1467–72.

40. Hsiao S-M, Su T-C, Chen C-H, Chang T-C, Lin H-H. Autonomic dysfunction and arterial stiffness in female overactive bladder patients and antimuscarinics related effects. Maturitas. 2014;79:65–9.

41. Choi JB, Kim YB, Kim BT, Kim YS. Analysis of heart rate variability in female patients with overactive bladder. Urology. 2005;65:1109–12.

42. Ben-Dror I, Weissman A, Leurer MK, Eldor-Itskovitz J, Lowenstein L. Alterations of heart rate variability in women with overactive bladder syndrome. Int Urogynecol J. 2012;23:1081–6.

43. Van Kerrebroeck P, Andersson KE. Terminology, epidemiology, etiology, and pathophysiology of nocturia. Neurourol Urodyn. 2014;33:S2–5.

44. Blackman MR. Age-related alterations in sleep quality and neuroendocrine function: interrelationships and implications. Jama. 2000;284:879–81.

45. Bonnemeier H, Wiegand UK, Brandes A, Kluge N, Katus HA, Richardt G, et al. Circadian profile of cardiac autonomic nervous modulation in healthy subjects: differing effects of aging and gender on heart rate variability. J Cardiovasc Electrophysiol. 2003;14:791–9.

46. Vaz Fragoso CA, Gill TM. Sleep complaints in community-living older persons: a multifactorial geriatric syndrome. J Am Geriatr Soc. 2007;55:1853–66 1882-3.

47. Wyman JF, Klutke C, Burgio K, Guan Z, Sun F, Berriman S, et al. Effects of combined behavioral intervention and tolterodine on patient-reported outcomes. Can J Urol. 2010;17:5283–90.

48. Wyman JF, Burgio KL, Newman DK. Practical aspects of lifestyle modifications and behavioural interventions in the treatment of overactive bladder and urgency urinary incontinence. Int J Clin Pract. 2009;63:1177–91.

49. Peters KM, MacDiarmid SA, Wooldridge LS, Leong FC, Shobeiri SA, Rovner ES, et al. Randomized trial of percutaneous tibial nerve stimulation versus extended-release tolterodine: results from the overactive bladder innovative therapy trial. J Urol. 2009;182:1055–61.

50. Cho JL, Lee EN, Lee MS. Effects of tai chi on symptoms and quality of life in women with overactive bladder symptoms: a non-randomized clinical trial. Eur J Integr Med. 2017;12:189–95.

51. Martin SA, Appleton SL, Adams RJ, Taylor AW, Catcheside PG, Vakulin A, et al. Nocturia, other lower urinary tract symptoms and sleep dysfunction in a community-dwelling cohort of men. Urology. 2016;97:219–26.

52. Lowenstein L, Kenton K, Brubaker L, Pillar G, Undevia N, Mueller ER, et al. The relationship between obstructive sleep apnea, nocturia, and daytime overactive bladder syndrome in women. Am J Obstet Gynecol. 2008;198:598–e1–5.

53. Coyne KS, Payne C, Bhattacharyya SK, Revicki DA, Thompson C, Corey R, et al. The impact of urinary urgency and frequency on health-related quality of life in overactive bladder: results from a national community survey. Value Health. 2004;7:455–63.

54. Wein AJ, Kavoussi LR, Campbell MF. Campbell-Walsh urology. Drake M, editor. USA: Elsevier; 2012.

55. Zdanys KF, Steffens DC. Sleep disturbances in the elderly. Psychiatr Clin North Am. 2015;38:723–41.

56. Stanley N. The physiology of sleep and the impact of ageing. Eur Urol Suppl. 2005;3:17–23.

57. Nesvold A, Fagerland MW, Davanger S, Ilingsen Ø, Solberg EE, Holen A, et al. Increased heart rate variability during nondirective meditation. Eur J Prev Cardiol. 2012;19:773–80.

26

Cost comparison between open radical cystectomy, laparoscopic radical cystectomy and robot-assisted radical cystectomy for patients with bladder cancer: A systematic review of segmental costs

Yasuhiro Morii[1], Takahiro Osawa[2], Teppei Suzuki[3,4], Nobuo Shinohara[2], Toru Harabayashi[5], Tomoki Ishikawa[4,6], Takumi Tanikawa[7], Hiroko Yamashina[4] and Katsuhiko Ogasawara[4*]

Abstract

Background: Robot-assisted radical cystectomy is becoming a common treatment for bladder carcinoma. However, in comparison with open radical cystectomy, its cost-effectiveness has not been confirmed. Although few published reviews have compared total costs between the two surgical procedures, no study has compared segmental costs and explained their impact on total costs.

Methods: A systematic review was conducted based on studies on the segmental costs of open, laparoscopic, and robot-assisted radical cystectomy using PubMed, Web of Science, and Cochrane Library databases to provide insight into cost-effective management methods for radical cystectomy. The segmental costs included operating, robot-related, complication, and length of stay costs. A sensitivity analysis was conducted to determine the impact of the annual number of cases on the per-case robot-related costs.

Results: We identified two studies that compared open and laparoscopic surgeries and nine that compared open and robotic surgeries. Open radical cystectomy costs were higher than those of robotic surgeries in two retrospective single-institution studies, while robot-assisted radical cystectomy costs were higher in 1 retrospective single-institution study, 1 randomized controlled trial, and 4 large database studies. Operating costs were higher for robotic surgery, and accounted for 63.1–70.5% of the total robotic surgery cost. Sensitivity analysis revealed that robot-related costs were not a large proportion of total surgery costs in institutions with a large number of cases but accounted for a large proportion of total costs in centers with a small number of cases.

Conclusions: The results show that robot-assisted radical cystectomy is more expensive than open radical cystectomy. The most effective methods to decrease costs associated with robotic surgery include a decrease in operating time and an increase in the number of cases. Further research is required on the cost-effectiveness of surgeries, including quality measures such as quality of life and quality-adjusted life years.

* Correspondence: oga@hs.hokudai.ac.jp
[4]Faculty of Health Sciences, Hokkaido University, N12-W5, Kitaku, Sapporo, Hokkaido, Japan
Full list of author information is available at the end of the article

Background

Radical cystectomy is a standard surgical technique for non-metastatic muscle-invasive bladder carcinoma [1]. Open radical cystectomy (ORC) has been the gold standard treatment method, while laparoscopic radical cystectomy (LRC) has also been used. The safety and efficacy of LRC have been well-documented [2]. Recently, robot-assisted radical cystectomy (RARC) has become increasingly common [3, 4]. The safety and efficacy of RARC compared to those of ORC have also been reported [4–6]. In addition, previous randomized controlled trials (RCTs) have reported no significant differences in 2-year progression-free survival rates [7] and quality of life (QOL) scores between ORC and RARC [8, 9]. Comparing the perioperative outcomes of ORC and RARC, Tang et al. [10] conducted a meta-analysis of several RCTs and reported significantly lower estimated blood loss (EBL), lower transfusion rates, longer operative times, and larger quantities of anesthesia used with RARC. Although surgical outcomes are important, cost-effectiveness is also of great significance if RARC is to be widely adopted [11]. In addition, as bladder carcinoma is reported to have the highest lifetime treatment costs per patient among all malignancies [12], the cost-effectiveness of bladder carcinoma treatments needs to be evaluated. Smith et al. conducted a cost analysis between ORC and RARC [11], and the results show a total cost advantage of $1630/case for RARC. In contrast, the cost-analysis by Bansal et al. showed a total cost advantage of approximately $1945/case for ORC [13]. Michels et al. [14] conducted a cost simulation of ORC and RARC and found that RARC costs €3365 more than ORC at 30 days. These studies indicated that operative time, length of stay (LOS), and the number of annual cases were key drivers of costs [14]. However, consensus regarding the most cost-effective surgical approach is yet to be reached. Although some reviews have been published on cost comparisons between surgical procedures [15, 16], they do not clarify the cost structure or focus on the total cost and not on segmental costs or cost-effective measures for robotic surgery. For hospitals, identification of the cost components that influence the total cost is crucial to make RARC more cost-effective. Therefore, we conducted a systematic review on the segmental costs of ORC, LRC, and RARC. This study aimed to provide cost-effectiveness data for ORC, LRC, and RARC and provide insights for the effective management of treatments and applicability of RARC for patients with bladder cancer. This study also aimed to clarify the current available knowledge to identify any gaps in order to promote future research.

Methods

Study selection and risk of bias assessment

This review was conducted according to the guidelines from the Preferred Reporting Items for Systematic Review and Meta-Analysis [17]. Two reviewers (Y.M. and T.O.) independently identified potentially relevant studies. The search was conducted using PubMed, Web of Science, and Cochrane Library databases on April 26, 2018. The search term was a combination of (bladder cancer) AND (radical cystectomy OR open radical cystectomy OR laparoscopic radical cystectomy OR robot-assisted radical cystectomy OR robotic radical cystectomy) AND (cost OR cost analysis OR cost-effectiveness OR cost utility analysis OR health technology assessment OR incremental cost effectiveness ratio OR ICER). The search terms were identified from "all texts." Studies comparing costs for ORC to RARC or ORC to LRC in the form of full articles written in English were included. Simulation studies and studies with cost analysis not from a hospital perspective were excluded. When there was a difference of opinion regarding the inclusion of an article, it was resolved by other coauthors. To evaluate potential bias in included studies, "risk of bias" analysis of the included non-database studies was performed using the Cochrane Risk of Bias Tool [18].

Data extraction and outcomes of interest

The reviewers independently extracted the following data (whenever available), including the first author, year of publication, country, study period, study design (whether the article was an RCT or a retrospective study), database used (in cases of database research), types of surgical procedure, number of patients who underwent ORC, LRC or RARC; type of urinary diversion (intracorporeal or extracorporeal), procedure for lymph node dissection, robot used for RARC, amortization period for the robot, and annual number of robotic cases. Perioperative outcomes were extracted from non-database studies, such as operative time, operating room occupancy time, EBL, blood transfusion rate, LOS, and complication rates. The extracted outcome measures (whenever data was available) included: types of cost, what the cost included, quality of life (QOL), quality-adjusted life years (QALY), and incremental cost effectiveness ratio (ICER). The data on perioperative cost was classified into four groups: operating, complication, total LOS, and robot-related costs. Operating costs included costs related to surgery (surgical equipment, personnel, operating room occupancy, and anesthesia). Complication costs included any cost related to perioperative complications within 90 days after surgery (including costs for complication treatments, readmission due to complication, and transfusion). Robot-related costs consisted of the initial robot purchase and annual maintenance fees. Per-case robot-related costs were also extracted. A sensitivity analysis on the per-case robot-related cost was conducted to analyze the effect of the number of cases on the total RARC costs. The costs were converted to US dollars using the currency exchange rate as of August 29, 2018. Next, the contribution of each cost segment to the total cost was calculated whenever possible. When there was incomplete or missing data essential for the systematic review, the reviewers attempted to contact the corresponding author of the article.

Results
Study selection
A flow chart of study selection is shown in Fig. 1. We initially identified 315 studies from PubMed, Web of Science, and Cochrane Library databases. Of the 315 studies, 11 were included in this study [11, 13, 19–27]. The characteristics of the included studies are listed in Table 1. Two studies compared ORC to LRC [19, 20], and nine compared ORC to RARC [11, 13, 21–27]. Of the studies that compared ORC to RARC, four were single-institutional retrospective studies [11, 13, 21, 22], one was a single-institutional RCT [23], and the remaining four were administrative large database studies [24–27]. The QOL was measured in one study [23] and no significant difference in QOL scores between ORC and RARC was found. No research was done using QALY or ICER. Intracorporeal urinary diversion was performed in the study by Bansal et al., while all other studies reported on extracorporeal urinary diversion. The rates of urinary diversion types performed are shown in Table 2.

Risk of bias evaluation
The results of the "risk of bias" evaluation are shown in Fig. 2. All studies but one were considered "High risk" in "Random sequence generation" and "Allocation concealment" as they were retrospective studies. Blinding of participants and personnel was considered "Low risk" because blinding cannot be achieved in operation theatre settings, and allocation does not affect outcomes. Four articles were considered "High risk" in "Selective reporting" because of missing primary outcomes or cost data. For example, Martin et al. did not publish the exact cost data in their article for proprietary reasons [21], and Smith et al. did not include surgeon fees in their analysis [11].

ORC vs LRC
Two studies compared ORC with LRC [19, 20]. According to a study by Hermans, cost did not significantly differ between ORC and LRC [19]. The mean and median

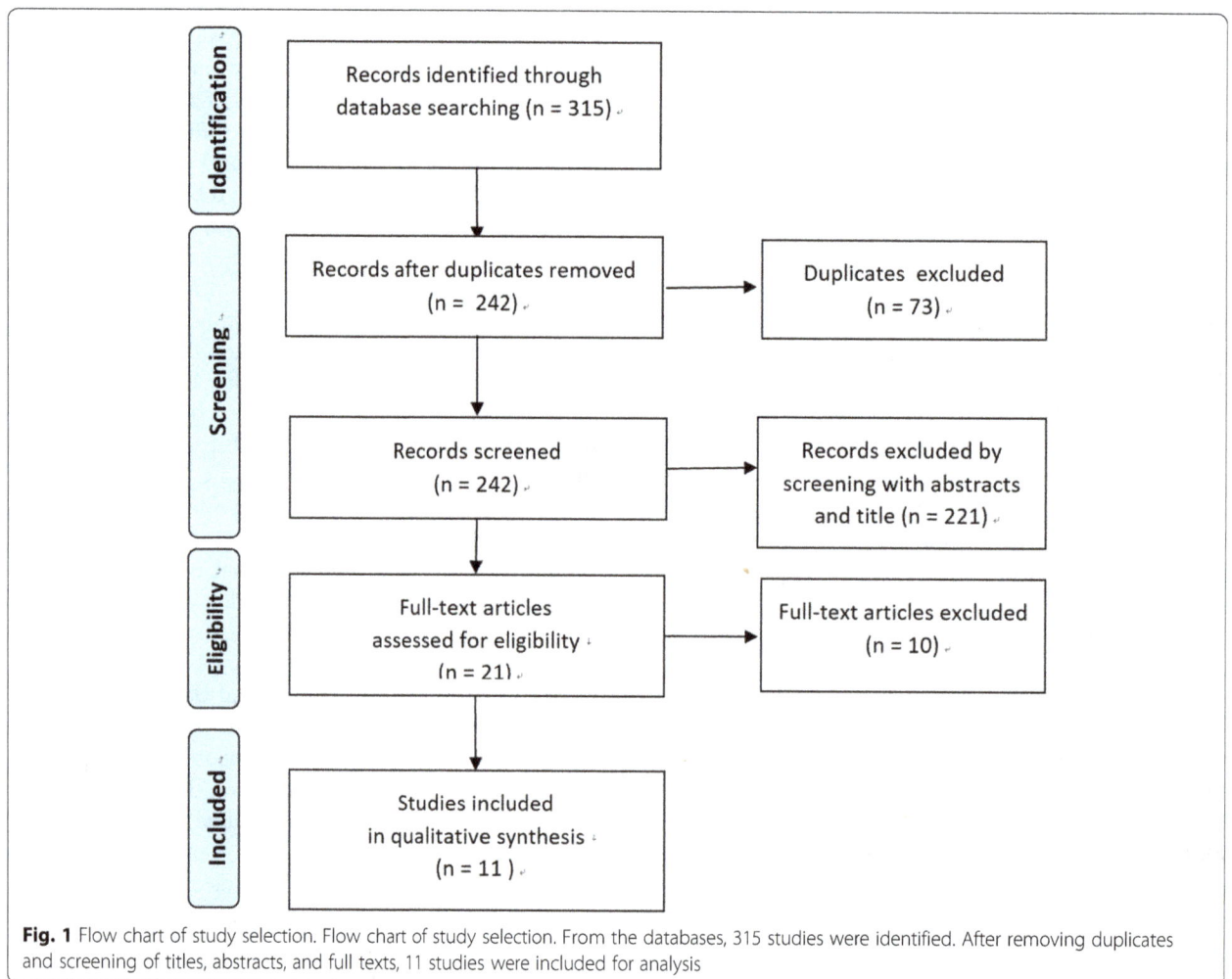

Fig. 1 Flow chart of study selection. Flow chart of study selection. From the databases, 315 studies were identified. After removing duplicates and screening of titles, abstracts, and full texts, 11 studies were included for analysis

Table 1 Characteristics of the included studies

Author	Country	Year	# of ORC case	# of LRC case	# of RARC case	Study Period	Study type (The name of databases used)
Bansal [13]	UK	2017	68		221	2011–2016	Single-institutional retrospective study
Bochner [23]	USA	2014	58		60	2010–2013	Single-institutional RCT
Martin [30]	USA	2011	14		19	2006-	Single-institutional retrospective study
Lee [22]	USA	2010	103		83	2002–2009	Single-institutional retrospective study
Smith [11]	USA	2010	20		20	2006-	Single-institutional retrospective study
Hermans [19]	Netherlands	2014	44	42		2005–2012	Single-institutional retrospective study
Zheng [20]	China	2012	65	45		2004–2011	Single-institutional retrospective study
Yu [26]	USA	2012	1444		224	2009	Administrative database study (Nationwide Inpatient Sample)
Leow [24]	USA	2014	34,672		2101	2004–2010	Administrative database study (Premier Perspective Darabase)
Hu [25]	USA	2016	7308		439	2002–2012	Administrative database study (Surveillance, Epidemiology, and End Results Program and Medicare linked data)
Monn [27]	USA	2014	25,986		3733	2009–2011	Administrative Database study (Nationwide Impatient Sample)

The characteristics of the 11 studies that compared ORC to LRC or ORC to RARC. The studies consisted of six single-institutional retrospective studies, a single-institutional RCT, and four database studies. The characteristics included information on authors, countries where the studies were performed, year of publication, number of cases (ORC, LRC or RARC), study periods, and study types. *RCT* Randomized controlled trial

direct healthcare costs per patient (operating room occupation, disposable surgical equipment, blood transfusions, and hospital stay costs) were $21,177 and $19,941 in the LRC group, and $26,914 and $19,214 in the ORC group, respectively. Mean operating time was significantly shorter with ORC, resulting in a lower operating room occupation cost ($6273 for ORC, and $7740 for LRC). LRC was associated with significantly lower costs of packed cells, ($878 vs $175), nursing ($12,066 vs $8211), and intensive care ($5417 vs $1177). Zheng et al. analyzed the total costs and found that LRC was significantly more expensive in comparison to ORC ($9993 vs $8197) [20].

Table 2 Per-case total costs and urinary diversion types performed

Author	Urinary diversion type (ORC) (% of total cases)	Urinary diversion type (RARC) (% of total cases)	Total cost (ORC)	Total cost (RARC)	Cost advantage for RARC
Bansal [13]	Ileal conduit (100%), Orthotopic neobladder (0%), Other (0%)	Ileal conduit (91.4%), Orthotopic neobladder (7.7%), Other (0.9%)	$13,512	$16,060	-$2548
Bochner [23][a]	Ileal conduit (45%)	Ileal conduit (40%)	$16,648	$18,388	-$1740
	Orthotopic neobladder (55%)	Orthotopic neobladder (55%)	$15,311	$19,231	-$3920
Martin [21]	Ileal conduit (100%)	Ileal conduit (100%)	N.A. (for institutional reason)		
Lee [22] [b]	Ileal conduit (50%)	Ileal conduit (57%)	$25,505	$20,659	$4846
	Continent cutaneous (22%)	Continent cutaneous (12%)	$22,697	$22,102	$595
	Orthotopic neobladder (28%)	Orthotopic neobladder (31%)	$20,719	$22,695	-$1976
Smith [11]	N.A.	N.A.	$16248[c]	$14608[c]	$1640
Yu [26][b]	Ileal conduit (76.4%) Other (23.4%)	Ileal conduit (75.7%) Other (24.3%)	$28100[d]	$34303[d]	-$6203
Leow [24]	Ileal conduit (93.9%), Continent (6.1%)	Ileal conduit (91.5%), Orthotopic Continent (8.5%)	$26679[d]	$30974[d]	-$4295
Hu [25]	Incontinent (81.3%) Continent (4.1%)[e]	Incontinent (80.5%) Continent (5.0%)[e]	$32521[d]	$36121[d]	-$3600
Monn [27]	N.A.	N.A.	$25098[d]	$30272[d]	-$5174

Per-case total costs of ORC and RARC and the types and rates of urinary diversions performed in the included studies [a]Patients with continent cutaneous tracts were not included in the analysis; [b]no significant differences in the rates of urinary diversion types performed between ORC and RARC groups; [c]surgeon fees were not included; and [d]significant cost differences existed between ORC and RARC [e]the rest is unknown

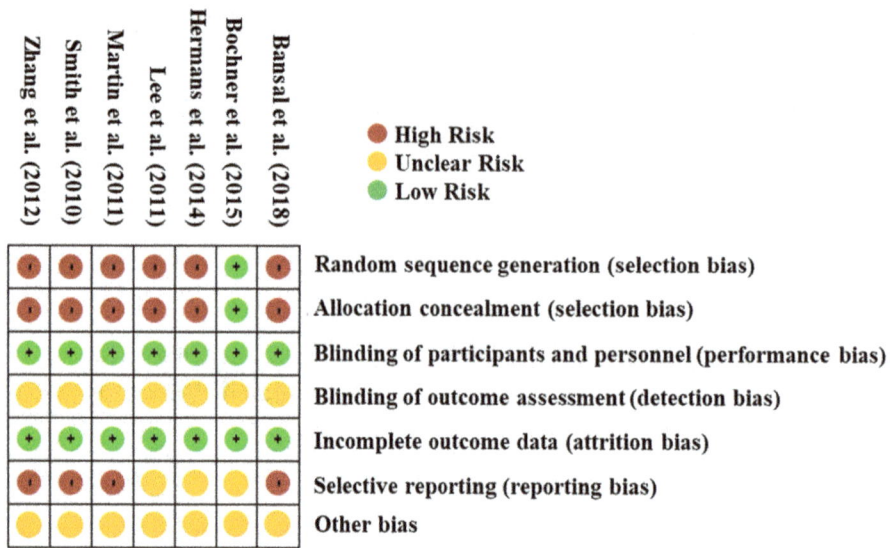

Fig. 2 Result of risk of bias evaluation. The results of "risk of bias" assessment conducted using the Cochrane Risk of Bias Tool [18]

ORC vs RARC

Total costs

The information regarding per-case total costs is summarized in Table 2. Total costs and the segmental costs are shown in Fig. 3. A single-institutional retrospective study reported that ORC had a cost advantage of $2548 [13], while two single-institutional retrospective studies reported that RARC had a cost advantage [11, 21]. Martin et al. published that RARC was 38% less expensive than

ORC although their research did not publish the exact cost data for proprietary reasons [21]. The results from one RCT and 4 database studies showed that RARC was $1740–$6203 more expensive [23–27]. Lee et al. subdivided their cohorts into radical cystectomy with ileal conduit, orthotopic neobladder, and cutaneous continent diversion subgroups, and compared the costs between ORC and RARC for these three subgroups [22]. In their research, RARC was less expensive than ORC for the ileal

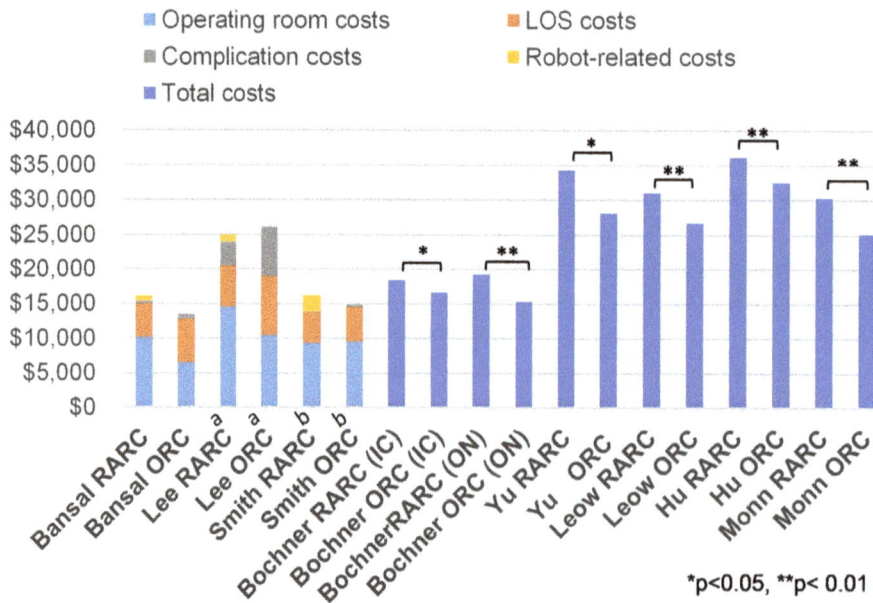

a: the median costs were used, b: surgeon fee was not included

Fig. 3 Summary of total costs and segmental costs for ORC and RARC. Summary of segmental and total costs in the included studies. Segmental costs are included whenever available; otherwise, total costs are shown. IC: Ileal conduit; ON: Orthotopic Neobladder

conduit, and cutaneous continent diversion subgroups; although, RARC was more expensive for the orthotopic neobladder subgroup.

Robot-related costs

The data on robot-related cost is presented in Table 3. In most studies, maintenance and purchase costs were not available. Robot purchase cost was shown only in one article (da Vinci© Surgical System: $1,650,000) [22]. Different amortization periods were used in the studies (5–10 years). The annual number of robotic-surgery cases varied from 288 to 400, and some included cases of other surgeries such as prostatectomies [11]. The per-case robot-related costs ranged from $766 to $2303 and were affected by amortization periods and the number of annual robot-surgery cases. The robot-related costs accounted for 4.8% of the total costs according to Bansal et al. [13], 4.8% of ileal conduit costs according to Lee et al. [21], and 15.8% according to Smith et al. [11]. Figure 4 shows the results of sensitivity analysis to clarify the effect of the annual number of cases on per-case robot-related costs. For example, when the annual number of cases was 50, the per-case robot-related cost would be $6128 of the total costs in the study by Bansal et al. (28.6% of the total RARC costs) [13], $6768 in the study by Martin et al. [21], $7220 in the study by Lee et al. (25.0–26.9%) [22], and $13,265 in the study by Smith et al. (51.9%) [11]. When the annual number of cases was 400, the per-case robot-related cost was $766 in the study by Bansal et al. (4.8% of the total RARC costs) [13], $846 in the study by Martin et al. [21], $903 in the study by Lee et al. (4.0–4.4%) [22], $1658 in the study by Smith et al. (11.9%) [11]. Per-case robot-related costs differed greatly depending on the annual number of cases.

Complication costs

The data on perioperative complication costs are presented in Table 4. Complication rates were higher for ORC in two retrospective single-institutional studies [13, 22]. Although Bochner et al. did not publish complication costs, complication rates did not significantly differ between the two groups in their RCT. In addition, a database study did not show a significant difference in complication rates between ORC and RARC [23]. Complication costs were published in two single-institutional retrospective studies [13, 22], which reported that complication costs were higher in ORC. Moreover, although Martin et al. did not publish data on cost for proprietary reasons in their single-institutional retrospective study [21], the results indicated that the average complication cost associated with RARC was 60% less than that for ORC.

Transfusion rates [13] and EBL [21, 23] were higher in ORC. Transfusion-associated costs were available in only two studies [11, 13], in which transfusion costs for ORC were more expensive than those of RARC ($115 vs. $28 and $322 vs. $107), and accounted for 0.2–2.0% of the total costs. Data on complication-associated costs based on the Clavien-Dindo grade were not available in any of the studies.

Operating costs

The data on operating costs is presented in Table 5. The mean operative time ranged from 228 to 420 min for ORC, and from 192 to 456 min for RARC. Operative time was longer for RARC, and operating costs were higher for RARC in all but one study [20]. Operating room occupancy time was not reported in the included studies. Operating costs accounted for 40.7–57.3% and 58.5–70.3% of the total costs of ORC and RARC, respectively. Lee et al. presented operating costs as median costs. Smith et al. did not include surgeon fees in their analysis. In the studies, no significant difference was found in the number of lymph nodes dissected. An RCT by Bochner et al. included patients who underwent standard or extended lymph node dissections, and the rates of patients who underwent extended dissections were matched between groups [22].

Length of stay cost

Data on LOS costs are presented in Table 6. The mean LOS ranged from 3.5–12.5 days and 3–10 days for ORC and RARC, respectively. The mean LOS did not differ in the RCT by Bochner et al. [23]. LOS costs were lower for RARC in all single-institutional studies. LOS costs accounted for approximately 30.7–46.7% and 26.0–30.2%

Table 3 Robot-related costs

Author	Purchase cost	Amortization period	Annual maintenance cost	# of case per year	Total per-case cost
Bansal [13]	N.A.	10-year	$323/case	400	$766
Bochner [23]	N.A.	N.A.	N.A.	N.A.	N.A.
Martin [21]	N.A.	7-year	N.A.	300	$1128
Lee [22]	$1,650,000	7-year	$125,000 (347$/case)	361	$1000
Smith [11]	N.A.	5-year	N.A.	288 (including prostatectomy cases)	$2303

Robot-related cost data of the included studies. Robot-related costs included robot purchase costs and annual maintenance costs. The robot-related costs were calculated using the amortization periods and the annual number of cases in the institutions. The data on amortization periods and annual number of cases are also listed in this table

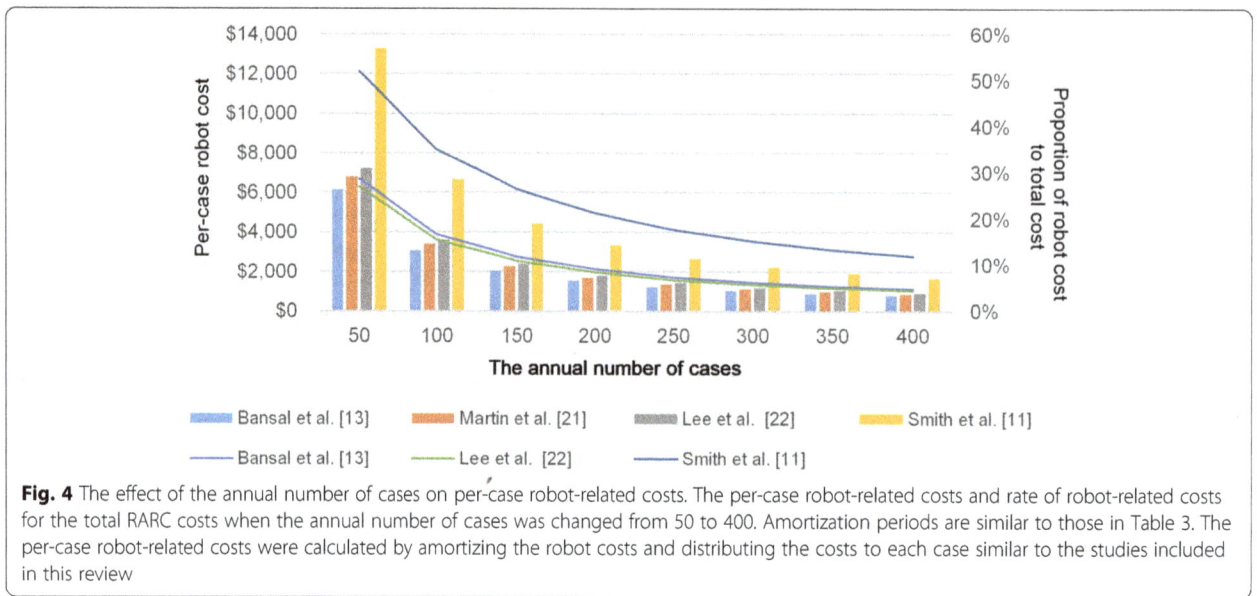

Fig. 4 The effect of the annual number of cases on per-case robot-related costs. The per-case robot-related costs and rate of robot-related costs for the total RARC costs when the annual number of cases was changed from 50 to 400. Amortization periods are similar to those in Table 3. The per-case robot-related costs were calculated by amortizing the robot costs and distributing the costs to each case similar to the studies included in this review

of the total costs for ORC and RARC, respectively. Lee et al. used median costs [22]. Bansal et al. used NHS reference costs to estimate the costs for excess bed days [13].

Discussion

Only one of the included single-institutional studies comparing ORC and RARC was an RCT while the other four were retrospective studies. In addition, the "risk of bias" evaluation showed that some studies could have "High risk" of "Selective reporting" as these studies did not report parts of the primary outcomes. Therefore, although these studies are important due to the lack of large studies comparing surgical procedures, more evidence from high quality studies (e.g. RCT) is required. Nevertheless, the results from single-institutional studies can provide insights on cost structures through interpretation with the included large database studies, which reflect the general cost trends.

Two single-institutional retrospective studies reported total cost advantages for RARC over ORC [21, 22]; another single-institutional retrospective study, one RCT, and four database studies showed total cost advantages for ORC [13, 22–26]. Considering the quality of the studies, the results indicated that, in general, RARC was more likely to be expensive. Michels et al. conducted a cost simulation of ORC and RARC using data from a literature review and reported that RARC was more expensive [14], similar to our study result. Leow et al. reported that the cost advantage in ORC was due to the additional costs of purchasing and maintaining robots and longer operative times for RARC [24, 28]. However, on the other hand, Martin et al. reported that the cost advantage in RARC was due to the lower complication rates [21]. These conflicting findings indicate that RARC cost-effectiveness was institution-dependent. Leow et al. reported that the surgical approach (robot-assisted vs

Table 4 Perioperative complication costs and proportion of the costs in the total costs

Author	Urinary diversion	Complication cost (ORC) (%)	Complication cost (RARC) (%)	Transfusion costs (ORC) (%)	Transfusion costs (RARC) (%)
Bansal [13]	Ileal conduit	$619 (5.1%)	$289 (2.3%)	$115 (0.9%)	$28 (0.2%)
Bochner [23]	Ileal conduit, Orthotopic neobladder	Included in the total cost		Included in the total cost	
Martin [21]	Ileal conduit	N.A. (for institutional reason)		N.A. (for institutional reason)	
Lee [22]	Ileal conduit	$7202 (28.2%)	$1624 (7.9%)	N.A	
	Orthotopic neobladder	$1663 (7.3%)	$1823 (8.2%)	N.A	
	Continent cutaneous	$2520 (12.2%)	$,911 (8.4%)	N.A	
	Total	$7103	$3482	N.A	
Smith [11]	N.A.	Not included in the analysis		$322 (2.0%)	$107 (0.7%)

Complication rates and costs, and the proportion of the total costs. The complication costs included complication treatment, readmission, and transfusion costs

Table 5 Operating costs

Author	Urinary diversion	Operating cost (ORC) (%)	Operating cost (RARC) (%)	ORC mean operating time (min)	RARC mean operating time (min)
Bansal [13]	Ileal conduit, Orthotopic neobladder	$6464 (47.8%)	$10,140 (63.1%)	192[a]	265[a]
Bochner [23]	Ileal conduit, Orthotopic neobladder	included in total cost		330[b]	464[b]
Martin [21]	Ileal conduit	N.A. (for institutional reason)		320[a]	280[a]
Lee [22][c]	Ileal conduit, Orthotopic neobladder, Continent cutaneous	$10,384 (40.7–50.1%)	$14,556 (64.1–70.5%)	420[d]	444
Smith [11]	N.A.	$9304 (57.3%)	$9527 (65.3%)	228[e]	246[e]

Operating costs, proportion of the costs to the total cost, and operative time of the included studies. The operating costs included operating room occupation costs, personnel fee, disposable equipment, and anesthesia. [a]No statistical comparison; [b] significantly different between ORC and RARC; [c]presented as median costs; [d]surgeon fees not included; and [e]occupancy time was reported

open) was neither a major factor on cost variations nor associated with high costs [28]. Therefore, focusing on the segmental costs, such as operating costs and robot costs, is necessary to figure out how each aspect contributes to the total cost. The results of segmental costs from this study are of great importance for improving cost-effectiveness of RARC compared to that of ORC, from the hospital's perspective. Per-case robot costs were calculated by amortizing the robot-related costs and dividing the costs by the annual number of cases in the subject hospitals, including cases of other surgeries such as prostatectomy. According to a previous study, robot equipment costs were attributed to higher costs in RARC [21]. Although robots were an expensive initial investment for an institution, the per-case robot-related costs accounted for only 4.8–15.8% of the total costs (Table 3) [11, 13, 22] because the included single-institutional studies were conducted in high volume hospitals (288–400 cases per year). On the other hand, sensitivity analysis (Fig. 4) revealed that per-case robot-related costs differed greatly depending on the annual number of cases. High-volume centers were more likely to have lower

per-case robot-related costs [24], while these costs tended to be higher in low-volume institutions.

The complication costs were higher for ORC in three single-institutional retrospective studies [13, 21, 22], accounting for 1.9% [13] and 16.7% [22] of the total costs. On the other hand, Bochner et al. showed in an RCT that there was no significant difference in perioperative complication rates between ORC and RARC, although the research did not report segmental costs for complications [23]. A previous meta-analysis of four RCTs by Tang et al. revealed no significant differences between groups in the occurrence rates of patients with Clavien-Dindo grade 2–5 or 3–5 [10]; therefore, complication costs may not differ between groups. Although complication costs differ with Clavien-Dindo grades, none of the included studies showed complication costs according to the Clavien grade at 90 days, which is a standard method of reporting postoperative complications. Further studies on complication costs are required with a high-level of evidence. Additionally, it is recommended that future studies focus on complication costs according to the Clavien-Dindo grade.

Table 6 Length of Stay costs

Author	Urinary diversion	Length of stay cost (ORC)	Length of stay cost (RARC)	Mean length of stay (ORC) (days)	Mean length of stay (RARC) (days)
Bansal [13]	Ileal conduit, Orthotopic neobladder	$6314 (46.7%)	$4836 (30.1%)	12.5	8.8
Bochner [23]	Ileal conduit, Orthotopic neobladder	N.A. (included in total cost)		8	8
Martin [21]	Ileal conduit	N.A. (included in total cost)		10	5
Lee [22][b]	Ileal conduit, Orthotopic neobladder, Continent cuteneous	$8592 (33.7–41.5%)	$5907 (26.0–28.6%)	8[a]	5.5[a]
Smith [11]	N.A.	$4982 (30.7%)	$4418 (30.2%)	5.3[b]	4.7[b]

LOS and related costs, and the proportion of the total costs in the included studies. [a]Significantly different between ORC and RARC; [b]costs are presented as median costs

Complication costs can differ among countries. A multi-institutional study by Osawa et al. reported that causes of complications differed between the USA and Japan [30]. International comparisons of complication costs also need to be conducted carefully.

Differences in transfusion rates between ORC and RARC have been reported in various studies [10]. However, our results showed that even though transfusion rates were clinically essential, the difference did not largely affect the total costs.

The operating costs of RARC were higher in all studies due to longer operative times, which was similar to previous reports [10]. Operating costs accounted for approximately 63.1–70.5% of the total RARC cost (Table 5 and Fig. 3). Most of the operating time costs were attributed to operating room occupation and surgeon fees which are dependent on the operative time. Therefore, if an institution succeeds in shortening the operating time, it would effectively reduce the total cost. Operative time has been reported to decrease significantly with increased surgeon experience [31] and hospital volume [29]. Leow et al. reported that although total costs were significantly higher in the RARC group, the difference did not exist between high-volume surgeons (≥7 cases per year in their study) and hospitals (≥19 cases per year) [24]. Large institutions can benefit from shorter operative times, lower complication rates, cheaper per-case robot costs, and therefore, achieve more cost-effective RARC. Patient centralization to high-volume centers has been suggested as an effective way for cost-effective RARC surgeries [24], which is supported by our results. However, further research is required to reveal the relationship between a surgeons' learning curve and cost-effectiveness of RARC.

Most studies were analyzed using operative time [13, 21, 22], except which used operating room occupancy time (utilization time) [11]. Operating rooms are essential for hospital profitability and thus, longer operating room occupation is associated with higher costs. For accurate cost estimations, it is recommended that these two parameters should be recorded and analyzed.

Urinary diversion types chosen can also influence the total cost. The results by Lee et al. showed that RARC was more cost-efficient for ileal conduit ($4846), while the cost benefit diminished for cutaneous continent diversion ($609), and was absent for orthotopic neobladder (–$1966; Table 2) [22]. This is one of the few studies that compare ORC with RARC by urinary diversion types. Current evidence on the impact of urinary diversion types on the costs is inadequate.

Recently, intracorporeal urinary diversions have become increasingly common [32]. Only one article included in this study was conducted with an intracorporeal urinary diversion [13]. Further studies are necessary to evaluate whether an intracorporeal or extracorporeal urinary diversion can influence operative time, and subsequently, the total costs.

Lymph node dissections differ depending on the surgeon and institution. Bochner et al. included patients who had undergone standard or extended lymph node dissections. In their RCT, the rates of patients who underwent extended dissections were matched between the ORC and RARC groups [23]. Lymph node dissections should be included when comparing ORC and RARC costs because extended dissections can lead to longer operating times and higher costs.

Three retrospective studies reported lower LOS costs for RARC. LOS costs also accounted for a large proportion of the total costs, following operating costs. However, Tang et al. conducted a meta-analysis of four RCTs and found no significant difference in LOS for ORC and RARC [10]. Of the studies included in this study, an RCT by Bochner et al. reported no significant difference of LOS between ORC and RARC. A database study by Leow et al. reported that while LOS differed significantly between ORC and RARC, LOS-related costs did not differ since most of the costs were due to surgery and intensive care unit admission [24]. Therefore, it is likely that LOS costs do not necessarily have a large impact on the differences between ORC and RARC costs.

LOS differs greatly between countries. Sugihara et al. compared the LOS of radical cystectomy patients in Japan and the USA and reported shorter durations in the USA (8 [7–11] days vs 32 [21–44] days) [33]. The effects of LOS changes should be considered with each country's healthcare system [34].

Few studies mention the perioperative protocols used in their studies (e.g. ERAS protocols), making it difficult to compare results between studies. Nabhani et al. reported that using the ERAS protocol led to a cost saving of $4488/procedure [35]. Future studies are expected to be conducted under standardized protocols for more generalizable results.

One study measured QOL for ORC and RARC patients and found no significant difference between groups. This finding supports the results of Messer et al. and Khan et al. [8, 9]. None of the included studies analyzed cost-effectiveness using quality measurements, such as QALY; therefore, it is recommended that future studies should focus on cost-effectiveness.

Comparison of ORC and LRC was done in only two studies that had differing conclusions on which procedure was more expensive. Further studies are required to clarify and confirm which procedure is more cost-effective.

This is the first systematic review on the segmental costs of radical cystectomy to identify which cost segments impact the total cost. Therefore, the results of this research are significant to understand cost structure and consider how RARC can be cost-effective. However, this research has several limitations. First, medical systems differ to certain extent between countries [34]. Therefore, the results should be interpreted along with each country's healthcare system. Correcting the segmental costs with references (e.g. NHS reference costs) will enable cost differences between institutions to be partially. Second, although clinical practice such as the use of surgical equipment could differ among institutions and surgeons, the information (e.g. number or quantity of equipment used) was not explained in detail. However, we included the database studies [24–27], which allows for some generalizability of the surgeons and institutions. Finally, the study periods were up to 90 days postoperatively. Bladder carcinomas have the highest lifetime treatment cost per patient out of all malignancies [12]. Therefore, future research on the lifetime costs would be valuable.

Conclusion

In this study, we systematically reviewed studies that compared costs of ORC, LRC, and RARC and segmented the costs into four groups to provide useful data for administrative purposes. The results revealed RARC to be more expensive. The results from the segmented costs indicated that RARC operating costs were higher and accounted for the largest proportion of total RARC costs. Sensitivity analysis revealed that the annual number of cases largely affected the per-case robot costs, and subsequently affected the total costs. Therefore, to make RARC cost-effective, a short operative time and high number of cases would be the most efficient method. Further studies focusing on complication costs with a high level of evidence is required. Data from this research can be used to make RARC more cost-effective than ORC. Future studies need to focus on the cost-effectiveness of ORC and RARC by using quality measurements, such as QALY; standardizing the methods of complication costs analyses (e.g. per Clavien-Dindo grade), and adopting standardized perioperative protocols, such as ERAS.

Abbreviations

EBL: Estimated blood loss; ICER: Incremental Cost Effectiveness Ratio; LOS: Length of stay; LRC: Laparoscopic radical cystectomy; ORC: Open radical cystectomy; QALY: Quality-adjusted life years; RARC: Robot assisted radical cystectomy; RCT: Randomized controlled trial

Authors' contributions

YM and TO made substantial contributions to the acquisition of data, conducting the search, analyzing data, and research design. TS, TI, KO, TT, and HY made substantial contributions to conception, design, interpretation, and manuscript review. NS and TH made substantial contributions to research design, interpretation of the data, and manuscript review. All authors have read and approved of the final version of the manuscript.

Author details

[1]Graduate school of Health Sciences, Hokkaido University, N12-W5, Kitaku, Sapporo, Hokkaido, Japan. [2]Department of Renal and Genitourinary Surgery Graduate School of Medicine, Hokkaido University, N14, W5, KitaKu, Sapporo, Hokkaido, Japan. [3]Hokkaido University of Education, Art, and Sports Business, Sapporo, Hokkaido, Japan. [4]Faculty of Health Sciences, Hokkaido University, N12-W5, Kitaku, Sapporo, Hokkaido, Japan. [5]Department of Urology, Hokkaido Cancer Center, 3-54, Kikusui 4-2, Shiroishiku, Sapporo, Hokkaido, Japan. [6]Institute for Health Economics and Policy, No.11 Toyo-kaiji Bldg, 1-5-11, Nishi-Shimbashi,Minato-ku, Tokyo, Japan. [7]Faculty of Health Sciences, Hokkaido University of Science, 7-Jo 15-4-1 Maeda, Teine, Sapporo, Hokkaido, Japan.

References

1. Stenzl A, Cowan NC, De Santis M, et al. The updated EAU guidelines on muscle-invasive and metastatic bladder cancer. Eur Urol. 2009;55:815–25.
2. Tang K, Li H, Xia D, Hu Z, Zhuang Q, Liu J, et al. Laparoscopic versus open radical cystectomy in bladder Cancer: a systematic review and meta-analysis of comparative studies. PLoS One. 2014;9(5):e95667.
3. Stein JP, Lieskovsky G, Cote R, Groshen S, Feng A, Boyd S, et al. Radical Cystectomy in the Treatment of Invasive Bladder Cancer : Long-Term Results in 1 , 054 Patients. J Clin Oncol. 2001;19:666–75.
4. Pruthi RS, Nielsen ME, Nix J, Smith A, Schultz H, Wallen EM, et al. Robotic radical cystectomy for bladder Cancer: surgical and pathological outcomes in 100 consecutive cases. J Urol. 2010;183:510–5.
5. Styn NR, Montgomery JS, Wood DP, Hafez KS, Lee CT, Tallman C, et al. Matched comparison of robotic-assisted and open radical cystectomy. Urology. 2012;79:1303–8.
6. Ishii H, Rai BP, Stolzenburg JU, Bose P, Chlosta PL, Somani BK, et al. Robotic or open radical cystectomy, which is safer? A systematic review and meta-analysis of comparative studies. J Endourol. 2014;28:1215–23.
7. Parekh DJ, Reis IM, Castle EP, Gonzalgo ML, Woods ME, Svatek RD, et al. Robot-assisted radical cystectomy versus open radical cystectomy in patients with bladder cancer (RAZOR): an open-label, randomised, phase 3, non-inferiority trial. Lancet. 2018;391:2525–36.
8. Messer JC, Punnen S, Fitzgerald J, Svatek R, Parekh DJ. Health-related quality of life from a prospective randomised clinical trial of robot-assisted laparoscopic vs open radical cystectomy. BJU Int. 2014;114:896–902.
9. Khan MS, Gan C, Ahmed K, Ismail AF, Watkins J, Summers JA, et al. A single-Centre early phase randomised controlled three-arm trial of open, robotic, and laparoscopic radical cystectomy (CORAL). Eur Urol. 2015;69:613–21.
10. Tang JQ, Zhao Z, Liang Y, Liao G. Robotic-assisted versus open radical cystectomy in bladder cancer: a meta-analysis of four randomized controlled trails. Int J Med Robot. 2018;14:e1867.
11. Smith A, Kurpad R, Lal A, Nielsen M, Wallen EM, Pruthi RS, et al. Cost analysis of robotic versus open radical cystectomy for bladder Cancer. J Urol. 2010; 183:505–9.
12. Sievert KD, Amend B, Nagele U, Schilling D, Bedke J, Horstmann M, et al. Economic aspects of bladder cancer: What are the benefits and costs? World J Urol. 2009;27:295–300.
13. Bansal SS, Dogra T, Smith PW, Amran M, Auluck I, Bhambra M, et al. Cost analysis of open radical cystectomy versus robot-assisted radical cystectomy. BJU Int. 2018;121:437–44.
14. Michels UTJ, Wijburg CJ, Witjes JA, Rovers MM, Grutters JPC. A cost-effectiveness modeling study of robot-assisted (RARC) versus open radical cystectomy (ORC) for bladder cancer to inform future research. Eur Urol Focus. 2018. https://doi.org/10.1016/j.euf.2018.04.014.
15. Attalla K, Kent M, Waingankar N, Mehrazin R. Robotic-assisted radical cystectomy versus open radical cystectomy for management of bladder cancer: review of literature and randomized trials. Future Oncol. 2017 Jun; 13:1195–204.
16. Mmeje CO, Martin AD, Nunez-Nateras R, Parker AS, Thiel DD, Castle EP. Cost analysis of open radical cystectomy versus robot-assisted radical cystectomy. Curr Urol Rep. 2013;14:26–31.
17. Moher D, Liberati A, Tetzlaff J, Altman DG, Altman D, Antes G, et al. Preferred reporting items for systematic reviews and meta-analyses: The PRISMA statement. PLoS Med. 2009;6(7):e1000097.
18. The Cochrane Collaboration. Cochrane Handbook for Systematic Reviews of Interventions version 5.1. Part 2–8. Available at http://handbook-5-1.cochrane.org/ (Accessed on 29 May 2019).

19. Hermans TJ, Fossion LM. What about conventional laparoscopic radical cystectomy? Cost-analysis of open versus laparoscopic radical cystectomy. J Endourol. 2014;28:410–5.

20. Zheng W, Li X, Zhang Z, Yu W, Gong K, Yi S. Comparison of laparoscopic and open cystectomy for bladder cancer: a single center of 110 cases report. Transl Andorol Urol. 2012;1:4–8.

21. Martin AD, Nunez RN, Castle EP. Cystectomy versus open radical cystectomy: a complete cost analysis. Urology. 2011;77:621–5.

22. Lee R, Ng CK, Shariat SF, Borkina A, Guimento R, Brumit KF, et al. The economics of robotic cystectomy: cost comparison of open versus robotic cystectomy. BJU Int. 2011;108:1886–92.

23. Bochner BH, Dalbagni G, Sjoberg DD, Silberstein J, Keren Paz GE, Donat S, et al. Comparing open radical cystectomy and robot-assisted laparoscopic radical cystectomy: a randomized clinical trial. Eur Urol. 2015;67:1043–50.

24. Leow JJ, Reese SW, Jiang W, Lipsitz SR, Bellmunt J, Trinh QD, et al. Propensity-matched comparison of morbidity and costs of open and robot-assisted radical cystectomies: a contemporary population-based analysis in the United States. Eur Urol. 2014;66:569–76.

25. Hu JC, Chughtai B, O'Malley P, Halpern JA, Mao J, Scherr DS, et al. Perioperative outcomes, health care costs, and survival after robotic-assisted versus open radical cystectomy: a National Comparative Effectiveness Study. Eur Urol. 2016;70:195–202.

26. Yu HY, Hevelone ND, Lipsitz SR, Kowalczyk KJ, Nguyen PL, Choueiri TK, et al. Comparative analysis of outcomes and costs following open radical cystectomy versus robot-assisted laparoscopic radical cystectomy: results from the US Nationwide inpatient sample. Eur Urol. 2012;61:1239–44.

27. Monn MF, Cary KC, Kaimakliotis HZ, Flack CK, Koch MO. National trends in the utilization of robotic-assisted radical cystectomy: an analysis using the Nationwide inpatient sample. Urol Oncol. 2014;32:785–90.

28. Leow JJ, Cole AP, Seisen T, Bellmunt J, Mossanen M, Menon M, et al. Variations in the costs of radical cystectomy for bladder Cancer in the USA. Eur Urol. 2018;73:374–82.

29. Leow JJ, Chung B, Chang S. Trends in surgical approach and outcomes for radical cystectomy: a contemporary population-based analysis. J Urol. 2018; 197(4):e725.

30. Osawa T, Lee CT, Abe T, Takada N, Hafez KS, Montgomery JS. A multi-center international study assessing the impact of differences in baseline characteristics and perioperative care following radical cystectomy. Bladder Cancer. 2016;2:251–61.

31. Leow JJ, Reese S, Trinh QD, Bellmunt J, Chung BI, Kibel AS, et al. Impact of surgeon volume on the morbidity and costs of radical cystectomy in the USA: A contemporary population-based analysis. BJU Int. 2015;115:713–21.

32. Gorin MA, Kates M, Mullins JK, Pierorazio PM, Matlaga BR, Schoenberg MP, Bivalacqua TJ. Impact of hospital volume on perioperative outcomes and costs of radical cystectomy: analysis of the Maryland health services cost review commission database. Can J Urol. 2014;21:7102–7.

33. Hussein AA, May PR, Jing Z, Ahmed YE, Wijburg CJ, Canda AE. Outcomes of Intracorporeal urinary diversion after robot-assisted radical cystectomy: results from the international robotic cystectomy consortium. J Urol. 2018; 199:1302–11.

34. Sugihara T, Yasunaga H, Horiguchi H, Fushimi K, Dalton JE, Schold J, et al. Performance comparisons in major uro-oncological surgeries between the USA and Japan. Int J Urol. 2014;21:1145–50.

35. Hashimoto H, Ikegami N, Shibuya K, Izumida N, Noguchi H, Yasunaga H, et al. Cost containment and quality of care in Japan: is there a trade-off? Lancet. 2011;378:1174–82.

36. Nabhani J, Ahmadi H, Schuckman AK, Cai J, Miranda G, Djaladat H, et al. Cost analysis of the enhanced recovery after surgery protocol in patients undergoing radical cystectomy for bladder Cancer. Eur Urol Focus. 2016;2:92–6.

Permissions

All chapters in this book were first published by BioMed Central; hereby published with permission under the Creative Commons Attribution License or equivalent. Every chapter published in this book has been scrutinized by our experts. Their significance has been extensively debated. The topics covered herein carry significant findings which will fuel the growth of the discipline. They may even be implemented as practical applications or may be referred to as a beginning point for another development.

The contributors of this book come from diverse backgrounds, making this book a truly international effort. This book will bring forth new frontiers with its revolutionizing research information and detailed analysis of the nascent developments around the world.

We would like to thank all the contributing authors for lending their expertise to make the book truly unique. They have played a crucial role in the development of this book. Without their invaluable contributions this book wouldn't have been possible. They have made vital efforts to compile up to date information on the varied aspects of this subject to make this book a valuable addition to the collection of many professionals and students.

This book was conceptualized with the vision of imparting up-to-date information and advanced data in this field. To ensure the same, a matchless editorial board was set up. Every individual on the board went through rigorous rounds of assessment to prove their worth. After which they invested a large part of their time researching and compiling the most relevant data for our readers.

The editorial board has been involved in producing this book since its inception. They have spent rigorous hours researching and exploring the diverse topics which have resulted in the successful publishing of this book. They have passed on their knowledge of decades through this book. To expedite this challenging task, the publisher supported the team at every step. A small team of assistant editors was also appointed to further simplify the editing procedure and attain best results for the readers.

Apart from the editorial board, the designing team has also invested a significant amount of their time in understanding the subject and creating the most relevant covers. They scrutinized every image to scout for the most suitable representation of the subject and create an appropriate cover for the book.

The publishing team has been an ardent support to the editorial, designing and production team. Their endless efforts to recruit the best for this project, has resulted in the accomplishment of this book. They are a veteran in the field of academics and their pool of knowledge is as vast as their experience in printing. Their expertise and guidance has proved useful at every step. Their uncompromising quality standards have made this book an exceptional effort. Their encouragement from time to time has been an inspiration for everyone.

The publisher and the editorial board hope that this book will prove to be a valuable piece of knowledge for researchers, students, practitioners and scholars across the globe.

List of Contributors

Ferdinando Fusco, Massimiliano Creta and Francesco Mangiapia
Dipartimento di Neuroscienze e Scienze Riproduttive ed Odontostomatologiche, Università Degli Studi Di Napoli Federico II, Via Pansini, 5, 80131 Naples, Italy

Cosimo De Nunzio
Dipartimento di Urologia, Ospedale Sant'Andrea, Università Degli Studi di Roma "La Sapienza", Rota, Italy

Valerio Iacovelli and Enrico Finazzi Agrò
Dipartimento di Medicina Sperimentale e Chirurgia, Università Degli Studi di Roma "Tor Vergata", Roma, Italy

Vincenzo Li Marzi
Dipartimento di Urologia, Ospedale Careggi, Università Degli Studi di Firenze, Firenze, Italy

Sally Temraz, Yolla Haibe, Maya Charafeddine, Omran Saifi, Deborah Mukherji and Ali Shamseddine
Department of Internal Medicine, American University of Beirut Medical Center, Riad El Solh, Riad El Solh, Beirut 110 72020, Lebanon

Qingwei Wang, Tao Zhang, Junwei Wu, Deshang Tao, Tingxiang Wan and Wen Zhu
Department of Urology, The First Affiliated Hospital of Zhengzhou University, Zhengzhou 450052, Henan, China

Jianguo Wen
Department of Urology, The First Affiliated Hospital of Zhengzhou University, Zhengzhou 450052, Henan, China
Department of Pediatric Surgery, The First Affiliated Hospital of Xinxiang Medical University, Xinxiang 453100, Henan, China

M-M Qin, G. Feng, X-N Li, J. Zhang, R. Zheng, X-C Liu and C. Pu
Clinical Laboratory, The First Affiliated Hospital of Wannan Medical College, No.2, West Zheshan Road, Wuhu 241001, Anhui, China

X. Chai and H-B Huang
Department of Urology, The First Affiliated Hospital of Wannan Medical College, Wuhu 241001, Anhui, China

Jing Sun
Department of Pathology, Xuan Wu Hospital, Capital Medical University, Beijing, China
Department of Pathology, Capital Medical University, Beijing, China

Dandan Wang, Leiming Wang, Lan Zhao and Lianghong Teng
Department of Pathology, Xuan Wu Hospital, Capital Medical University, Beijing, China

Jiangtao Wu
Department of Urology, Xuan Wu Hospital, Capital Medical University, Beijing, China

Cheng Wang
Department of Pathology and Laboratory Medicine, Dalhousie University, Nova Scotia, Canada

Mieke Van Hemelrijck
King's College London, School of Cancer and Pharmaceutical Sciences, Translational Oncology and Urology Research (TOUR), London SE1 9RT, UK

Francesco Sparano, Francesco Cottone and Fabio Efficace
Data Center and Health Outcomes Research Unit, Italian Group for Adult Hematologic Disease (GIMEMA), Rome, Italy

Debra Josephs
King's College London, School of Cancer and Pharmaceutical Sciences, Translational Oncology and Urology Research (TOUR), London SE1 9RT, UK
Guy's and St Thomas' NHS Foundation Trust, Medical Oncology, London, UK

Mirjam Sprangers
Department of Medical Psychology, Location AMC, Amsterdam University Medical Centers, Amsterdam, The Netherlands

Tian-Wei Wang
Nanjing Medical University, 101 Longmian Rd, Nanjing 211166, China

Hui Yuan, Wen-Li Diao, Rong Yang, Xiao-Zhi Zhao and Hong-Qian Guo
Department of Urology, Nanjing Drum Tower Hospital, Medical School of Nanjing University, 321 Zhongshan Rd., Nanjing 210008, China

Dalia F. El Agamy and Yahya M. Naguib
Clinical Physiology Department, Faculty of Medicine, Menoufia University, Menoufia, Egypt

Jameel Nazir
Astellas Pharma Europe Ltd, 2000 Hillswood Drive, Chertsey KT16 0PS, UK

Zalmai Hakimi
Astellas Pharma Europe B.V, Leiden, the Netherlands

Florent Guelfucci
Creativ-Ceutical Ltd., London, UK

Amine Khemiri
Creativ-Ceutical Ltd., Tunis, Tunisia
Present Address: Keyrus Biopharma, Tunis, Tunisia

Francis Fatoye
Manchester Metropolitan University, Manchester, UK

Ana María Mora Blázquez and Marta Hernández González
Astellas Pharma S.A., Madrid, Spain

A. Ivchenko and A. Wiedemann
Department of Urology, Evangelisches Krankenhaus-Witten gGmbH, UniversityWitten/Herdecke, Pferde-bachstrasse 27, 58455 Witten, Germany

R.-H. Bödeker
Department of Statistics, Institute of Medical Informatics, University Clinic Giessen, Rudolf-Buchheim-Strasse 6, 35392 Gießen, Germany

C. Neumeister
Department of Medical Science/Clinical Research, Dr. R. Pfleger GmbH, Dr.-Robert-Pfleger-Strasse 12, 96052 Bamberg, Germany

Zhenxing Yang, Luqiang Zhou, Jie Xu and Zhenqiang Fang
Department of Urology, Second Affiliated Hospital, Third Military Medical University, Chongqing 400037, China

Bingqiang Fu
SurExam Bio-Tech Co, Guangzhou 510663, Guangdong, China

Ping Hao
Department of Oncology, Second Affiliated Hospital, Third Military Medical University, Chongqing 400037, China

Hui Shan and Xiao-Dong Zhang
Department of Urology, Beijing Chaoyang Hospital, Capital Medical University, No.8 Gongti South Road, Beijing 100020, China

Er-Wei Zhang
Department of Urology, The First Affiliated Hospital of Zhengzhou University, Zhengzhou, China

Peng Zhang
Department of Urology, China Meitan General Hospital, Beijing, China

Ning Zhang, Peng Du and Yong Yang
Department of Urology, Beijing Cancer Hospital, Beijing, China

Haiwen Huang, Libo Liu, Han Hao and Zhijun Xi
Department of Urology, Peking University First Hospital, 8 Xishiku Street, Xicheng District, Beijing 100034, China
Institute of Urology, Peking University, National Urological Cancer Center, 8 Xishiku Street, Xicheng District, Beijing 100034, China

Bing Yan
Department of Urology, Xingtai People's Hospital, 16 Hongxing Street, Qiaodong District, Xingtai 054001, China

Meixia Shang
Department of Medical Statistics, Peking University First Hospital, 8 Xishiku Street, Xicheng District, Beijing 100034, China

Meenal Sharma and Zhiming Yang
Department of Pathology and Laboratory Medicine, University of Rochester Medical Center, Rochester, NY, USA

Takuro Goto
Department of Pathology and Laboratory Medicine, University of Rochester Medical Center, Rochester, NY, USA
James P. Wilmot Cancer Institute, University of Rochester Medical Center, Rochester, NY, USA

Hiroshi Miyamoto
Department of Pathology and Laboratory Medicine, University of Rochester Medical Center, Rochester, NY, USA
James P. Wilmot Cancer Institute, University of Rochester Medical Center, Rochester, NY, USA
Department of Urology, University of Rochester Medical Center, Rochester, NY, USA

Yun-Sok Ha, Sang Won Kim, So Young Chun, Jae-Wook Chung, Seock Hwan Choi, Jun Nyung Lee, Bum Soo Kim, Hyun Tae Kim, Eun Sang Yoo, Tae Gyun Kwon and Tae-Hwan Kim
Department of Urology, School of Medicine, Kyungpook National University, Daegu, South Korea
Department of Urology, School of Medicine, Kyungpook National University, Kyungpook National University Hospital, Daegu, South Korea

Won Tae Kim and Wun-Jae Kim
Department of Urology, Chungbuk National University College of Medicine, Cheongju, South Korea

Gerardo Bosco, Alex Rizzato and Matteo Paganini
Environmental and Respiratory Physiology Laboratory, Department of Biomedical Sciences, University of Padova, Padova, Italy

Edoardo Ostardo
Unità Operativa di Urologia, Azienda Ospedaliera Santa Maria degli Angeli, Pordenone, Italy

Giacomo Garetto
ATIP Centro di Medicina Iperbarica, Padova, Italy

Giorgio Melloni
Department of Statistics, Harvard School of Medicine, Boston, MA, USA

Giampiero Giron, Lodovico Pietrosanti and Ivo Martinelli
OTI Services, Centro di Medicina Iperbarica, Venezia, Italy

Enrico Camporesi
TEAMHealth Research Institute, TGH, Tampa, Florida, USA

Mingchen Ba, Shuzhong Cui, Yuanfeng Gong, Yinbing Wu, Kunpeng Lin, Yinuo Tu, Bahuo Zhang and Wanbo Wu
Intracelom Hyperthermic Perfusion Therapy Center, Cancer Hospital of Guangzhou Medical University, No. 78 Hengzhigang Road, Guangzhou, Guangdong 510095, People's Republic of China

Hui Long
Department of Pharmacy, Guangzhou Dermatology Institute, Guangzhou, Guangdong, People's Republic of China

Ricardo H. Pineda, Joseph Hypolite, Nao Iguchi and Anna P. Malykhina
Division of Urology, Department of Surgery, University of Colorado Denver, Anschutz Medical Campus, 12700 E 19th Ave, M/S C317, Aurora, CO 80045, USA

Sanghee Lee
Department of Urology, University of California San Diego, 3855 Health Science Drive, Room 4345, Bay 4LL, La Jolla, CA 92093, USA

Alonso Carrasco Jr
Children's Mercy Hospital, 2401 Gillham Rd, Kansas City, MO 64108, USA

Randall B. Meacham
Division of Urology, Department of Surgery, University of Colorado Denver, Academic Office One Bldg., Rm 5602, 12631 East 17th Ave., M/S C319, Aurora, CO 80045, USA

Guoqing Chen and Limin Liao
Department of Urology, China Rehabilitation Research Center, Beijing 100068, China
Department of Urology, Capital Medical University, Beijing, China

Fei Zhang
Department of Urology, Baotou Central Hospital, Baotou 014040, China

Yasushi Hayashida and Keisuke Taniguchi
Department of Urology, National Hospital Organization Ureshino Medical Center, 2436 Shimosyuku, Ureshino 843-0393, Japan

Yasuyoshi Miyata, Tomohiro Matsuo, Kojiro Ohba and Hideki Sakai
Department of Urology, Nagasaki University Graduate School of Biomedical Sciences, 1-7-1 Sakamoto, Nagasaki 852-8501, Japan

Mitsuru Taba and Shinji Naito
Department of Pathology, National Hospital Organization Ureshino Medical Center, 2436 Shimosyuku, Ureshino 843-0393, Japan

Itamar Getzler, Zaher Bahouth, Ofer Nativ and Sarel Halachmi
Department of Urology, Bnai Zion Medical Center, Faculty of Medicine, Technion - Israel Institute of Technology, Golomb 47, 31048 Haifa, Israel

Jacob Rubinstein
Department of Mathematics, Technion - Israel Institute of Technology, Haifa, Israel

Palma Maurizi, Michele Antonio Capozza, Silvia Triarico and Antonio Ruggiero
Pediatric Oncology Unit, Foundation "A. Gemelli" Hospital IRCCS – Catholic University of Sacred Hearth, Largo A. Gemelli 8, 00168 Rome, Italy

Maria Luisa Perrotta and Vito Briganti
Pediatric Surgery Unit, San Camillo Forlanini Hospital, Rome, Italy

Wasilijiang Wahafu, Sai Liu, Mengtong Wang, Qingbao He, Liming Song, Mingshuai Wang and Yinong Niu
Institute of Urology, Capital Medical University, Department of Urology, Capital Medical University Beijing Chao-Yang Hospital, Beijing 100020, China

Feiya Yang and Nianzeng Xing
Institute of Urology, Capital Medical University, Department of Urology, Capital Medical University Beijing Chao-Yang Hospital, Beijing 100020, China
Department of Urology, National Cancer Center/ National Clinical Research Center for Cancer/Cancer Hospital, Chinese Academy of Medical Sciences and Peking Union Medical College, Beijing 100021, China

Wenbin Xu and Lin Hua
School of Biomedical Engineering, Capital Medical University, Beijing 100069, China

Andrew T. Lenis, Nicholas M. Donin and Karim Chamie
David Geffen School of Medicine at the University of California Los Angeles, 300 Stein Plaza, Suite 348, Los Angeles, California 90095, USA
Department of Urology, Health Services Research Group, David Geffen School of Medicine at UCLA, Los Angeles, California, USA
Jonsson Comprehensive Cancer Center, David Geffen School of Medicine at UCLA, Los Angeles, California, USA

Kian Asanad
David Geffen School of Medicine at the University of California Los Angeles, 300 Stein Plaza, Suite 348, Los Angeles, California 90095, USA

Maher Blaibel
Riverside School of Medicine, University of California, Riverside, California, USA

Jooyeon Park, Sang-Eun Jun, Eun-Ju Lee and Nahyun Kim
College of Nursing, Keimyung University, Daegu, Republic of Korea

Choal Hee Park
Department of Urology, Keimyung University School of Medicine, Daegu, Republic of Korea

Seung Wan Kang
College of Nursing, Seoul National University, Seoul, Republic of Korea

Yasuhiro Morii
Graduate school of Health Sciences, Hokkaido University, N12-W5, Kitaku, Sapporo, Hokkaido, Japan

Takahiro Osawa and Nobuo Shinohara
Department of Renal and Genitourinary Surgery Graduate School of Medicine, Hokkaido University, N14, W5, KitaKu, Sapporo, Hokkaido, Japan

Teppei Suzuki
Hokkaido University of Education, Art, and Sports Business, Sapporo, Hokkaido, Japan
Faculty of Health Sciences, Hokkaido University, N12-W5, Kitaku, Sapporo, Hokkaido, Japan

Hiroko Yamashina and Katsuhiko Ogasawara
Faculty of Health Sciences, Hokkaido University, N12-W5, Kitaku, Sapporo, Hokkaido, Japan

Toru Harabayashi
Department of Urology, Hokkaido Cancer Center, 3-54, Kikusui 4-2, Shiroishiku, Sapporo, Hokkaido, Japan

Tomoki Ishikawa
Faculty of Health Sciences, Hokkaido University, N12-W5, Kitaku, Sapporo, Hokkaido, Japan
Institute for Health Economics and Policy, No.11 Toyo-kaiji Bldg, 1-5-11, Nishi-Shimbashi, Minato-ku, Tokyo, Japan

Takumi Tanikawa
Faculty of Health Sciences, Hokkaido University of Science, 7-Jo 15-4-1 Maeda, Teine, Sapporo, Hokkaido, Japan

Index